The Athletic Trainer's Guide to

Psychosocial Intervention and Referral

The Athletic Trainer's Guide to

Psychosocial Intervention and Referral

JAMES M. MENSCH, PhD, ATC

ATHLETIC TRAINING PROGRAM DIRECTOR
UNIVERSITY OF SOUTH CAROLINA
COLUMBIA, SC

GARY M. MILLER, PhD, NCC

UNIVERSITY OF SOUTH CAROLINA
COLUMBIA, SC

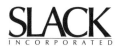

SLACK
INCORPORATED

*Delivering the best in health care information
and education worldwide*

www.slackbooks.com

ISBN: 978-1-55642-733-6

Copyright © 2008 by SLACK Incorporated

The Athletic Trainer's Guide to Psychosocial Intervention and Referral Instructor's Manual
is also available from SLACK Incorporated. Don't miss this important companion to
The Athletic Trainer's Guide to Psychosocial Intervention and Referral.
To obtain the Instructor's Manual, please visit http://www.efacultylounge.com.

The procedures and practices described in this book should be implemented in a manner consistent with the professional standards set for the circumstances that apply in each specific situation. Every effort has been made to confirm the accuracy of the information presented and to correctly relate generally accepted practices. The authors, editor, and publisher cannot accept responsibility for errors or exclusions or for the outcome of the material presented herein. There is no expressed or implied warranty of this book or information imparted by it. Care has been taken to ensure that drug selection and dosages are in accordance with currently accepted/recommended practice. Due to continuing research, changes in government policy and regulations, and various effects of drug reactions and interactions, it is recommended that the reader carefully review all materials and literature provided for each drug, especially those that are new or not frequently used. Any review or mention of specific companies or products is not intended as an endorsement by the author or publisher.

SLACK Incorporated uses a review process to evaluate submitted material. Prior to publication, educators or clinicians provide important feedback on the content that we publish. We welcome feedback on this work.

Contact SLACK Incorporated for more information about other books in this field or about the availability of our books from distributors outside the United States.

Published by: SLACK Incorporated
                  6900 Grove Road
                  Thorofare, NJ 08086 USA
                  Telephone: 856-848-1000
                  Fax: 856-853-5991
                  www.slackbooks.com

Library of Congress Cataloging-in-Publication Data

The athletic trainer's guide to psychosocial intervention and referral / [edited by] James M. Mensch, Gary M. Miller.
    p. ; cm.
  Includes bibliographical references and index.
  ISBN 978-1-55642-733-6 (alk. paper)
  1. Athletes--Mental health. 2. Athletes--Psychology. 3. Athletic trainers. 4. Medical referral. 5. Sports--Psychological aspects. 6. Sports--Social aspects. I. Mensch, James. II. Miller, Gary M.
  [DNLM: 1. Physical Education and Training. 2. Sports--psychology. QT 255 A871 2008]

RC451.4.A83A84 2008
617.1'027--dc22

                            2007030568

Printed in the United States of America.

Last digit is print number: 10 9 8 7 6 5 4 3 2 1

Dedication

To my wife Laurene, thanks for your love and support and
for putting up with me for all these years.
To my parents, any success I have had in life is the direct result
of your love and support.
James M. Mensch, PhD, ATC

This book is dedicated to my wife Lynda A. Neese and
our three grandsons, Harry, Brandon and Owen.
Gary M. Miller, PhD, NCC

Contents

Acknowledgments

Almost 4 years ago, we developed the idea of publishing a small handbook for athletic trainers to assist them in dealing with the psychosocial issues of their athletes and patients. With the encouragement of John Bond of SLACK Incorporated, we decided to develop a textbook in this area, requiring us to expand the project. We were able to contact and gain the assistance of a widely diverse group of professionals for their assistance in completing this assignment and thank all of them for their contributions to this book.

We also wish to thank April Billick at SLACK Incorporated for assisting us in the process of finalizing this book. Her encouragement and efforts have helped make this process flow to completion. We also thank Natalie G. Bennett for her assistance as we examined each chapter of the book prior to finalizing it.

James M. Mensch and Gary M. Miller

About the Authors

James M. Mensch, PhD, ATC received a Bachelor of Science degree in Kinesiology from Temple University, a Master's of Science degree in Pedagogy from Louisiana State University, and a Doctor of Philosophy degree in Kinesiology from the University of Maryland. Currently, Dr. Mensch is Director of the Graduate Athletic Training Program at the University of South Carolina. Dr. Mensch has published articles in the *Journal of Athletic Training, Research Quarterly for Exercise and Sport,* and *Athletic Therapy Today.* He currently serves as an associated editor for *Athletic Therapy Today,* a site-visitor for CAATE, and a reviewer for the NATA-REF grant program. Dr. Mensch's current work is centered around a research grant with the Department of Defense and the Army Military Base at Fort Jackson, SC.

He lives with his wife (Laurene) and 2 children (Jack—7 years old and Anna Grace—4 years old) in Ballentine, SC.

Gary M. Miller, PhD, NCC completed his Bachelor's of Science degree in Health and Physical Education from Slippery Rock State College in 1962. He completed his Master of Education degree in School Counseling at Duquesne University in 1964 and his Certificate of Advances Studies in Counselor Education from Kent State University in 1966. His PhD was completed in 1969 at Case Western Reserve University and he took his first teaching position at Eastern Michigan University in the Department of Counseling that same year. He has been on the faculty of the University of South Carolina since 1975, teaching in counselor education. A specific area of interest he has developed involves counseling student athletes, and it is through this interest that he has been educating athletic trainers regarding interpersonal skills and competencies for their work with student athletes.

His wife, Dr. Lynda A. Neese, is a middle school counselor. Their blended family includes Derek M. Miller, Kevin J. Miller, Dr. Brent Driggers, their wives, and three grandsons, Harry Driggers, Brandon Miller, and Owen Driggers.

Dr. Miller has been an active counselor educator, serving as the editor for *Spectrum,* the international newsletter of the Association for Counselor Education and Supervision and the president of the Southern Association for Counselor Education and Supervision. In addition, he has served as a site visitor on numerous accreditation visits for the Council for the Accreditation of Counseling and Related Educational Programs. He is also a Natinoal Certified Counselor.

Contributing Authors

Thomas D. Armsey, MD joined Midlands Orthopaedics on July 10, 2006. He received his undergraduate degree from Xavier University in Cincinnati and his medical degree from Wright State University School of Medicine in Dayton, OH. His residency was in family medicine at Long Beach Memorial Medical Center at the University of California, Irvine, and his fellowship work was in sports medicine at the University of California and Center for Health Sciences in Los Angeles. Dr. Armsey is a member of the American Academy of Family Physicians, American Medical Society of Teachers of Family Medicine, and the Kentucky Academy of Family Physicians. Dr. Armsey serves as a team physician for football, basketball, and nonrevenue sports at UCLA, the University of Kentucky and most recently, the University of South Carolina, where he was director of primary care sports medicine.

John P. Batson, MD, FAAP is board certified in pediatrics and holds a certificate of added qualification in primary care sports medicine. He has been in private practice for the past 5 years and has served as a Clinical Associate Professor with USC School of Medicine. He has been selected to serve on multiple state-wide taskforce panels related to adolescent athletic health and pediatric physical activity/health promotion. He has received a special achievement award from the American Academy of Pediatrics for his work with overweight youth. In addition, he was selected to serve on the National American Heart Association Spokespersons Panel related to childhood physical activity and obesity. Currently he is completing a 1-year accredited fellowship in interventional spine care. He will return to private practice upon completion of this training, specializing in adult and pediatric sport and spine medicine

Mark E. Cole, MS, ATC, LAT, CSCS is a doctoral student in the College of Health Sciences at the University of Wisconsin-Milwaukee studying sport psychology and the sociology of sport. His research interests include the perception, understanding, utilization, and management of emotion in sport; disordered eating in athletes; and sociocultural bias in sports medicine. He has been a certified athletic trainer since 1991, a certified strength and conditioning coach since 1999, and is licensed to practice athletic training in the state of Wisconsin. As an athletic trainer, Mark has worked extensively at the scholastic, collegiate, Olympic, and professional levels.

Teresa B. Fletcher, PhD, LPC, NCC is an assistant professor in the department of psychology and sociology at North Georgia College and State University. She played volleyball at Loyola University in Chicago and later coached at the University of Evansville prior to earning a Master's degree in Community Counseling at Northeastern Illinois University. She received her doctorate in Counseling and Counselor Education at the University of North Carolina at Greensboro (family counseling emphasis, sport psychology cognate). Dr. Fletcher's work is informed by reality and strategic family therapies and intelligence theory. Dr. Fletcher is a licensed professional counselor and her interests include eating and lifestyle behaviors among individuals and athletes as well as emotional intelligence in counseling and sport.

Bryan D. Fox, PhD is the Director of Special Projects with the Addiction Recovery Services at Palmetto Health. He has over 12 years of counseling experience, working with adults and adolescents in both inpatient and outpatient settings. He has taught courses on addiction treatment and prevention and provided clinical instruction for medical residents specific to treating adolescents. In addition, Dr. Fox has been a frequent guest lecturer, helping athletic training students learn how to identify clinical issues in athletes and make appropriate referrals. Dr. Fox earned a Bachelor of Arts degree in Psychology from Furman University, a Master of Education degree in Rehabilitation Counseling, and a Doctor of Philosophy degree in Motor Development from the University of South Carolina.

Jeffery A. Guy, MD, a native of California, received his medical degree, magna cum laude, from Harvard University School of Medicine in Boston, MA in 1994. Prior to a sports medicine fellowship at the American Sports Medicine Institute in Birmingham, AL (2000-2001), he held two fellowships in Boston, which included a trauma fellowship at Massachusetts General Hospital (1999) and a pediatric sports medicine fellowship at Children's Hospital (2000). In 2001, Dr. Guy became Assistant Professor of Orthopaedic Surgery at the University of South Carolina School of Medicine. Dr. Guy's sports medicine experience includes a long list of athletic coverage, including assistant team physician for Auburn University and the University of Alabama. Dr. Guy is currently company physician for the Columbia City Ballet and is the founder of the South Carolina SMART program (Sports Medicine for Athletes and Recreational Teams), which serves more than 25 high schools and middle schools in the greater Columbia area. Dr. Guy is currently team physician and orthopaedic surgeon for several high school and college teams, most notably the University of South Carolina Gamecocks. He currently serves as Medical Director for the University of South Carolina athletic programs.

Daniel B. Kissinger, PhD, LPC, NCC is an Assistant Professor and coordinator of the community counseling specialization in the counselor education program at the University of Arkansas, Fayetteville. He holds a Master of Science degree in counseling from Clemson University and a Master of Science degree in kinesiology from the University of Nevada, Las Vegas. He received his doctoral degree in counselor education from the University of South Carolina, Columbia. He is a licensed professional counselor and nationally certified counselor, and holds the supervision specialization in Arkansas. His research focuses on the phenomenological experiences of counselors-in training, counselors, and student athletes.

Matthew E. Lemberger, PhD is an Assistant Professor in the Division of Counseling and Family Therapy at the University of Missouri—St. Louis. Dr. Lemberger has worked in both school and community-based settings as a counselor and in other related human service roles. His research focuses on areas such as counselor training, school counseling issues (e.g., closing the achievement gap), cultural issues in counseling, counseling supervision, and individual psychology. His contribution to this text comes from both his experience as a professional counselor and as an athlete in a variety of sports.

Timothy D. Malone, MD attended the College of Charleston (obtaining a Bacherlor of Arts degree in Physics) and the University of South Carolina School of Medicine. He completed his residency in General Psychiatry and Child and Adolescent Psychiatry program at William S. Hall Psychiatric Institute, Columbia, SC. He is board certified in general psychiatry, child and adolescent psychiatry, forensic psychiatry, and addiction medicine by the American Society of Addiction Medicine. He is the Clinical Professor for Child and Adolescent Psychiatry at the University of South Carolina, Medicine, Child and Adolescent Professor Addiction Medicine and the Director of Wellness for Sports Medicine at the University of South Carolina. He was Chief of Psychiatry at Palmetto

Health Alliance (2004 and 2005) and a nominated teacher of the year by the Child and Adolescent Residents for 2005, 2006, and 2007.

Barbara B. Meyer, PhD is an Associate Professor in the Department of Human Movement Sciences at the University of Wisconsin-Milwaukee. She received her Doctor of Philosophy degree in Health Education, Counseling Psychology, and Human Performance (sport psychology emphasis, counseling cognate) from Michigan State University. Dr. Meyer's interest in applied sport psychology is informed by social psychology theory, intelligence theory, and cognitive behavioral therapy. Current research is focused on (a) the assessment of emotional intelligence in athletic populations; (b) the description of emotional intelligence in athletes and coaches; and (c) the relationship between emotional intelligence, sport participation, sport performance, and satisfaction with the sport experience. Dr. Meyer's research and knowledge of theory serve as a foundation for her ongoing work as a performance enhancement consultant to world class athletes, performing artists, and corporate groups.

Eva V. Monsma, PhD is an Associate Professor in the Department of Physical Education at the University of South Carolina. She received her doctorate from Michigan State University in 1999 in the psychosocial aspects of physical activity. Her research interests include imagery use by children, injured athletes, and allied health professionals as well as biological and psychological characteristics of aesthetic sport athletes. She teaches psychology of sport and injury rehabilitation; the art and science of coaching; child and adolescent growth, development, and measurement; and evaluation and research in physical education. As a sport psychology consultant and former figure skating coach, she has nearly 20 years of experience applying principles of sport psychology with athletes.

Ashley Mulvey, MS, ATC completed her contributions while attending the University of South Carolina where she received a master of science degree in 2006. Preceding her education at University of South Carolina she attended Marshall University where she earned a Bachelors degree in athletic training. Ashley's passion for athletic training began in her home town of Danbury, CT where she had opportunities for further education in athletic training. Ashley is currently working for Merck and Co as a pharmaceutical representative.

Joshua Scott, MD, FACSM received his undergraduate Bachelor of Science degree in Health Sciences at Clemson University. He continued onto medical school and completed his residency in Pediatrics at the Medical University of South Carolina. Upon completion of medical school, Dr. Scott began work at Fellowship in Primary Care Sports Medicine at the University of South Carolina. Dr. Scott currently works in Private Practice Pediatrics and Sports Medicine in Los Angeles where he lives with his wife, Lyne.

Jason J. Stacy, MD was educated at the University of Wisconsin, Madison, WI. Dr. Stacy received a Bachelor of Science degree in Zoology. He earned a doctor of medicine from the Medical College of Wisconsin, Milwaukee. He completed a residency at Baptist Lutheran Medical Center Family Practice, Kansas City, MO. Dr. Stacy joined the faculty of the University of South Carolina School of Medicine in 2004 after completing a primary care sports medicine fellowship at Palmetto Health Richland. He is currently a team physician for the University of South Carolina Athletics.

Laura J. Veach, PhD, LPC, LCAS, CCS, NCC is an Associate Professor in the Department of Counseling at Wake Forest University. She is licensed both as a professional counselor (LPC) and clinical addiction specialist (LCAS). She graduated with a Doctor of Philosophy degree in Counselor Education with her cognate in Health Promotion and Human Performance from the University of New Orleans. She has over 25 years of clinical and management experience in various clinical settings, such as psychiatric hospitals, university counseling centers, Employee Assistance Programs, and addiction treatment centers. She specializes in counseling and research in the areas of substance use disorders, careers, and relationship issues. Dr. Veach has written various articles and chapters pertaining to community counseling issues published. Dr. Veach is the current Past-President of the International Association of Addictions and Offender Counseling (IAAOC), a division of the American Counseling Association.

H. Ray Wooten, PhD is a professor and Graduate Program Director in the Department of Counseling and Human Services at St. Mary's University in San Antonio, TX. Interests and writing include student athletes and psychosocial difficulties, as well as the use of alternative and complimentary therapies.

Introduction

This book was developed through careful consideration of the current National Athletic Trainers' Association (NATA) Educational Competencies, which were released in 2006. However, the emergence of this book began in 2003 when Gary Miller was asked to speak in a seminar class lead by Jim Mensch for his athletic training students at the University of South Carolina. As topics were discussed, these two professionals decided to develop a book focusing on the psychosocial competencies required in the education of professional athletic trainers. The readers of this book will see how these have been addressed in each chapter throughout the book and will benefit by participating in the activities presented at the conclusion of each chapter.

Drs. Mensch and Miller recognized the need to have input from other professionals with expertise in the specific topics presented in the book. They enlisted the assistance of colleagues who prepared information in concert with the NATA educational competencies. These individuals are thanked for their contributions and are listed in the Contributing Authors section of the book.

Chapter 1 provides an overview of the background influencing the development of psychosocial competencies for the profession of athletic training. Information is presented that sets the stage for the chapters that follow.

An introduction of the basic skills of communication for interacting with a patient are provided in Chapter 2. Throughout the chapter, there are skills presented along with ways to understand and motivate individuals. A protocol, HOPE, for use with patients along with the SPORT model of goal setting is also presented.

Being able to make a positive psychosocial referral of an individual is the principal topic of Chapter 3. In addition to the model presented, information regarding the various mental health professionals to whom a referral may be made is presented.

Substance abuse information is found in Chapter 4. The commonly abused substances are presented as well as signs and symptoms one can look for in the abusing patient. Intervention strategies are also found in this chapter.

In Chapter 5, disordered eating issues are addressed. Warning signs and prevention strategies are provided along with current information about prevention strategies that may be useful for the professional athletic trainer to consider.

The psychological response to one's injury is the featured topic of Chapter 6. Life-stress and injury models are presented as well as motivational and anxiety theories that impact the patient.

Additional mental health issues are presented in Chapter 7. The author discusses the positive benefits of athletic involvement and mental health risks along with clarifying specific mental health disorders.

Catastrophic injuries are presented throughout Chapter 8. A section clarifying the differences between normal and pathological responses to injury is presented. Also, a discussion of the necessary aspects of the therapeutic relationship and the professional athletic trainer is included.

Nutritional supplements are the topic in Chapter 9. The issue of anabolic steroids is addressed as are the legal and physiological implications of the use of supplements. There is also a focus on healthy eating as an ergogenic aid for patients.

The psychological impact of sports on children and adolescents is examined in Chapter 10. The authors pinpoint principles of normal growth and the problems that can emerge for youth participating in competitive athletics. Interventions and strategies for the professional athletic trainer are also included.

Chapter 11 examines psychological issues and trends facing the professional athletic trainer. The author incorporates a perspective that includes psychosocial issues relating to physical and psychological health. Also addressed are lifestyle choices individuals make along with ways to look at patients from a holistic point of view. In this chapter, the author also examines gender issues relevant to the professional athletic trainer.

We hope that you find this book beneficial in your professional preparation and that you will keep it as a source in your professional library for years to come. It has truly been a team effort in completing this and we wish you well in your career.

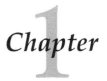

Chapter

ATHLETIC TRAINING AND PSYCHOSOCIAL ISSUES

James M. Mensch, PhD, ATC

Chapter Objectives

- ❖ Identify specific psychosocial issues.
- ❖ Provide a historical overview of the evolution of psychosocial issues in athletic training.
- ❖ Identify the current required psychosocial competencies and proficiencies for athletic training education programs as outlined in the new 2006 National Athletic Trainers' Association (NATA) *Educational Competencies*.
- ❖ Outline specific knowledge and skills related to psychosocial issues that athletic trainers need to be competent professionals as outlined in the 2004 National Athletic Trainers' Association Board of Certification (NATABOC) *Role Delineation Study*.
- ❖ Discuss the role of athletic trainers in treating psychosocial issues in nontraditional settings.

NATA Educational Competencies

PROFESSIONAL DEVELOPMENT AND RESPONSIBILITY DOMAIN

1. Differentiate the essential documents of the national governing, certifying, and accrediting bodies, including (but not limited to) the *Athletic Training Educational Competencies, Standards of Practice, Code of Ethics, Role Delineation Study,* and the *Standards for the Accreditation of Entry-Level Athletic Training Education Programs.*

2. Summarize the current requirements for the professional preparation of the athletic trainer.

3. Summarize the history and development of the athletic training profession.

A certified athletic trainer (ATC) is described as the individual most directly responsible for all phases of health care in an athletic environment (Prentice, 2006). The roles and responsibilities of athletic trainers are very broad, encompassing a variety of specialties encompassed under the sports medicine umbrella. Specific responsibilities for athletic trainers include injury prevention, first aid and injury management, injury evaluation, and rehabilitation. However, the specific roles and responsibilities of an athletic trainer will to some degree be defined by and vary according to the clinical setting in which they work (NATABOC, 2004). Some areas of emphasis common throughout all levels of competition for athletes and physically active individuals are the issues relevant to psychosocial and mental wellness. Athletic trainers in all settings will be required to interact with athletes and physically active individuals suffering from some type of psychosocial or emotional problem.

All athletes and physically active individuals are influenced to some degree by different psychosocial issues that may enhance or deter aspects of their participation in athletics or recovery from an injury. Identifying allied heath personnel that understand psychosocial issues and support athletes from all levels of participation is often difficult. Each of the following sports medicine professionals has some level of training and obligation to provide athletes/patients with appropriate treatment and referral for a wide variety of psychosocial issues:

- Athletic trainer
- Nurse
- Physician
- Physical therapist
- Strength and conditioning specialist
- Exercise physiologists
- Nutritionist
- Physician's assistant
- Counselor
- Sports psychologist
- Clinical psychologist

Determining which allied health professional is in the best position to provide appropriate care to an athlete/patient suffering from a psychosocial issue or emotional problem is not easy. In addition, universities, colleges, high schools, and sports medicine clinics may not have the most appropriate resources (e.g., a clinical psychologist or counselor) to help support individuals suffering from different psychosocial issues. The role many allied health professionals play in supporting athletes/physically active individuals suffering from these psychosocial issues is dictated by their educational training and state licensing agencies and/or practice acts. Athletes, coaches, parents, and support staff may not be familiar with the level of training each allied health professional has related to dealing with psychosocial issues. Since laws and supervision of allied health professionals vary from state to state, it is difficult for anyone to understand the specific roles that each professional is legally permitted to play in treating physically active individuals or athletes. In no other area of athletics or health care is the role of a sports medicine professional as vague and undefined as it is with psychosocial issues. The purpose of this chapter is to outline specific psychosocial issues relevant to athletes and physically active individuals, as well as discuss the educational training and expectations for ATCs confronted with these problems in their employment setting.

What Are Psychosocial Issues?

Psychosocial issues are not tangible. Unlike a fracture or shoulder dislocation, psychosocial issues cannot be diagnosed with an x-ray or magnetic resonance image (MRI). It is not possible to look inside an athlete's mind and determine the best course of action. It may not be possible to see the pain or understand the etiology behind a psychosocial issue. Instead, allied health professionals, including athletic trainers, must rely on self-reported information from the patient and inferences from his or her behavior that many times may be inaccurate or biased. Unless the athlete or patient is willing to open up and discuss his or her problems truthfully, it is impossible to know what is going on inside his or her head. Subsequently, the most debilitating injury or illness for an athlete may not come from a fractured leg or torn ligament, but rather a psychosocial issue that remains hidden from all members of the sports medicine team. Since athletic trainers have frequent contact with athletes both before and after injuries, they are in a unique position to closely examine the physical and mental well-being of athletes as well as make any necessary referrals (Etzel, Ferrante, & Pinkney, 1991). Whether or not they are trained or legally/ethically permitted to care for an athlete/patient suffering from a psychosocial disorder, ATCs are often asked and expected to counsel patients through these issues.

Psychosocial is a wonderful "label" for educators and practicing professionals to characterize issues outside of the traditional sports medicine realm. Psychosocial is defined as issues or situations "involving both psychological and social aspects" (Dirckx, 2001). The combination of two broad disciplines (psychology and sociology) results in a myriad of problems that may influence athletic performance and/or medical treatment of a patient. A clearer understanding of how each construct relates to athlete performance and potential injury/illness is critical to managing psychosocial issues for athletes and physically active individuals.

PSYCHOLOGICAL INFLUENCE

Issues pertaining to psychology and mental health have a long-standing history and relationship with athletes and sports performance. Today many athletes and coaches look to sports psychologists for a variety of reasons in the hope they may enhance performance in sports and exercise. Sports psychology is broadly defined as "a science in which the principles of psychology are applied in a sport or exercise setting" (Cox, 1998). The Association for the Advancement of Applied Sports Psychology (AAASP) emphasizes the intervention, performance enhancement, and health psychology and their relationship with sport and exercise (Ray, Terrell, & Hough, 1999). At the present time, it is common for a sports psychologist to be intimately involved with athletes from all levels (professional, college, high school, recreation) of athletic competition. The enhanced recognition of athletes and role of sports in the lives of spectators and participants has been accompanied by increased interest into the psychological well-being of athletes (Storch, Storch, Killiany, & Roberti, 2005). At each level of competition there are a variety of different situations pertaining to mental health and psychosocial issues that may warrant appropriate counseling from a trained professional.

Literature examining various psychological issues and aspects of sports, athletic performance, and medicine is extremely common (Andersen, 2000; Gieck, 1994 Robertson & Newton, 2005; Roh & Perna, 2000; Udry & Andersen, 2002;). Traditionally, sports medicine professionals have primarily concerned themselves with the physical readiness of injured athletes to return to competition. The most common interaction athletic trainers will have with psychological issues and athletes will occur during rehabilitation from injury. Optimal injury rehabilitation requires athletic trainers to consider a holistic approach, combining both the physical and psychological aspects influencing the rehabilitation process. However, injured athletes are not the only individuals that benefit from an appropriate psychosocial intervention and referral. Individuals benefiting from an increased awareness of skills and strategies related to different psychological constructs include:

- *Athletes in competitive sports (professional, college, high school, youth).* Athletes can be counseled to use a variety of psychological constructs to enhance their athletic performance.
- *Recreational athletes.* Recreational athletes can benefit from training in many of the same psychological constructs used by competitive athletes.
- *Injured athletes at all levels of competition.* Athletic trainers and other sports medicine professionals will play a significant role in providing injured athletes at all levels with the skills necessary to cope with specific psychosocial issues.
- *Coaches.* Coaches will attempt to implement any specific psychological skill/strategy that may assist athletes in reaching their highest athletic potential.
- *Parents and significant others.* Family plays an important role in the sports culture for many athletes, specifically when the athlete becomes injured. Parents and significant others have a great deal of influence over an athlete and must be involved in managing specific psychosocial issues that may negatively affect performance or recovery from an injury.

COMMON PSYCHOLOGICAL CONSTRUCTS

Expectations from coaches, parents, and athletes to provide support in areas pertaining to psychosocial intervention and referral have forced educators and practitioners to re-evaluate the roles they play in these difficult situations. Despite the lack of appropriate training, state laws, and specific practice acts, many sports medicine professionals and nonprofessionals have no problem with offering suggestions and/or treatment relative to a wide variety of psychological constructs. Many of these constructs appear nonevasive, and therefore allied health professionals often do not consider the consequences of potentially inappropriate guidance or counseling. Many psychosocial issues emerge on a daily basis where athletic trainers and other allied health professionals become personally involved with the athlete/patient. Examples of typical psychological constructs relevant to sports and athletes/physically active individuals are listed as follows:

- *Achievement motivation.* An athlete's predisposition to approach or avoid a competitive situation, including the concept of desire or desire to excel (Cox, 1998). Example: An athlete with a career-ending knee injury needs to begin a tough 9-month rehabilitation program. How will motivation play a role in his or her rehabilitation and successful return to play?

- *Anxiety.* A negative emotional state with feelings of nervousness, worry, and apprehension associated with achievement or arousal of the body (Weinberg & Gould, 1995). Example: An athlete has been released to full-contact and will be ready to play in the next game. This will be the first game since tearing his or her anterior cruciate ligament (ACL) several months ago. The athlete is extremely nervous and worries that the knee will not hold up in a real game.

- *Imagery.* Creating or recreating an experience in the mind (Weinberg & Gould, 1995). Example: Two athletes have the same exact injury. One has been taught specific skills in imagery as part of the rehabilitation protocol. The other athlete follows the same rehabilitation protocol, minus the imagery skills. Can imagery play a role in enhancing therapeutic rehabilitation and a successful return to sports participation?

- *Self-efficacy.* The perception of one's ability to perform a task successfully (Bandura, 1986). Example: An athlete involved in a rehabilitation program has completed 95% of the required treatments. As he or she enters the functional phase and return to play, the athlete begins to discuss his or her concerns about returning to full participation. The athlete cites concerns regarding his or her ability to successfully compete at the same level prior to the injury.

- *Attribution theory.* A cognitive approach to motivation in which perceived causation plays an important role in explaining behavior (Heider, 1944). Example: A tennis player who is unranked with a record of 3 wins and 15 losses beats our best player (Nancy) who is ranked #3 in the country with a record of 17 wins and 1 loss. Nancy has been suffering from a sore shoulder and blames the loss on her shoulder and the athletic trainer.

- *Burnout.* A psychological, emotional, and sometimes physical withdrawal from an activity in response to excessive stress or dissatisfaction (Smith, 1986). Example: A fifth year senior with four prior surgeries is contemplating quitting the team. The coach and other teammates are pressuring him or her to have a fifth surgery, but the athlete has told you he or she is burned out.

- *Locus of control.* The extent to which people believe they are responsible for their behavioral outcomes (Rotter, 1966). Example: Part of the rehabilitation program for an athlete with a post-surgical ACL repair is to strengthen the quadriceps muscles. The athlete would like to strengthen the quadriceps by performing exercises in the pool, but the athletic trainer would rather have the athlete perform leg extensions in the weight room. What is the problem/benefit of allowing the athlete to decide?

- *Addiction.* Habitual psychological and physiological dependence on a substance or practice that is beyond voluntary control (Dirckx, 2001). Example: After several surgical procedures to repair a fractured/dislocated hip, you discover the athlete is addicted to pain medication.

PSYCHOLOGICAL RESPONSE

The psychological response of an athlete to different aspects of sports (e.g., winning, losing, injury, big games, poor performance) can be unpredictable. It is imperative that sports medicine team members understand the impact of an athlete's psychological response on his or her physical and mental health and return to competition. For example, an athlete that returns to competition after an injury with anxiety and tension related to the injury may be predisposed to one or more of the following (Williams & Scherzer, 2006):

- Re-injury
- Injury to another body part
- Lowered confidence resulting in a temporary performance decrement
- Lowered confidence resulting in a permanent performance decrement
- General depression and fear of further injury, which can sap motivation and the desire to return to competition

A clearer understanding of how each psychological construct may be related to some aspect of an athlete's health care and subsequent performance is critical for athletic trainers. A major purpose of this book is to help clarify the role athletic trainers and other members of the sports medicine team play in supporting athletes with specific problems related to many of the psychological constructs (see Chapters 4 through 11).

SOCIOLOGICAL INFLUENCES

The previous section outlines specific examples of psychological influences that impact directly on the individual (healthy and injured athletes). Psychological constructs such as motivation, anxiety, imagery, self-efficacy, burnout, and locus of control all apply to the individual. Sociological issues also have a long-standing association with athletes and sports. However, sociology of sport is a discipline that focuses on social relations, group interactions, and sports-related social phenomena (Cox, 1998). Since groups and relationships are composed of individuals, sometimes it is difficult to understand and determine differences between psychological and social issues. To help clarify and categorize issues that combine both psychological and sociological issues, educators and practitioners have created the term *psychosocial* or *social psychology*. Most allied health professionals are more familiar with the physical nature of injuries and illnesses and less equipped to deal with sociological factors that may play a role in the care and prevention of sports injuries.

COMMON EXAMPLES OF A SPORTS CULTURE

Many of the societal problems associated with athletes are the result of a sports culture that perpetuates the importance of individual athletic performance and winning. A "win at all cost" attitude is a reflection of a sports culture that socializes athletes to adopt specific attitudes and values that in some cases may be detrimental and unhealthy. Frey (1991) suggests that a "culture of risk" adopts beliefs and a mentality that encourages athletes to play with pain and injuries and those who play with pain are glorified by coaches and fans. For example, an athlete may be afraid of being labeled weak or soft and continues to play through severe pain, risking permanent injury. A sports culture that perpetuates negative behaviors results in a variety of sociological issues that may require some type of intervention, potentially from a ATC. Specific examples of these sociological/cultural issues include:

- *Ethics/morality.* Example: You find out an athlete has been cheating the drug testing protocol and in fact has taken steroids the entire year.
- *Sexual orientation issues.* Example: During a 9-month rehabilitation for an injured leg, a football player confides in you that he is a homosexual but is not willing to "come out" for fear of retribution from teammates.
- *Gender issues.* Example: It has become evident that the female athletes at this university do not receive the same level of medical attention as the males. The facilities and sports medicine equipment are substandard. All male sports are covered by an ATC and equivalent female sports are covered by an uncertified student.
- *Youth and adolescent issues.* Example: A 13-year-old baseball pitcher begins rehabilitation from an ulnar collateral ligament repair. After a few weeks you learn that the athlete's parent encouraged him to throw through the elbow pain in the hopes that surgery would be required so the physician could "tighten up all the ligaments and muscles" in an attempt to increase the speed of his fastball.
- *Society expectations.* Example: A freshmen swimmer begins to struggle with an eating disorder. She is unable to cope with the expectations of the coach, teammates, and media for being labeled the next great national champion for the best swimming team in the country.
- *Racial issues.* Example: Less than 10% of the athletic training membership is ethnically diverse, as opposed to the higher percentage of athletes under a ATC's care. Establishing a relationship across cultural and racial lines is critical for athletic trainers.
- *Aggression.* Example: A very intense football player is unable to control his aggression off the field. You learn he takes out his aggression on his girlfriend and is both physically and mentally abusive.

Despite the fact that many of these sociological issues are beyond their daily practice and job responsibility, athletic trainers often become the first individual an athlete will confide in. Athletes are often reluctant to confide in a coach or teammate for fear of punishment and losing their standing (position) within the team. As a result, athletic trainers must be equipped to care for athletes dealing with a wide span of sociological problems. Prior to learning general counseling skills, intervention strategies, and referral guidelines, it is critical for athletic trainers to become more aware of different psychosocial issues that affect athletes.

Many sociological issues associated with sports stem from larger societal problems. For example, cheating and racism are common throughout all aspects of life and society, not just sports/athletics. Understanding how sociological issues influence the potential health and performance of an athlete or physically active individual requires a more in-depth understanding of the athlete and the problem. For example, an athlete may present with a number of abnormal signs and symptoms related to depression but go untreated because no sports medicine professional was able to intervene on behalf of the athlete. Sports medicine professionals, including athletic trainers, should not be asked to be responsible for every psychological and sociological problem athletes and other physically active individuals encounter. However, it is reasonable to expect that the individuals closest to athletes, specifically injured athletes, have specific "helping skills" to help initiate the appropriate care for all individuals suffering from both psychological and sociological problems. Chapters 2 and 3 in this book will provide appropriate intervention/counseling strategies, and Chapters 4 through 11 will provide referral techniques specific to the role of the ATC to initiate recovery for any athlete/patient suffering from specific psychosocial issues outlined in Chapters 4 through 11.

RESPONDING TO PSYCHOSOCIAL ISSUES

Many of the psychological and sociological issues facing athletes and physically active individuals are interrelated. Typically, psychosocial issues are attempted to be resolved by a variety of different individuals, some with little or no training. The attitude that psychosocial issues can be resolved by a good conversation with someone or getting a "good night's sleep" results in a disservice to the athlete/patient with the problem. Athletic trainers are in a unique position to provide a wide variety of services to healthy and injured athletes. The large amount of time spent with athletes at practice, games, travel, and meals provides athletic trainers with insight and a chance to know each athlete at a more intimate level than any other allied health professional. As a result, athletic trainers have been asked to provide specific levels of support for athletes and physically active individuals suffering from a wide variety of psychosocial issues. The expectation for athletic trainers to become trained with the knowledge and skills to treat and refer athletes dealing with psychosocial issues has increased dramatically over the past 10 years, and today has become a large component of the didactic and clinical educational requirements for athletic training education programs.

For many years after the establishment of the NATA, practicing athletic trainers were not viewed as legitimate allied health care professionals. The educational and clinical preparation of athletic trainers, specifically pertaining to psychosocial issues, was suspect and questioned for a long time. A clearer understanding of the evolution of psychosocial issues in athletic training education is helpful for students as they formulate a perspective of the roles and responsibilities of athletic trainers. A historical perspective of athletic training education is identified as a specific cognitive competency required by accredited athletic training education programs. Educating current students on historical issues related to education reform (clinical and didactic) creates the educated and well-informed professionals needed to advance the standing of the athletic training profession within the allied health community.

Evolution of Psychosocial Issues in Athletic Training Education

For many years, educational experiences for athletic trainers covering specific knowledge and skills related to psychosocial issues was basically nonexistent. From the establishment of the NATA in 1950 until the late 1990s, very little attention was given to psychosocial issues in athletic training education. Today many athletic trainers acknowledge they lack the appropriate skills and training necessary to treat and counsel athletes on issues related to psychosocial well-being (Larson, Starkey, & Zaichkowsky, 1996; Moulton, Molstad, & Turner, 1997; Wiese, Wiese, & Yukelson, 1991). Studies indicate that athletic trainers are unaware of on-campus support services and do not refer a significant number of injured athletes with pronounced psychological distress for counseling (Larson et al., 1996). A brief historical overview of an athletic trainer's educational training and role in dealing with psychosocial issues and counseling will explain why many current athletic trainers feel uncomfortable in many of these situations as well as why this information is a critical component of a student's educational experience within accredited programs.

Table 1-1
1959 Athletic Training Curriculum Model (Suggested Courses)

- Physical therapy school prerequisites (minimum 24 semester hours)
- Biology/zoology (8 semester hours)
- Physics and/or chemistry (6 semester hours)
- Social sciences (10 semester hours)
- Electives (e.g., hygiene, speech)
- Specific course requirements (if not included above): anatomy, physiology, physiology of exercise
- Applied anatomy and kinesiology
- Laboratory physical science (6 semester hours, chemistry and/or physics)
- Psychology (6 semester hours)
- Coaching techniques (9 semester hours)
- First aid and safety
- Nutrition and foods
- Remedial exercise
- Organization and administration of health and physical education
- Personal and community hygiene
- Techniques of athletic training
- Advanced techniques of athletic training
- Laboratory practices (6 semester hours or equivalent)
- Recommended courses: general physics, pharmacology, histology, pathology

EARLY ATHLETIC TRAINING EDUCATION

During the early years of athletic training in the late 1950s and early 1960s, education requirements were designed based on meeting prerequisites for physical therapy preparation and secondary-level teacher certification (Schwank & Miller, 1971). There was no specific focus on content related to athletic training or injured athletes except for two courses: basic and advanced athletic training. In addition, there was no formal course related to clinical experiences, and clinical skills were learned during field experiences under the guidance of a ATC. Skills for managing all problems associated with an injured athlete were learned "on-the-job" during interactions with more experienced ATCs. The initial athletic training guidelines consisted of 6 hours of education in psychology, thus limiting the preparation of athletic trainers to support athletes/patients facing various psychosocial issues. An example of an athletic training curriculum during the early years of the profession is provided in Table 1-1 (Delforge & Behnke, 1999).

The athletic training curriculum model during the 1970s was very similar to that of the late 1950s. Two major changes to athletic training education programs were to 1) drop the requirement of prerequisites for physical therapy school, and 2) add a minimum number of clinical hour experiences (600 hours) under the direct supervision of a ATC. These changes were an attempt to remove irrelevant or minimally relevant material from the curriculum and narrow the focus of athletic training education to a core of courses (Delforge & Behnke, 1999). In the late 1960s, an effort was made by the NATA Certification Committee to develop a national certification exam. The purpose of a standardized exam was to ensure that all ATCs had met some set of minimal competencies for practice in the profession. The first national certification exam for athletic trainers was administered in 1970. Despite continued growth in athletic training education and certification requirements during the

Table 1-2
Mid-1970s Athletic Training Curriculum Model

- Anatomy (1 course)
- Physiology (1 course)
- Physiology of exercise (1 course)
- Applied anatomy and kinesiology (1 course)
- Psychology (2 courses)
- First aid and safety (1 course)
- Nutrition (1 course)
- Remedial exercise (1 course)
- Personal, community, and school health (1 course)
- Basic athletic training (1 course)
- Advanced athletic training (1 course)
- Laboratory or practical experiences in athletic training to include a minimum of 600 total clock hours under the direct supervision of an NATA-ATC

1970s, the educational experiences specific to psychosocial issues remained as 6 hours of coursework in psychology. An example of an athletic training curriculum during the mid-1970s is provided in Table 1-2 (Delforge & Behnke, 1999).

The athletic training curriculum models of the 1950s, 1960s, and 1970s basically prepared students to be athletic trainers as apprenticeships with classes centered on teacher preparation and physical therapy (Delforge & Behnke, 1999). There was always a requirement of two psychology courses, but no mention of specific skills or training related to dealing with psychosocial issues in an athletic/sports context. During this time there was no structure to incorporate the clinical experiences students obtained under a ATC with any required course in the curriculum. There was no chance for athletic training students to integrate clinical experiences associated with psychosocial issues with their required psychology courses.

THE 1980S AND 1990S: EDUCATIONAL COMPETENCIES

During the early years of the 1980s, the NATA implemented education reform that eliminated the requirement of specific courses in athletic training education programs. The new standards required athletic training education programs to implement specific subject matter (not specific courses) into the curriculum, which provided more flexibility in the development of educational experiences. In 1983, the NATA published *The Guidelines for Development and Implementation of NATA Approved Undergraduate Athletic Training Programs*, which contained the standards for development of athletic training academic majors (Delforge & Behnke, 1999). The specific subject matter requirements for athletic training education programs as outlined in the 1983 guidelines are listed in Table 1-3.

In addition to the new requirement of specific subject matter for athletic training education programs, the 1983 guidelines also established competencies in athletic training. These educational competencies were based on the results of the first *Role Delineation Study* (NATABOC, 1982), which identified specific performance domains of ATCs. The purpose of the *Role Delineation Study* and educational competencies was to identify the job responsibility of athletic trainers and subsequent knowledge and skills needed to fulfill these responsibilities. The 1983 guidelines included educational competencies specific to psychosocial intervention and referral, which meant practicing athletic trainers identified

> ### Table 1-3
> ## *1983 Athletic Training Curriculum Subject Matter Requirements*
>
> - Prevention of athletic injuries/illnesses
> - Evaluation of athletic injuries/illnesses
> - First aid and emergency care
> - Therapeutic modalities
> - Therapeutic exercise
> - Administration of athletic training programs
> - Human anatomy
> - Human physiology
> - Exercise physiology
> - Kinesiology/biomechanics
> - Nutrition

specific knowledge and skills within this domain as a significant component of a ATC's job. The initial educational competencies related to psychosocial issues and required of accredited athletic training education programs were very vague and included within the following domain (NATA, 1983):

1983 COUNSELING AND GUIDANCE EDUCATIONAL COMPETENCIES

Provides health care information and advises and counsels athletes, parents, and coaches on matters pertaining to the physical, psychological, and emotional health and well-being of the competitive athlete.

Specific knowledge and intellectual skills related to psychosocial issues are:

- Physiological effects of physical activity on menstruation (oligomenorrhea, amenorrhea, dysmenorrheal) and associated psychological considerations.

- Prevailing misconceptions regarding the proper utilization of foodstuffs as related to common food fads and fallacies, dietary supplements, and nutritional needs of the competitive athlete.

- Physiological processes and time factors involved in the digestion, absorption, and assimilation of various foodstuffs as related to the design and planning of pre-game/event meals, including consideration of menu content, time scheduling, and the effect of pre-event tension and anxiety.

- The effects of commonly abused drugs and other substances on the athlete's physical and psychological health and athletic performance (alcohol, tobacco, stimulants, steroids, narcotics, etc.).

- Commonly available school health services, community health agencies, and community-based psychological and social services.

- The role and function of various community-based medical/paramedical specialists (orthopedists, neurologists, internists, etc.) and other health care providers (psychologists, counselors, social workers, etc.).

- Common signs and indications of mental disorders (psychoses, etc.), emotional disorders (neurosis, anxiety, depression, etc.), or personal/social conflict (family problems, school-related stress, etc.).

- Accepted protocol governing the referral of athletes for personal health, psychological, or social services.

Affective domains (attitudes and values) are:

- Acceptance of the professional, ethical, and legal parameters which define the proper role of the ATC in providing health care information and counseling.
- Acceptance of the responsibility to provide health care information and counseling consistent with the ATC's professional training and expertise.

The 1983 *Competencies in Athletic Training* was revised several times in the 1990s and more specific knowledge and skills related to psychosocial issues and referral became integrated into the professional preparation of athletic trainers. As a result of educational reform in athletic training, entry-level athletic training education programs now require specific educational competencies to be covered in the didactic and clinical experiences of the program, including a specific domain to cover psychosocial intervention and referral. The fourth edition of *Athletic Training Educational Competencies* was released in February 2006 (NATA, 2006).

REMOVAL OF THE BOARD OF CERTIFICATION INTERNSHIP TO CERTIFICATION

In 2004, the NATA and the Board of Certification (BOC) instituted a requirement to eliminate the internship (apprenticeship) route to BOC certification, thus requiring all candidates seeking BOC certification to complete an accredited entry-level athletic training education program. The internship route leading to certification from the BOC was a model designed to allow future professionals in athletic training the chance to learn specific knowledge and skills "on-the-job" and under the tutelage of an experienced ATC. The internship route to certification was a common practice for students to meet eligibility requirements for the BOC certification examination from the inaugural certification exam in 1970 (Westphalen & McLean, 1978) up until the removal of the internship route to certification in 2004. The internship route to BOC certification was characterized by different didactic and clinical portions of athletic training education that varied across programs and therefore experiences pertaining to psychosocial issues could not be planned. Removal of the internship route to BOC certification in 2004 helped to standardize athletic training education and enhance consistency with professional preparation in other allied health disciplines. After 2004, all educational competencies (including psychosocial competencies) became a more regular component of the didactic and clinical experiences of athletic training students.

2006 NATA Educational Competencies

Entry-level athletic training education is competency based. The NATA Education Council created a list of specific educational competencies and clinical proficiencies required for effective performance as an entry-level ATC. The educational competencies are used to do the following:

- Develop curriculum and educational experiences within accredited athletic training education programs (the knowledge and skills in the educational competencies document serve as the core content of athletic training education).

- Assist athletic training students, approved clinical instructors (ACIs), and clinical supervisors in clearly identifying the knowledge and skills to be practiced and taught as part of clinical education.
- Serve as a guide for the development of educational experiences in preparation for the BOC examination.

The educational competencies and proficiencies are categorized according to 12 specific domains. The 12 domains outline the general education requirements to be taught in both the classroom and clinical setting. The competencies and proficiencies in the 2006 *Athletic Training Educational Competencies* were created to help standardize the educational experiences of students in accredited athletic training education programs and enhance the overall quality of athletic training professionals. The athletic training required educational competencies are divided into 12 domains:

1. Risk Management and Injury Prevention
2. Pathology of Injuries, Illnesses, and Disease
3. Orthopedic Assessment and Evaluation
4. Acute Care of Injury and Illness
5. Pharmacology
6. Therapeutic Modalities
7. Therapeutic Exercise
8. Medical Conditions and Disabilities
9. Nutritional Aspects of Injuries and Illnesses
10. Psychosocial Intervention and Referral
11. Health Care Administration
12. Professional Development and Responsibilities

PSYCHOSOCIAL INTERVENTION AND REFERRAL DOMAIN

One of the 12 education domains identified by the NATA is psychosocial intervention and referral. Specific knowledge and skills pertaining to psychosocial issues are now required by entry-level athletic training education programs and expected of practicing ATCs. Education programs are required to integrate knowledge, skills, and values associated with recognition, intervention, and referral of appropriate psychosocial issues as outlined in the 2006 *Athletic Training Educational Competencies*. The psychosocial intervention and referral domain identifies 14 comprehensive cognitive competencies, 2 clinical proficiencies, and a list of core values to be integrated into the didactic and clinical experiences of athletic training students in entry-level athletic training education programs. The latest edition of the *Athletic Training Educational Competencies* outlines the knowledge, skills, and values that entry-level ATCs must possess. It incorporates the recognition, intervention, and referral necessary when psychosocial aspects impact the athlete/patient. The following is a list of the cognitive educational competencies related to psychosocial issues (NATA, 2006) along with an example related to athletic training and the chapters in this book in which they are addressed.

Cognitive Competencies

- Explain the psychosocial requirements (i.e., motivation and self-confidence) of various activities that relate to the readiness of the injured or ill individual to resume participation (Chapters 3 and 6). *Example: At what point is an athlete who has recovered from an ACL injury ready to return to play? Does he or she trust the knee without a brace? How does an athletic trainer know if the athlete is mentally ready?*

- Explain the stress-response model and the psychological and emotional responses to trauma and forced inactivity (Chapter 6). *Example: Why are two athletes with the same exact injury responding so different to the rehabilitation? Why is Kent so emotional about a simple ankle sprain?*

- Describe the motivational techniques that the athletic trainer must use during injury rehabilitation and reconditioning (Chapter 6). *Example: Sidney refuses to give 100% during the rehabilitation of his ankle. I do not think he is lazy, but I have tried everything I know to get him to complete his exercises. I wish I could get across to him.*

- Describe the basic principles of mental preparation, relaxation, visualization, and desensitization techniques (Chapter 6). *Example: Bobby indicates that he is having a hard time concentrating at home plate while batting as a result of getting hit in the head by a pitch a few weeks ago. His batting average has dropped 50 points in the last week. He asks you for help.*

- Describe the basic principles of general personality traits, associated trait anxiety, locus of control, and patient and social environmental interactions (Chapters 6 and 7). *Example: What type of preparation is needed for the first day of rehabilitation for a freshmen athlete far from home who had up to this point never been hurt a day in his life?*

- Explain the importance of providing health care information to patients, parents/guardians, and others regarding the psychological and emotional well-being of the patient (Chapters 2 and 3). *Example: No one seems to understand why Jenny, the star athlete, committed suicide yesterday. Many believe it had something to do with her struggles with an eating disorder.*

- Describe the roles and function of various community-based health care providers (to include, but not be limited to psychologists, counselors, social workers, human resources personnel) and the accepted protocols that govern the referral of patients to these professionals (Chapter 3). *Example: It is clear that the recently certified graduate assistant athletic trainer needs help in dealing with an athlete on the team who was diagnosed as clinically depressed back in high school.*

- Describe the theories and techniques of interpersonal and cross-cultural communication among athletic trainers, their patients, and others involved in the health care of the patient (Chapter 2). *Example: It was easy to see why the coach was so upset. After all, the athletic trainer told Suzy she could not practice at all for 2 weeks even though she had not been seen by a physician. Suzy is the type of athlete who will shut down while she is injured.*

- Explain the basic principles of counseling (discussion, active listening, and resolution) and the various strategies that ATCs may employ to avoid and resolve conflicts among superiors, peers, and subordinates (Chapter 2). *Example: All the coach does is complain about the athletes who are injured on the team and cannot play. Like it is my fault (athletic trainer) that he practices his or her athletes too hard and then they get injured.*

- Identify the symptoms and clinical signs of common eating disorders and the psychological and sociocultural factors associated with these disorders (Chapter 5). *Example: I had no idea that Jenny the star athlete was suffering from an eating disorder. All of my experiences up until this year have been with male sports and they do not have those types of problems.*

- Identify and describe the sociological, biological, and psychological influences toward substance abuse, addictive personality traits, commonly abused substances, signs and symptoms associated with the abuse of these substances, and their impact on an individual's health and physical performance (Chapter 4 and 9). *Example: I know Pat liked to party and Mark was in the weight room all the time, but no one seemed to have any idea that Pat was abusing alcohol and Mark was taking steroids.*

- Describe the basic signs and symptoms of mental disorders (psychoses), emotional disorders (neuroses, depression), or personal/social conflict (family problems, academic or emotional stress, personal assault or abuse, sexual assault, sexual harassment), as well as the contemporary personal, school, and community health service agencies, such as community-based psychological and social support services, that treat these conditions and the appropriate referral procedures for accessing these health service agencies (Chapters 3 and 7). *Example: I think John the basketball player might be bipolar. He is acting like the individual I saw on TV who had it. He is always acting weird.*

- Describe the acceptance and grieving processes that follow a catastrophic event and the need for a psychological intervention and referral plan for all parties affected by the event (Chapters 3, 6, and 8). *Example: It seems as though the entire team, athletic department, and coaches have not recovered from the sudden death of Jenny the star athlete. I did not know what to do to help.*

- Explain the potential need for psychosocial intervention and referral when dealing with populations requiring special consideration (to include but not limited to those with exercised-induced asthma, diabetes, seizure disorders, drug allergies and interactions, unilateral organs, physical and/or mental disability) (Chapters 3 and 10). *Example: I know that Chris is a diabetic, but it is not my job to monitor his diet 24 hours a day. I do not have time to check his blood sugar every hour for the entire season.*

- Describe the psychosocial factors that affect persistent pain perception (i.e., emotional state, locus of control, psychodynamic issues, sociocultural factors, and personal values and beliefs) and identify multidisciplinary approaches for managing patients with persistent pain (Chapter 11). *Example: Lisa is an emotional wreck. She has had plenty of diagnostic tests including an MRI, bone scan, and x-ray and they cannot find anything structurally wrong with her leg. She continues to complain about her leg and when I tell the coaches nothing is wrong with her—they ride her even harder. I give up with her.*

The educational competencies specific to psychosocial issues and referral present unique challenges to ATCs. Having appropriate knowledge and skills to intervene in specific situations is vital to the health care and well-being of the athlete. The expectation for athletic trainers to address these issues has evolved over the past 50 years. Currently, athletic trainers are expected to possess specific knowledge, skills, and competence related to a variety of psychosocial issues.

Clinical Proficiencies

Clinical proficiencies are commonly identified as the decision-making process and application of specific skills in a real scenario (NATA, 2006). Clinical proficiencies measure a student's ability to apply certain knowledge and skills to solve a specific problem. Clinical proficiencies serve as a guide and athletic trainers must be able to integrate basic knowledge and skills across the different employment settings in which athletic trainers are employed. The 2006 *Athletic Training Educational Competencies* requires students to demonstrate an ability to solve problems using skills across educational domains and different disciplines. The required clinical proficiencies from the psychosocial intervention and referral domain are described as follows.

- *Clinical Proficiency #1.* Demonstrate the ability to conduct an intervention and make the appropriate referral of an individual with a suspected substance abuse or mental health problem. Effective lines of communication should be established to elicit and convey information about the patient's status. While maintaining patient confidentiality, all aspects of the intervention and referral should be documented using standardized record-keeping methods.

- *Clinical Proficiency #2.* Demonstrate the ability to select and integrate appropriate motivational techniques into a patient's rehabilitation program. This includes, but is not limited to, verbal motivation, visualization, imagery, and desensitization. Effective lines of communication should be established to elicit and convey information about the techniques. While maintaining patient confidentiality, all aspects of the program should be documented using standardized record-keeping methods.

The clinical proficiencies relating to psychosocial issues and referral are meant to be a culminating event where students must access multiple skills and knowledge to recognize, intervene, and refer specific pathological problems. Students in athletic training education programs must first acquire specific knowledge related to psychosocial issues and referral, and then practice these skills through scenarios, exercises, and case studies. The following are two key components of the clinical proficiencies associated with psychosocial intervention and referral:

1. The ability to conduct an appropriate intervention
2. Integrating motivational techniques into an injury rehabilitation

Additional Educational Competencies

Problems associated with the physical and mental health of an athlete do not fit perfectly into specific educational domains. Athletic trainers must be able to integrate skills and knowledge across specific educational domains to provide a more holistic treatment plan for athletes and physically active individuals. The 2006 *Athletic Training Educational Competencies* includes additional knowledge and skills related to psychosocial interventional and referral issues not listed within that specific domain. The following is a list of additional cognitive educational competencies related to psychosocial issues (NATA, 2006), along with an example related to athletic training and the chapters in this book in which they are addressed. The number listed before the competency represents the actual cognitive competency listed in the 2006 *Athletic Training Educational Competencies*.

MEDICAL CONDITIONS AND DISABILITIES DOMAIN

10. Explain the possible causes of sudden death syndrome (Chapter 8). *Example: Only after the sudden death of one of our athletes did we think to have an action plan in place.*

18. Describe and know when to refer common psychological medical disorders from drug toxicity, physical and emotional stress, and acquired disorders (e.g., substance abuse, eating disorders/disordered eating, depression, bipolar disorder, seasonal affective disorder, anxiety disorders, somatoform disorders, personality disorders, abusive disorders, and addiction (Chapters 3, 4, 5, 7, and 11). *Example: It seems as though Bill is always stressed about something and now I think it is beginning to affect his playing. I think he needs to talk with a professional counselor.*

NUTRITIONAL ASPECTS OF INJURIES AND ILLNESSES DOMAIN

9. Describe the principles, advantages, and disadvantages of ergogenic aids and dietary supplements used in an effort to improve physical performance (Chapter 9). *Example: Everyday after practice I see empty cans of creatine on the floor. Yesterday one of my high school athletes asked if it was safe to take it. I told him no, but I am not sure. I told him to ask Betty the school dietician.*

12. Explain the principles of weight control for safe weight loss and weight gain, and explain common misconceptions regarding the use of food, fluids, and nutritional supplements in weight control (Chapters 5 and 9). *Exercise: I thought Debbie and her coach were smarter than that. Can you believe they both think all nutritional supplements are monitored by the Food and Drug Administration (FDA) and that creatine will actually help Debbie lose weight?*

14. Describe disordered eating and eating disorders (i.e., signs, symptoms, physical and psychological consequences, referral systems) (Chapters 3 and 5). *Example: I wish I would have known more about disordered eating prior to the tragedy with Jenny.*

ACUTE CARE OF INJURIES AND ILLNESSES DOMAIN

27. Identify the signs, symptoms, possible causes, and proper management of the following: toxic drug overdose (Chapter 4). *Example: I just found Don passed out in the weight room. His teammates said he did not look right and he has not acted right all day.*

30. Identify information obtained during the examination to determine when to refer an injury or illness for further or immediate medical attention (Chapters 2 and 3). *Example: Even after I evaluated John's knee for 20 minutes, I still was not sure whether I should send him to the physician. He seemed to be OK.*

PATHOLOGY OF INJURIES AND ILLNESSES DOMAIN

4. Identify the normal acute and chronic physiological and pathological responses (e.g., inflammation, immune response, and healing process) of the human body to trauma, hypoxia, microbiological agents, genetic derangements, nutritional deficiencies, chemicals, drugs, and aging to the musculoskeletal system adaptations to disuse (Chapters 4 and 9). *Example: What a shame. I do not think Cecil had any idea about the extent of damage his dependency on drugs and disordered eating would cause.*

RISK MANAGEMENT AND INJURY PREVENTION DOMAIN

14. Explain the precautions and risks associated with exercise in special populations (Chapter 10). *Example: I cannot believe the pee wee football coach who works at the recreation center is making his 10-year-old players lift weights, especially squats!*

HEALTH CARE ADMINISTRATION DOMAIN

20. Differentiate the roles and responsibilities of the athletic trainer from those of other medical and allied health personnel who provide care to patients involved in physical activity, and describe the necessary communication skills for effectively interacting with these professionals (Chapter 3). *Example: The day after an injured athlete from my high school was improperly removed from the field, I scheduled a meeting with the physicians, EMS personnel, physical therapist, coaches, nurses, and*

*administrators from my high school. It is important for us to outline an appropriate proto-
col for dealing with an injured athlete on the field.*

21. Describe the role and functions of various community-based medical, para-
    medical, and other health care providers and protocols that govern the referral of
    patients to these professionals (Chapter 3). *Example: Fred on the track team told me
    yesterday he was thinking about killing himself. I need to get him help right now, but who
    should I call—a psychologist, psychiatrist, or counselor? What is the difference?*

PROFESSIONAL DEVELOPMENT AND RESPONSIBILITY DOMAIN

5. Differentiate the essential documents of the national governing, certifying, and
   accrediting bodies, including (but not limited to) the *Athletic Training Educational
   Competencies, Standards of Practice, Code of Ethics, Role Delineation Study*, and the
   Standards for the Accreditation of Entry-Level Athletic Training Education Programs
   (Chapters 1 and 12). *Example: My boss is trying to fire me and have my BOC credential
   revoked because I gave an athlete a "sample" of Vioxx (Merck & Co., Whitehouse Station,
   NJ). He says I violated state law and some code of ethics. They cannot fire me for this. I
   know the athlete has taken Vioxx before.*

8. Summarize the current requirements for the professional preparation of the athletic trainer (Chapter 1). *Example: Sally had no idea that athletic trainers were responsible for so many different competencies and proficiencies. Her perception of athletic trainers
   has changed since joining the program.*

16. Summarize the history and development of the athletic training profession
    (Chapter 1). *Example: Tony did not understand why some states regulated the practice of
    athletic training and others did not. When asked for his opinion on current educational
    reform and the progress of the athletic training profession over the last 50 years, he had
    very little to say.*

17. Describe the theories and techniques of interpersonal and cross-cultural com-
    munication among athletic trainers, patients, administrators, health care profes-
    sionals, parents/guardians, and other appropriate personnel (Chapter 11). *Example:
    Fran just does not get along with Brian (an injured athlete). I think he may be offended
    by some of the jokes Fran will tell—many of them make fun of religion and are culturally
    insensitive.*

Core Values in Athletic Training

Early versions of the educational competencies included a large number of effective
competencies that were by their very nature hard to assess. In the 2006 edition of the
Athletic Training Educational Competencies, the affective portion of the competencies were
integrated into a common set of "core values" in athletic training. These core values com-
prise many of the necessary skills for athletic trainers when dealing with psychosocial
issues in athletes and physically active individuals. The NATA (2006) indicates these core
values permeate every aspect of professional practice and should be incorporated into
instruction in every part of the educational (didactic and clinical) program. Table 1-4
identifies the application of specific core values only relevant to psychosocial issues and
required as part of an entry-level athletic training education program (NATA, 2006).

Many of the core values in athletic training are directly related to the care, prevention,
and treatment of athletes suffering from some type of psychosocial disorder. The core

Table 1-4

NATA Core Values Associated With Psychosocial Issues

Teamed Approach to Practice

- Recognize the unique skills and abilities of other health care professionals
- Understand the scope of practice of other health care professionals
- Understand the scope of practice of athletic trainers
- Include the patient (and family, where appropriate) in the decision-making process
- Demonstrate the ability to work with others in affecting positive patient outcomes

Legal Practice

- Know, comply, and document compliance with the laws that govern athletic training
- Practice athletic training in a legally compliant manner
- Understand the consequences of violating the laws that govern athletic training

Ethical Practice

- Understand and comply with the NATA's *Code of Ethics* and the BOC's *Standard of Practice*
- Understand and comply with other codes of ethics, as applicable

Cultural Competence

- Understand the cultural differences in attitudes and behaviors toward health care

values are broad, providing flexibility for their incorporation into athletic training education programs.

Role Delineation Study and Psychosocial Issues

In the early 1980s, the BOC completed the first *Role Delineation Study* to identify a comprehensive list of professional skills to be completed by ATCs (Delforge & Behnke, 1999). The *Role Delineation Study* is deigned to create consistency between the BOC certification exam and the actual skills identified by practicing ATCs. The *Role Delineation Study* ensures that the BOC examination has content validity. The 2004 *Role Delineation Study* (4th ed.) is organized into six domains:

1. Prevention
2. Clinical evaluation and diagnosis
3. Immediate care
4. Treatment, rehabilitation, and reconditioning
5. Organization and administration
6. Professional responsibility

Within each domain, specific tasks, knowledge, and skills are outlined and evaluated by experts (ATCs). A sample of 5,000 ATCs was asked to evaluate the importance and criticality for the domains and tasks identified within the *Role Delineation Study* (NATABOC, 2004). Tasks, knowledge, and skills specific to psychosocial issues and referral are integrated throughout the six domains of the *Role Delineation Study*. It is clear that ATCs identify a variety of skills and knowledge related to psychosocial issues and referral that are a necessary component of current practice in athletic training. Specific tasks, knowledge, and skills related to psychosocial issues and referral identified in the 2004 *Role Delineation Study* (4th ed.) are listed in Table 1-5 (NATABOC, 2004).

It is clear that a variety of tasks, knowledge, and skills related to psychosocial issues and referral is important and a part of the expectant role for practicing athletic trainers. The 2004 *Role Delineation Study* suggests that knowledge and skills related to psychosocial issues and referral should be incorporated into the educational experiences within accredited programs and tested information in the BOC examination. While it is clear that psychosocial issues and referral are an important component of a ATC's education (*Athletic Training Educational Competencies*) and job (Role Delineation Study), it is unclear how these skills and knowledge are implemented into practice in a variety of settings.

Defining the Role of the Athletic Trainer in Psychosocial Issues

The role ATCs play in supporting athletes/patients suffering from an assortment of psychosocial issues and referral has become much clearer and more standardized. The skills and knowledge associated with psychosocial issues and referral are important to ATCs in three ways: 1) cognitive and clinical competencies from the psychosocial intervention and referral domain are a required component in both the didactic and clinical component of athletic training education programs (NATA, 2006), 2) a core set of values relevant to treating athletes with different psychosocial issues are to be included in all aspects of instruction in entry-level athletic training education programs, and 3) the *Role Delineation Study* used to identify the current practice of athletic trainers and provide the framework for the BOC certification exam clearly identifies specific knowledge and skills related to psychosocial issues necessary for entry-level ATCs (NATABOC, 2004).

Despite the increasing emphasis of psychosocial issues in education reform and professional practice, athletic trainers often feel unprepared and unqualified to handle these types of situations. Research suggests that ATCs are frequently exposed to and feel less prepared and trained to assist/counsel athletes experiencing psychosocial problems (Larson et al., 1996; Moulton et al., 1997; Wiese et al., 1991). Research in athletic training overwhelmingly supports the idea of providing athletic trainers with more knowledge and skills in the psychosocial intervention area. A study by Moulton et al. (1997) found that 79% of surveyed athletic trainers felt a need for more education and training in counseling. Larson et al. (1996) surveyed a national sample of athletic trainers and suggested that athletic trainers believe they are less trained in counseling than in other competencies. More than 70% of nationally surveyed athletic trainers identified a specific incident where an injured athlete encountered stress and anxiety. In addition, more than half (53%) of the same sample indicated athletes experienced significant levels of emotional distress and compliance with treatment appointments were common (Larson et al., 1996). Larson and colleagues (1996) also reported most (85%) ATCs felt a course in sports psychology was either "relatively important" or "very important" in the educational experiences of athletic training students. However, only 54% of the sampled ATCs had taken a formal course in sports psychology.

Table 1-5

Knowledge and Skills From BOC Role Delineation Study Associated With Psychosocial Issues

Prevention Domain

Facilitate healthy lifestyle behaviors using effective education, communication, and interventions to reduce the risk of injury and illness and promote wellness.

Knowledge of:
- Professional resources for stress management and behavior modification
- Predisposing factors for nutritional and stress-related disorders
- Appropriate use of exercise in stress management

Skill in:
- Recognizing signs and symptoms of nutritional and stress-related disorders
- Educating appropriate patients on nutritional disorders, maladaptation, substance abuse, and overtraining
- Communicating with appropriate professionals regarding referral and treatment for patients with nutritional and stress-related disorders

Clinical Evaluation and Diagnosis Domain

Obtain a history through observation, interview, and/or review of relevant records to assess current or potential injury, illness, or condition.

Skill in:
- Identifying psychosocial factors associated with injuries, illnesses, and conditions

Formulate a clinical impression by interpreting the signs, symptoms, and predisposing factors of the injury, illness, or condition to determine the appropriate course of action.

Knowledge of:
- Psychosocial dysfunction and implications associated with injuries, illnesses, and health-related conditions

Skill in:
- Interpreting the pertinent information from the evaluation
- Identifying the appropriate course of action

Educate the appropriate patient(s) regarding the assessment by communicating information about the current or potential injury, illness, or health-related condition to encourage compliance with recommended care.

Knowledge of:
- Communication skills and techniques
- Potential complications and expected outcomes

Skill in:
- Utilizing appropriate counseling techniques

Share assessment findings with other health care professionals using effective means of communication to coordinate appropriate care.

Knowledge of:
- Communication skills and techniques
- Role and scope of practice of various health care professionals

Skill in:
- Communicating with health care professionals
- Collaborating with health care professionals
- Directing a referral to other medical personnel   *(continued)*

Table 1-5 (continued)

Knowledge and Skills From BOC Role Delineation Study Associated With Psychosocial Issue

Immediate Care Domain

Facilitate the timely transfer of care for conditions beyond the scope of practice of the athletic trainer by implementing appropriate referral strategies to stabilize and/or prevent exacerbation of the condition(s).

Knowledge of:
- Conditions beyond the scope of the athletic trainer
- Roles of medical and allied health care providers

Skill in:
- Recognizing acute conditions beyond the scope of the athletic trainer
- Communicating with other medical and allied health care providers
- Managing life and non–life-threatening conditions until transfer to appropriate medical providers and facilities

Treatment, Rehabilitation, and Reconditioning Domain

Administer therapeutic and conditioning exercise(s) using standard techniques and procedures in order to facilitate recovery, function, and/or performance.

Knowledge of:
- Psychology related to treatment, rehabilitation, and reconditioning

Administer treatment for general illness and/or conditions using standard techniques and procedures to facilitate recovery, function, and/or performance.

Knowledge of:
- Psychological reaction to injuries, illnesses, and conditions

Skill in:
- Recognizing atypical psychosocial conditions

Educate the appropriate patient(s) in the treatment, rehabilitation, and reconditioning of injuries and illnesses and/or conditions using applicable methods and materials to facilitate recovery, function, and/or performance.

Knowledge of:
- Available psychosocial, community, family, and health care support systems related to treatment, rehabilitation, and reconditioning
- Learning process across the lifespan
- Ethnicity and culture

Skill in:
- Identifying appropriate patients to educate
- Disseminating information to patients at an appropriate level

Provide guidance and/or counseling for the appropriate patient(s) in the treatment, rehabilitation, and reconditioning of injuries, illnesses, and/or conditions through communication to facilitate recovery, function, and/or performance.

Knowledge of:
- Psychological effects related to rehabilitation, recovery, and performance
- Referral resources
- Psychological dysfunction

(continued)

Table 1-5 (continued)

Knowledge and Skills From BOC Role Delineation Study Associated With Psychosocial Issue

Skill in:
- Identifying appropriate patients for guidance and counseling
- Using appropriate psychosocial techniques (e.g., goal setting and stress management) in rehabilitation
- Referring to appropriate health care professionals
- Using effective communication skills
- Providing guidance/counseling for the patient during the treatment, rehabilitation, and reconditioning process

Professional Responsibility Domain

Adhere to statutory and regulatory provisions and other legal responsibilities relating to the practice of athletic training by maintaining and understanding of these provisions and responsibilities in order to contribute to the safety and welfare of the public.

Knowledge of:
- Criteria for determining the legal standard of care in athletic training (e.g., state statutes and regulations, professional standards and guidelines, publications, customs, practices, and societal expectations).

Skill in:
- Researching professional standards and guidelines

Group Discussion: How does the knowledge and skills pertaining to psychosocial issues outlined in the *Role Delineation Study* differ from those identified in the *Athletic Training Educational Competencies?*

IDENTIFYING A SUPPORT TEAM

A common theme related to psychosocial issues and identified throughout the *Athletic Training Educational Competencies* and *Role Delineation Study* was the ability of the athletic trainer to communicate with and understand the roles of various allied health professionals (NATA, 2006; NATABOC, 2004). It is imperative for athletic trainers to recognize the various members of the allied health community with appropriate training related to psychosocial issues. Athletes may also find themselves interacting with a large number of nonallied health professionals who have no training, but rather an opinion or past experience they feel entitles them to become involved with the athlete. These individuals may include a parent, significant other, teammate, strength and conditioning coach, friend, manager, or relative. Some of these individuals (e.g., significant other or friend) may be welcomed by the athlete while others (e.g., parents or teammates) may not be welcomed, but feel it necessary to become involved based on their relationship to the athlete and/or their situation. In many cases the athletic trainer serves as the gatekeeper to providing athletes with access to additional allied health professionals. Therefore, all athletic trainers should be familiar with appropriate referral protocols to assist and support athletes suffering from a psychosocial issue. (Chapter 3 provides a complete overview of issues related to referral.)

While all members identified previously may have some role in assisting an athlete with a psychosocial issue, clearly a major step in treating the problem is to identify a support team consisting of key personnel. This is not always an easy task. Levels of support for an athlete suffering from a psychosocial issue may vary based upon the available resources of a university or college, community, sports medicine clinic, athletic department, and family.

Each university is required to provide some type of mental health or wellness support for all students of the university. The amount of resources specified for athletes suffering from psychosocial issues will vary. Some athletic departments will have qualified professionals on staff while others will refer patients out into the community. Many athletic departments have specific protocols in place to deal with a variety of issues, including eating disorders, substance abuse, and catastrophic injuries. Other athletic departments and medical staff will deal with specific problems on a case-by-case basis.

THE RELATIONSHIP BETWEEN PSYCHOSOCIAL ISSUES AND ATHLETIC INJURIES

Based on current educational standards and the *Role Delineation Study,* athletic trainers play a critical role in dealing with psychosocial issues in a variety of athletic and health care settings. The relationship between injured athletes and psychosocial issues is the most significant and warrants special attention in this chapter. Current literature suggests that psychological issues are associated with aspects of injury/illness rehabilitation, including prediction of injury occurrence, rehabilitation adherence, compliance, and recovery (Brewer, 1998; Daly, Brewer, Van Raatle, Petitas, & Sklar, 1995; Davis, 1991; Taylor & Taylor, 1997). Roh and Perna's (2000) comprehensive overview of psychological and counseling issues related to athletic training suggested that 80% of the reported studies identified a link between specific psychosocial variables and occurrence of athletic injuries. A comprehensive analysis of research studies outlined by Roh and Perna (2000) indicated that stress and social support are clearly linked to athletic injuries. Additional psychological factors linked to the stress-injury relationship include personality constructs such as hardiness, locus of control, and competitive trait anxiety (Williams & Roepke, 1993). It is clear from the literature that psychosocial issues are directly related to a variety of aspects of athlete injuries and rehabilitation. Chapter 6 provides a more detailed analysis of the relationship between injured athletes, rehabilitation, and specific psychosocial issues.

CURRENT TEACHING PRACTICES

A track record in athletic training was clearly established over the first 50 years when psychosocial issues were not a major component of formal educational experiences. The sudden increase in expectations to integrate specific knowledge and skills into the educational experiences (didactic and clinical) of students has required athletic training educators to modify their curriculum. Many athletic training educators might not feel comfortable teaching the knowledge and skills related to psychosocial issues. When athletic training educators feel unprepared to appropriately cover psychosocial issues in athletic training, the content becomes diluted and only the most controversial and popular psychosocial issues such as eating disorders and substance abuse are thoroughly covered. Current educational standards dictate that athletic trainers will play a more prominent role in assisting athletes with a variety of psychosocial issues. Specific knowledge and skills to manage these types of situations must be clearly identified and thoroughly covered as part of their didactic and clinical experiences in athletic training education programs. It will take several years for practicing athletic trainers and educators to become more comfortable with the role they play in psychosocial issues and referral.

EMPLOYMENT SETTINGS FOR CERTIFIED ATHLETIC TRAINERS

The opportunity for ATCs continues to expand outside of the traditional employment settings (college, university, professional). Athletic trainers currently work in a variety of settings (Prentice, 2006):

- Secondary schools
- School districts
- Sports medicine clinics
- Corporate/industrial settings
- Colleges and universities
- College/university educator
- Military
- Professional sports
- Physicians extenders
- Medical supply/equipment sales
- Researcher
- Administrator

The movement of ATCs into nontraditional settings has forced athletic trainers to learn communication and counseling skills with an entirely different type of patient. The physical, mental, and emotional make-up of athletes is completely different than the patients in most of these nontraditional settings. For example, adolescent athletes are unable to physically or emotionally deal with issues (especially psychosocial issues) in the same manner as adults. Athletic trainers must be able to integrate common skills of counseling (see Chapter 2) and referral (see Chapter 3) to athletes/patients in a variety of nontraditional settings.

Knowledge and skills pertaining to psychosocial issues and referral are applicable to many different populations. Examples of different individuals include the following:

- Young athletes
- Military
- Hospice patients
- Elderly
- Corporate employees

Many of the communication and counseling skills required by athletic trainers to interact with a wide variety of patients remain fairly constant. Learning appropriate helping skills is necessary no matter what type of patient is suffering from a psychosocial problem. Referral skills are also necessary and remain rather constant regardless of the patient. There are cases where the differences in patients may require different techniques, but the principle remains constant. Two constant principles that athletic trainers must keep in mind are 1) provide optimal health outcomes for patients, and 2) demonstrate knowledge, attitudes, behaviors, and skills necessary to work respectfully and effectively in a diverse work environment. Consider the following examples of how the setting and type of athlete/patient may dictate the course of action by an athletic trainer:

- Joe from the plant is out on workers' compensation, but will not show up for treatment to the clinic. His feeling is that if you make him better, he will have to go back to work. He shows up enough to keep his worker's comp policy active, but does not do the exercises correctly and with any effort.

- Peter is a collegiate football player going to the National Football League (NFL) after the season. He is reluctant to push the rehabilitation of his knee to participate in the last game of the season and potentially damage his knee and his draft status. The team's record is 3-7 and they have no chance at postseason play.

- Helen is an elderly grandmother of five and comes to the clinic for rehabilitation of her knee. She suffers from osteoporosis and a degenerative knee. Her daughters have convinced her that holistic medicine, including putting castor oil patches and magnets on her knee, will help with the pain. She says it helps and asks your opinion.

- The CEO of a big company has asked you (an athletic trainer) to lead a fitness/exercise program for her employees. The program needs to be appropriate for a wide range of individuals with different physical, psychological, and emotional characteristics as well as different cultural and social backgrounds. The following is a list of personnel who will be attending the program.

    * Mitch smokes two packs of cigarettes a day and has asked for help to quit smoking and get back into shape.

    * Sally weighs 300 pounds and has never exercised a day in her life.

    * Bob is a former athlete and works out five times a week.

    * Cindy is taking medication for depression and wants to know how the drugs may interact with her work-out program.

    * Fred has hypertension and previous triple bypass surgery. He is anxious to begin but worried about his previous condition.

    * Sue has been fighting breast cancer and wants to know how the exercise program will work with her chemo and radiation therapy.

    * Patricia has been out of work for 2 weeks with carpal tunnel syndrome and will not engage in any exercise with her upper body.

- Tom is a military soldier at the local fort and is recovering from ACL surgery. As the athletic trainer on the military base, it is hard to hold him back. He is much too aggressive with his exercises and risks further injury. When you tell him, he replies that you do not understand the military.

- Jack is a 10-year-old boy playing little league and is in need of an ulnar collateral ligament repair. He will be coming to the clinic for rehabilitation after the surgery. His dad wants the accelerated protocol so that he can be ready for 11-year-old little league next summer. His dad shows up to rehab each session and takes charge of the home portion of the protocol.

- At the orthopedic office, the physician sends you into an exam room to assess the patient. When the patient finds out you are not a physician, he refuses to be examined by you and demands to see only an orthopedic surgeon. What do you say to the patient and the physician?

As athletic trainers enter into different employment settings, they are faced with new challenges to providing appropriate medical care to athletes/patients. In many settings athletic trainers are still developing their roles and relationships with patients and other health care professionals. The interactions athletic trainers have with patients and allied health personnel outside of the traditional athletic setting will ultimately determine the success athletic trainers have in those settings. The ability to manage a psychosocial issue is only a small component of the skills and knowledge necessary for athletic trainers to excel in nontraditional settings.

Conclusion

The knowledge and skills associated with psychosocial issues and referral are an important component of an athletic trainer's job. This chapter provides a historical perspective of an athletic trainers' role in the area of psychosocial issues and referral. It also provides specific requirements pertaining to psychosocial issues from two key documents: the *Athletic Training Educational Competencies* and the *Role Delineation Study*. The evolution of athletic training education suggests that ATCs will continue to play a more significant role in the mental health and well-being of athletes and physically active individuals. It is important for athletic trainers to be able to integrate the knowledge and skills related to psychosocial issues to an extensive population of patients. The settings in which athletic trainers provide these types of skills will also continue to expand outside of the traditional athletic environments. Although many athletic trainers and other allied health personnel lack confidence and formal training in treating psychosocial issues, they become the focal point in providing the appropriate treatment to the athlete or physically active individual suffering from a psychosocial issue. Therefore, it is important for athletic trainers to be prepared with specific helping/counseling skills (see Chapter 2) and strategies for referral (see Chapter 3). In addition, athletic trainers must be prepared to implement these skills and strategies into a variety of situations involving the physical, psychological, and emotional well-being of athletes and physically active individuals (see Chapters 4 through 11).

Chapter Exercises

1. Research the eligibility and/or regulation of the practice of ATCs within your own state. Discuss the regulation (licensure, certification, or registration) of ATCs as it pertains to counseling or treating psychosocial issues.

2. Provide a specific example of a situation related to an injury/illness (health care) involving an athlete and/or physically active individual and each of the above *psychological* constructs. See if you can think of both a personal contact and a more famous example (professional athlete).

3. Identify two to three additional psychological constructs (not listed previously) that may play a role in the health care of an athlete or physically active individual.

4. Provide a specific example of a situation in sports involving an athlete and/or physically active individual and each of the previous *sociological* issues. See if you can think of both a personal contact and a more famous example (professional athlete).

5. Explain how required knowledge and skills specific to psychosocial issues changed from the 1960s and 1970s to the requirements identified in the 1983 guidelines.

6. Identify the course(s) in your program where the content within each of the 12 domains is covered.

7. Explain how required knowledge and skills specific to psychosocial issues changed from the 1983 guidelines to the current requirements outlined in the 2006 educational competencies.

8. Break up into groups and provide additional examples of scenarios and situations in which athletic trainers are required to intervene and address issues related to each additional competency.

9. Provide an example of how each of the core values listed previously are valuable and/or necessary for athletic trainers in relation to the psychosocial issues intervention and referral educational domain.

10. Rank and then compare the following individuals according to who you feel is the most important individual to help the athlete based on the following short scenarios (1 = most important to 8 = least important):

   • Athlete feels rehabilitation of knee injury is not complete even though he or she has been cleared by a physician to return to play. Athlete feels the knee just will not be able to hold up in a game.

   ___Athletic trainer   ___Counselor
   ___Sports psychologist   ___Strength and conditioning coach
   ___Coach   ___Team captain
   ___Psychologist   ___Athlete with previous experience

   • Athlete thinks he or she may have an eating disorder.

   ___Athletic trainer   ___Counselor
   ___Sports psychologist   ___Strength and conditioning coach
   ___Coach   ___Psychologist
   ___Team captain   ___Athlete with previous experience

   • Athlete is unable to calm him- or herself down before games.

   ___Athletic trainer   ___Counselor
   ___Sports psychologist   ___Strength and conditioning coach
   ___Coach   ___Psychologist
   ___Nutritionist/dietician   ___Athlete with previous experience

   • Athlete is mentally depressed.

   ___Athletic trainer   ___Counselor
   ___Sports psychologist   ___Strength and conditioning coach
   ___Coach   ___Psychologist
   ___Team captain   ___Athlete with previous experience

11. Identify the protocol in your setting (if appropriate) that deals with the following issues: a) eating disorder, b) substance abuse, and c) catastrophic injury.

References

Andersen, M. (2000). *Doing sport psychology*. Champaign, IL: Human Kinetics.

Bandura, A. (1986). *Social foundations of thought and action: A social cognitive theory*. Englewoods Cliffs, NJ: Prentice-Hall.

Brewer, B. W. (1998). Adherence to sport injury rehabilitation programs. *Journal of Sports Psychology, 10,* 70-82.

Cox, R. H. (1998). *Sport psychology: Concepts and applications* (4th ed.). Boston, MA: McGraw-Hill.

Daly, J. M., Brewer, B. W., Van Raatle, J. L., Petitas, A. J., & Sklar, J. H. (1995). Cognitive appraisal, emotional adjustment, and adherence to rehabilitation following knee surgery. *Journal of Sport Rehabilitation, 5,* 175-182.

Davis, J. O. (1991). Sports injuries and stress management: An opportunity for research. *Sports Psychologist, 5,* 175-182.

Delforge, G. D., & Behnke, R. S. (1999). The history and evolution of athletic training education in the United States. *Journal of Athletic Training, 34*(1), 53-61.

Dirckx, J. H. (Ed.). (2001). *Stedman's concise medical dictionary for the health professions* (4th ed.). Baltimore, MD: Lippincott Williams & Williams.

Etzel, E. F., Ferrante, A. P., & Pinkney, J. (1991). *Counseling college student athletes: Issues and interventions.* Morgantown, WV: Fitness Information Technology.

Frey, J. (1991). Social risks and the meaning of sport. *Sociology of Sport Journal, 8,* 136-145.

Gieck, J. (1994). Psychological considerations for rehabilitation. In W. Prentice (Ed.), *Rehabilitation techniques in sports medicine* (pp. 238-252). St. Louis, MO: Mosby.

Heider, F. (1944). Social perception and phenomenal causality. *Psychological Review, 51,* 358-374.

Larson, G. A., Starkey, C., & Zaichkowsky, L. D. (1996). Psychological aspects of athletic injuries as perceived by athletic trainers. *Sports Psychologist, 10,* 37-47.

Moulton, M. A., Molstad, S., & Turner, A. (1997). The role of athletic trainers in counseling collegiate athletes. *Journal of Athletic Training, 32,* 148-150.

National Athletic Trainers' Association. (1983). *Competencies in athletic training.* Greenville, NC: NATA.

National Athletic Trainers' Association. (2006). *Athletic training educational competencies* (4th ed.). Dallas, TX: NATA.

National Athletic Trainers' Association Board of Certification. (1982). *Role delineation study* (1st ed.). Omaha, NE: Board of Certification.

National Athletic Trainers' Association Board of Certification. (2004). *Role delineation study* (4th ed.). Omaha, NE: Board of Certification.

Prentice, W. (2006). *Arnheim's principles of athletic training* (12th ed.). New York: McGraw-Hill.

Ray, R., Terrell, T., & Hough, D. (1999). The role of the sports medicine professional in counseling athletes. In R. Ray & D. Bjornstal (Eds.), *Counseling in sports medicine* (pp. 4-20). Champaign, IL: Human Kinetics.

Robertson, J. M., & Newton, F. B. (2005). Working with men in sports settings. In G. R. Brooks & G. E. Good (Eds.), *The new handbook of psychotherapy and counseling with men: A comprehensive guide to settings, problems, and treatment approaches (pp. xii, 443).* San Francisco, CA: Jossey-Bass

Roh, J. L., & Perna, F. M. (2000). Psychology/counseling: A universal competency in athletic training. *Journal of Athletic Training, 35,* 458-465.

Rotter, J. B. (1966). Generalized expectancies for internal versus external control of reinforcement. *Psychological Monographs: General and Applied, 80*(1, Whole No. 609).

Schwank, W. C., & Miller, S. J. (1971). New dimensions for the athletic training profession. *Journal of Health, Physical Education, and Recreation, September,* 41-43.

Smith, R. E. (1986). Toward a cognitive-affective model of athletic burnout. *Journal of Sport Psychology, 8,* 36-50.

Storch, E., Storch, J., Killiany, E., & Roberti, J. (2005). Self-reported psychopathology in athletes: A comparison of intercollegiate student-athletes and non-athletes. *Journal of Sports Behavior, 28*(1), 86-97.

Taylor, J., & Taylor, S. (1997). *Psychological approaches to sports injury rehabilitation.* Gaithersburg, MD: Aspen.

Udry, E., & Andersen, M. (2002). Athletic injury and sports behavior. In T. S. Horn (Ed.), *Advances in sport psychology* (2nd ed., pp. 529-553). Champaign, IL: Human Kinetics.

Weinberg, R. S., & Gould, D. (1995). *Foundations of sport and exercise psychology.* Champaign, IL: Human Kinetics.

Westphalen, S. W., & McLean, L. 1978. Seven years of certification by the NATA. *Athletic Training, 13,* 86-88,91.

Wiese, D. M., Wiese, S. R., & Yukelson, D. P. (1991). Sports psychology in the training room: A survey of athletic trainers. *Sports Psychologist, 5,* 15-25.

Williams, J., & Scherzer, C. (2006). Injury risk and rehabilitation: Psychological considerations. In J. Williams (Ed.), *Applied sport psychology* (5th ed., pp. 565-583). New York: McGraw Hill.

Williams, J. M., & Roepke, N. (1993). Psychology of injury and injury rehabilitation. In R. Singer, M. Murphey, & L. Tennant (Eds.), *Handbook of research in applied sport psychology.* (pp. 815-839). New York, NY: Macmillian.

Bibliography

Bramewell, S., Masuda, M., Wagner, N., & Holmes, T. (1975). Psychological factors in athletic injury: Development and application of the social and athletic readjustment scale (SARRS). *Journal of Human Stress, 1,* 6-20.

Ivey, A. E., & Ivey, M. B. (2003). *Intentional interviewing and counseling: Facilitating client development in a multicultural society* (5th ed.). Pacific Grove, CA: Thompson Brooks Cole.

Kerr, G., & Minden, H. (1988). Psychological factors related to the occurrence of athletic injuries. *Journal of Sport and Exercise Psychology, 10,* 167-173.

Passer, M. W., & Seese, M. D. (1983). Life stress and athletic injury: Examination of positive versus negative event and three moderator variables. *Journal of Human Stress, 9,* 11-16.

Petrie, T. A. (1993). The moderating effects of social support and playing status on the life-stress relationship. *Journal of Sports Psychology, 5,* 1-16.

Smith, R. E., Smoll, F. L., & Ptacek, J. T. (1990). Conjunctive moderator variables in vulnerability and resiliency research: Life stress, social support, and coping skills, and adolescent sports injuries. *Journal of Personality and Social Psychology, 58,* 360-370.

Chapter

HELPING APPROACHES, SKILLS, AND APPLICATIONS

Gary M. Miller, PhD, NCC

Chapter Objectives

❖ Provide a framework for understanding human behavior and human interactions.

❖ Provide a background of healthy psychological growth and information regarding the major theories of counseling, specifically behavioral and person-centered approaches to helping individuals.

❖ Outline choice theory (Glasser, 1998) and how it impacts the motivation of athletes.

❖ Explain the interpersonal skills of counseling, including cross-cultural communication ideas from the work of Ivey and Ivey (2003) that will be useful as athletic trainers interact with athletes, staff, and other personnel.

❖ Discuss the HOPE protocol.

❖ Present a goal-setting model (i.e., SPORT) for assisting athletic trainers in setting goals with patients.

NATA Educational Competencies

PSYCHOSOCIAL INTERVENTION AND REFERRAL DOMAIN

1. Explain the importance of providing health care information to patients, parents/guardians, and others regarding the psychological and emotional well-being of the patient.

2. Describe the theories and techniques of interpersonal and cross-cultural communication among athletic trainers, their patients, and others involved in the health care of the patient.

3. Explain the basic principles of counseling (discussion, active listening, and resolution) and the various strategies that certified athletic trainers may employ to avoid and resolve conflicts among superiors, peers, and subordinates.

ACUTE CARE OF INJURIES AND ILLNESSES DOMAIN

1. Identify information obtained during the examination to determine when to refer an injury or illness for further or immediate medical attention.

As noted in Chapter 1, the survey by Moulton, Molstad, and Turner (1997) of certified athletic trainers found that only 36% indicated that they were given sufficient training in counseling skills. Results from this study and others demonstrate the need for added training in counseling skills for athletic trainers to enhance their competencies in this area (Cramer Roh & Perna, 2000).

Athletic trainers need to understand that behavior is not a random reaction to a situation but is intentional and serves a purpose for the individual. In the following section, theories for working with individuals from three different perspectives will be presented.

Healthy Psychological Development

When considering the development of an individual's personality, it is useful to have a framework of the healthy personality versus the unhealthy one. Rather than place an emphasis on unhealthy psychological growth, in this chapter an emphasis will be on positive personality development. Psychological problem issues will be discussed later in Chapters 4, 5, and 7.

Douglas H. Heath wrote about healthy psychological development in 1980. In his article, he examined how individuals mature and develop healthy perspectives of life. He used the term *psychological sectors* to clarify the following five components of the healthy personality:

1. Symbolization
2. Allocentrism
3. Integration
4. Stability
5. Autonomy

SYMBOLIZATION

Heath (1980) notes that symbolization is one of the abilities of the mature person, suggesting that the mature person has the ability to accurately reflect on his or her cognitive processes. He believes that the mature individual is aware of the motives behind the behavior he or she demonstrates and is sensitive to his or her interpersonal relationships. The mature person is able to learn from past experiences and examine current situations in anticipation of future consequences. Heath indicates that to help a person mature, one needs assistance in the following areas: 1) developing clear goals, 2) having a model of a person to emulate, 3) being able to accept confrontation and challenges, and 4) being able to reflect on one's growth by learning about what healthy growth is, so the individual can change his or her behavior in a positive manner.

ALLOCENTRISM

Besides symbolization, Heath (1980) also notes that allocentrism represents another sign of healthy personality development. He suggests that healthy individuals move from being egocentric and narcissistic to becoming empathic and developing an understanding of others. As this occurs, the individual becomes more objective and can assess situations more analytically. Therefore, the person can more clearly predict the opinions others may have of him or her. In moving toward a more allocentric perspective, the person needs to experience the conditions of 1) trusting others to have open personal relationships with them, 2) expecting to participate in promoting the growth of other individuals, 3) learning the skills of caring and cooperating with others, and 4) having an opportunity to assume different roles in relationships with others.

INTEGRATION

According to Heath (1980), the healthy, maturing person becomes more integrated, having more consistent values along with the ability to be cooperative and reciprocal in relationships with others. To achieve this integration, it is essential that the person has 1) engaged in active involvement in his or her learning, 2) had the opportunities to reflect on what he or she has learned, and 3) been exposed to complex problems that require the ability to both synthesize and analyze information through induction and deduction.

STABILITY

The mature personality also shows the trait of stability (Heath, 1980). The person is not rigid and can efficiently think when faced with personally stressful situations. Even if the person's thinking does become impaired for a short period of time, he or she tends to be more resilient in his or her recovery than the immature person. In addition to his or her cognitive functioning, the stable person demonstrates a solid self-concept. Experiences that promote the development of stability include 1) being able to rehearse for an upcoming event, 2) being able to examine situations and learn how to correct one's actions, 3) being allowed to experience the consequences of his or her choices, and 4) being able to accept and affirm one's strengths.

AUTONOMY

The concluding component of the healthy person is autonomy (Heath, 1980). The healthy person is self-regulating, thus having control over one's self and demonstrating independence from external approval, pressures, and expectations. This person does not see his or her self-concept being based on others' views. In order to develop autonomy, one must have experienced 1) the belief that others trust him or her and see his or her potential to be self-regulating, 2) encouragement to be responsible early and consistently, 3) structures and expectations that are commensurate with one's abilities to develop one's autonomy, and 4) opportunities to transfer what one has learned to other situations, thus increasing the parameters for learning and growth.

When working with individuals and listening to how they discuss their situations, athletic trainers can consider Heath's (1980) sectors. If the patient seems to lack self-insight about how he or she needs to deal with his or her treatment plan, the athletic trainer may see this as a symbolization issue and re-examine the four points noted to promote growth in this sector. Perhaps the person needs to have expectations clarified or may need to be confronted with the fact that he or she is engaging in behaviors contrary to promoting successful recovery from an injury. The athletic trainer may also meet the individual who demonstrates apprehension and uncertainty about the work the athletic trainer is doing with him or her. Perhaps this patient is demonstrating a lack of maturity related to the allocentrism sector. The patient may need to develop a sense of trust prior to believing that the specific athletic trainer with which he or she is working is the one he or she believes capable of providing the most help to him or her. With this issue of trust, the athletic trainer needs to be aware of the work of Zunin and Zunin (1972) in which the authors note that the crucial formations of a relationship are established within the first 4 minutes of contact individuals have with each other. It is therefore imperative that the athletic trainer demonstrates sound interpersonal skills, which will be discussed later in this chapter, to promote an effective working alliance with the patient.

The next section of the chapter focuses on four specific developmental styles individuals have in describing their problems. This knowledge will help the athletic trainer focus on the cognitive levels used by their patients.

Developmental Counseling and Therapy

The most recent developments in developmental counseling and therapy (DCT) are found in the work of Ivey, Ivey, Myers, and Sweeney (2005). These authors note that the work of Piaget is the foundation of their efforts. They have developed the following four cognitive/emotional styles that people use as they interact with others:

1. Sensorimotor/elemental
2. Concrete/situational
3. Formal/operational
4. Dialectic/systemic

The first is the sensorimotor/elemental. Here the person can experience emotions and cognitions at the present moment. A patient may engage in random expression of both thoughts and feelings when describing a problem situation. Usually, the individual demonstrates a short attention span and cannot present information in a clear linear fashion. When speaking, the patient tends to be unfocused and "all over the place" in his or her conversations.

Ivey et al. (2005) cite the concrete/situational style as the second cognitive/emotional style. When a person is speaking from this framework, he or she is able to describe the problem in a clear, linear manner and can include numerous details for the athletic trainer to hear. Individuals functioning at this level will retell their story many times, yet are unable to pinpoint a specific pattern of their behavior. Individuals lacking verbal skills will often give short answers to questions. Patients who function from this style are action oriented and will take an active role in their work with the athletic trainer.

Formal/operational is the next cognitive/emotional style in DCT (Ivey et al., 2005). At this level, patients can discuss themselves and their feelings and sometimes can describe these from others' points of view. Unlike the sensorimotor/elemental, where one experiences numerous feelings, individuals at the formal/operational level talk about the feelings rather than actually experiencing them. Also, unlike the concrete/situational patient, they can recognize the patterns of their behavior but have difficulty giving specific examples regarding these patterns. These patients tend to be abstract in their discussions and often need to be asked to provide specific, clear examples of what is going on with them.

The fourth component of DCT cognitive/emotional styles (Ivey et al., 2005) is the dialectic/systemic. Patients functioning at this level are able to address problems from multiple points of view. Most people do not operate in this style. It is one in which a patient can deeply reflect on one's own and others' perspectives. Individuals who function at this level are great at analyzing their problems; however, getting them to act on their situation may be difficult. They can suffer from "paralysis from analysis." They talk but do not act. It is also likely that this patient has difficulty experiencing emotions as well as being able to accurately label them.

Understanding these styles can be very useful for the athletic trainer in communication and treatment planning with a patient. The athletic trainer who hears a patient describing a problem from the sensorimotor/emotional style may need to ask for some specific examples of what has happened, thus moving the discussion into the concrete/situational style in order to get a clearer picture of what is going on with the patient. Likewise, the athletic trainer may ask questions to try to determine if the patient is able to see the pattern in what he or she is doing (formal/operational) in an effort to help the patient with an issue. It may also be useful to help the patient take a more holistic view and describe the situation from the perspectives of others (dialectic/systemic). Using a holistic perspective in a team sport can be very useful to help the athlete examine one's rehabilitation program as it relates to the entire team and not just to him- or herself. For some athletes, this perspective can be useful in the rehabilitation process.

Having discussed some of the basics of DCT, the focus will now shift to the underpinnings of how athletic trainers may perceive the patients they help. The models of helping and coping will provide a perspective on this.

Helping and Coping

Brickman et al. (1982) address ways helpers view the situation of the patient. They address the attribution of responsibility people place on situations. They note, "We assign blame to people when we hold them responsible for having created problems. We assign control to people when we hold them responsible for influencing or changing events" (p. 369).

Of the four models Brickman et al. (1982) have developed, two (the moral and medical models) attribute the same individual for both the problem and its solution or for neither the problem nor its solution. The remaining two (the compensatory and enlightenment) models attribute responsibility for the solution to someone other than the principal party who is cited for causing the problem.

In the moral model (Brickman et al., 1982), the individual is seen as having responsibility for creating the problem and for subsequently being responsible for solving it.

From this perspective, the person alone must come to a resolution of the problem being experienced. Consequently, the patient is expected to be responsible for his or her own well-being. A dilemma resulting from this model is when the individual develops the thinking pattern that he or she is limitless and can achieve anything he or she chooses to undertake. Believing they are limitless, these patients begin to think that they do not need the assistance of others to succeed. Such thinking can result in them being isolated from positive relationships with others.

In the compensatory model, Brickman et al. (1982) discuss that although the person is not directly responsible for the dilemma being faced, he or she is responsible for developing a solution to the issue being faced. Others may see the individual as being deprived due to the failure of the environment in which he or she lives. In dealing with his or her situation, a patient can direct one's efforts toward trying to solve the problems and can enlist the help of others in resolving the issues at hand. From the compensatory perspective, the individual does not need to berate one's self for the situation but can take an active part in seeking a solution. A downside of this perspective is that the patient can experience a great amount of pressure in making efforts to resolve the multiple external situations that may be negatively impacting one's life. This can take its toll on the patient as he or she strives to deal with the many issues being faced. When one attempts to resolve problems created by others and does not find the success sought, it is not uncommon for the person to become hostile.

In their 1982 paper, Brickman and colleagues introduce the medical model as the third way an individual can be affected. This model suggests that the patient is neither the cause of the problem nor responsible for the solution of it. In their own eyes and in the eyes of others, people are seen as incapacitated due to forces beyond their control. Therefore, it is much easier to seek and obtain assistance from others. The patient is not blamed for the problem as others try to help him or her. However, a drawback to this perspective emerges if the person becomes dependent on others for assistance with things one can independently achieve. The medical model is the one usually incorporated in the work of the athletic trainer during the rehabilitation process of an individual.

Brickman et al. (1982) present the enlightenment model as one in which the individual is seen as being responsible for the problem being faced and yet not responsible for the solution. Because the solution of the issue is beyond the patient, he or she must maintain a relationship with an outside source for him or her to be successful in fully resolving the problem. Brickman et al. (1982) suggest that the person cannot control undesirable behaviors but through the affiliation with an outside source, he or she can gain some control over the situation. The 12-step approach used by Alcoholics Anonymous follows the enlightenment model, emphasizing a belief in a higher power as essential in the recovery process. Brickman et al. (1982) note that in this model the patient can become deeply attached to the external source of help and begin focusing one's entire life around it, consequently not believing that one can cope with life on a daily basis. There is a danger that the source of help can become all consuming for the person and that one may actually sacrifice his or her own beliefs and individuality to that person or organization that has helped the patient gain a better sense of control over various problems.

As the athletic trainer works with athletes and other physically active individuals, he or she needs to consider the framework the individual uses to explain the issue being presented. An athletic trainer may work with some patient who wants to take full responsibility for his or her rehabilitation and actually disregard the treatment plan designed for him or her. The patient may be seeing his or her injury from the moral model, in that he or she wants to override the athletic trainer's plans and take it upon him- or herself to be fully responsible for the treatment. Others, using the compensatory framework, may be so competitive that they want to rush the treatment plan so they can continue their normal activities. From this framework, they may push themselves and actually impede rehabilitation or worsen the injury. The athletic trainer may also work with the patient from the medical model who becomes overly dependent and will not make a move without the approval of the athletic trainer. This person contacts the athletic trainer about each and everything he or she is to do regarding the treatment plan, almost taking a passive role in his or her recovery. Finally, a patient may not follow the treatment plan set by the athletic trainer, but begin to rely on some enlightened external expert he or she may have found and may use this external advice and inhibit his or her treatment and progress. The patient may begin taking herbs and other supplements because some "highly respected" guru has promoted a specific product or treatment program. These patients, following the enlightenment model, may use this advice to treat themselves even though it is counterproductive to sound athletic training practice.

It can become difficult for the athletic trainer to work with individuals whose style of looking at their problem and whose method of coping can be counterproductive. It is suggested that the athletic trainer gain an understanding of the framework the person is using to describe his or her situation and how he or she plans to participate in their rehabilitation prior to initiating a treatment program. Having such an understanding may be useful to assuring that all parties are not working at cross-purposes.

Models of helping and coping are directly related to the transitions individuals experience in life. The following information relates to six specific transitions patients may experience in their lives.

Life Transitions

Throughout one's lifetime, an individual will experience a variety of events, some of which lead to significant transitions for them. Ivey et al. (2005, p. 81) present these in their work with DCT as follows:

- *Elected transitions:* Graduating from school, changing jobs, having a baby, retiring, moving, divorcing
- *Surprise transitions:* Car accident, death of a child, plant closing, an unexpected raise or significant promotion, a reduction by the state in welfare benefits for poor mothers
- *Nonevents (when the expected does not happen):* A couple experiences infertility, a promotion or raise does not come through, child does not leave home
- *Life on hold (occurs almost without your awareness):* Long engagement, waiting to die in a hospice, waiting for the "right person" to come along, waiting for an important other person to make a key decision
- *Sleeper transition (occurs almost without your awareness):* Becoming fat or thin, falling in love, getting bored at a job you once loved, gradually tiring of a relationship, a neighborhood deteriorating or becoming overrun with drugs
- *Double whammies:* Retiring and losing a spouse by death, having a baby and reverting to one income, caring for ill parents at home at the same time that one of your children divorces and moves back home, suffering through a house fire in the winter at the same time the welfare office has lost your file

As the athletic trainer listens to a patient, it is helpful to understand the transition stage the individual is facing. Obviously, the elected transitions may cause stress in the person's life, even though he or she has chosen for the transition to occur. One will hear patients speak of these events and oftentimes the stress is viewed as "good stress" for them. However, when the patient is dealing with a situation in which another must make a decision that will directly impact the patient, "bad stress" may be having a negative impact on the patient. When stress becomes too severe for the patient to deal with alone, there may be a need to refer the individual as discussed in Chapter 3.

In the following section of the chapter, various theories of counseling will be described. These are presented as an overview of the principal approaches used by professional helpers in the counseling profession. Keep in mind, professional counselors spend extensive time in developing an understanding of these prior to working with a client. In addition, professional counselors take clinical practicum and internship courses where they are supervised using these approaches prior to becoming certified or licensed to practice.

Cognitive Approaches

These approaches to counseling evolved in the United States during the 20th century. B. F. Skinner (Nye, 1975) believed that individuals could shape and influence the behavior of others through three major processes. First, if we reinforce the behavior of a person, we increase the probability that the reinforced behavior will continue. Secondly, if the person's behavior is demonstrated but not reinforced, there is strong probability that the behavior will be discontinued or extinguished. Lastly, through the process of punishing an individual whenever the behavior is exhibited, the behavior also has strong probabilities of not being repeated. A question often asked about these ideas is "Who determines which behaviors are appropriate and which are not and need to be stopped?" Consequently, individuals in the counseling profession have debated how such an approach could work well with human beings.

John Krumboltz (1966) made great strides in adapting the behavioral-scientific approach to counseling. During the decade of the 1970s, his ideas were adapted by many in the counseling profession. Two major points most behaviorist counselors follow are all behavior is learned and learning can change behavior.

To assist the individual in making changes, the behavioral counselor works at helping the person set goals that meet the following three criteria: 1) the goal must be one the individual seeks to attain, 2) the helper must be willing to assist the individual in reaching the goal, and 3) it is a goal that can be assessed in order to determine the level of achievement the individual has achieved (Krumboltz, 1966). Blackham and Silberman (1980) cite four steps in the goal-setting process that one needs to consider. First, they note that one must clearly define the problem in concrete terms. Next, one should try to determine the basis of the problem and how the individual dealt with past situations similar to it. Blackham and Silberman (1980) then suggest that a goal be set, keeping in mind the ideas presented by Krumboltz (1966). Lastly, Blackham and Silberman (1980) suggest the best methods for changing the behavior be selected and implemented. As can be seen, behavioral helpers use strategies to help individuals define goals, plan to change them, and then move ahead to attaining the goals that have been set.

The behavioral orientation to helping involves the use of a variety of techniques. Using positive reinforcement consists of having things such as social recognition to provide the incentive for the person completing the goal that has been set. Athletic trainers are often the sources of such recognition because they compliment and encourage patients in reaching their goals.

When assisting a person who is undergoing rehabilitation for an injury, athletic trainers often use shaping as a technique. This behavioral strategy involves helping the person make gradual improvements through making small, incremental steps that approximate the goal to be achieved. As each step is taken, behaviorists use the term *chaining* (i.e., the links come together and the goal is achieved). In such an approach, the athletic trainer and the individual need to follow an established sequence that leads to the goal. This sequence is important in helping link the behaviors together.

Using maintenance, the athletic trainer can incorporate a behavioral technique that promotes the self-management of the individual (Thorensen & Mahoney, 1974). When this occurs, the patient can observe the progress and become the monitor of one's own progress. Athletic trainers can have the patient keep an ongoing record or journal to chart the progress being made to achieve a goal.

The Rational-Emotive Behavior Approach

In addition to behavioral approaches to counseling and helping others, Albert Ellis developed a helping approach called Rational-Emotive Therapy (1958), which he reconfigured as Rational-Emotive Behavior Therapy (REBT) in 1994. This cognitive approach focuses on changing a person's thinking about a situation that he or she wants to change. Consequently, the person begins to behave and act according to the changes made. Ellis believes that individuals engage in thinking styles that are irrational and represent major factors in the person not living a full, productive life. For example, Ellis and Dryden (1997) identified five central dysfunctional ways of thinking:

1. It is necessary to be admired and loved by all of the important individuals in one's life. If not, one thinks, "Life is awful."

2. One is required to be fully competent in numerous undertakings to be considered a person of worth. If not, one thinks, "It is my fault."

3. There are some individuals who are bad and should be punished for their behavior. If so, one thinks, "I must get even."

4. It is wise to avoid responsibilities. If so, one thinks, "People do not care and it does not matter."

5. When things do not go as one wants them to, it is awful and catastrophic. If so, one thinks, "People and things around me should be as I want them; otherwise the situation is terrible."

When a patient engages in such self-talk, he or she creates a life that brings little joy and much frustration.

A way to examine how to deal with a situation is to help the person reconfigure the faulty thinking pattern. Ellis (1994) has noted that when an event happens at point A, an individual incorporates one of the faulty thinking patterns at point B and then at point C has an unhealthy emotional reaction to the situation, resulting in hurt feelings and disappointment in one's self and others. Ellis has been a supporter of helping the person learn new, more healthy ways of thinking at point B, which should result in a more rational and appropriate set of feelings at point C. He notes that a patient's beliefs about a situation (point B) result in emotional consequences (point C) about the event that has taken place at point A. Walen, DiGiuseppe, and Wessler (1980) added two additional components to the A-B-C approach of Ellis by including a point D where the individual learns to actively dispute the irrational beliefs at point B, thus moving onward in developing a more effective philosophy at point E, resulting in the development of more productive thoughts and behaviors for the person.

An example of this for the athletic trainer is when an injured patient does not take responsibility for following the rehabilitation program planned for her. An example follows: Point A, the rehabilitation program, has been planned for her; point B, she tries to avoid responsibility for following the program, believing that it does not matter to her coach if she recovers; point C, after few weeks of not following her program, she becomes upset with the athletic trainer and the coach because she is not getting the playing time she believes she deserves. This upset at point C could have been avoided had she taken the responsibility to follow the program set up for her with the belief at point B, therefore, disputing the irrational thinking with the following rational thinking: "Even if nobody notices, it does matter to the coach and the team that I work hard at getting better because I want to contribute to the efforts of the team." This new effective thinking (point E) can result in behaviors that are more productive and rewarding for the participant. When helping a patient using this approach, the athletic trainer needs to incorporate confrontation skills, which will be discussed later in the chapter.

The person-centered approach will be presented in the following section. It has basic foundations in the existential-humanistic perspective of working with individuals.

The Person-Centered Approach

The person-centered approach has evolved from the work of Carl R. Rogers. Rogers believed that humans are basically good individuals striving to move ahead in a positive manner. When his approach emerged in the 1950s, he influenced psychology that prior to his work placed major emphasis on mainly examining the behavioral and thought processes of human beings. Rogers took a more holistic perspective, viewing individuals not only as thinkers and behavior generators, but included the feelings and emotions experienced by the person as valid in the helping process.

Rogers described the 19 propositions upon which his theory of personality was based in his book, *Client-Centered Therapy* (1951, pp. 481-533):

1. Every individual exists in a continually changing world of experience of which he or she is the center.

2. The individual reacts to the field as it is experienced and perceived. This perceptual field is, for the individual, "reality."

3. The organism reacts as an organized whole to this phenomenal field.

4. The organism has one basic tendency and striving—to actualize, maintain, and enhance the experiencing organism.

5. Behavior is basically the goal-directed attempt of the organism to satisfy its needs as experienced in the field as perceived.

6. Emotion accompanies and in general facilitates such goal-directed behavior, the kind of emotion being related to the seeking versus the consummatory aspects of the behavior, and the intensity of the emotion being related to the perceived significance of the behavior for the maintenance and enhancement of the organism.

7. The best vantage point for understanding behavior is from the internal frame of reference of the individual him- or herself.

8. A portion of the total perceptual field gradually becomes differentiated as the self.

9. As a result of interaction with the environment, and particularly as a result of evaluation interaction with others, the structure of self is formed—an organized, fluid, but consistent conceptual pattern of perceptions of characteristics and relationships of the "I" or the "me," together with values attached to these concepts.

10. The values attached to experiences, and the values that are part of the self-structure, in some instances are values experienced directly by the organism, and in some instances are values introjected or taken over from others, but perceived in distorted fashion, as if they had been experienced directly.

11. As experiences occur in the life of the individual, they are either (a) symbolized, perceived, and organized into some relationship to the self, (b) ignored because there is no perceived relationship to the self-structure, or (c) denied symbolization or given a distorted symbolization because the experience is inconsistent with the structure of the self.

12. Most of the ways of behaving that are adopted by the individual are those which are consistent with the concept of self.

13. Behavior may, in some instances, be brought about by organic experiences and needs that have not been symbolized. Such behavior may be inconsistent with the structure of the self, but in such instances the behavior is not "owned" by the individual.

14. Psychological maladjustment exists when the organism denies awareness of significant sensory and visceral experiences, which consequently are not symbolized and organized into the gestalt of the self-structure. When this situation exists, there is a basis for potential psychological tension.

15. Psychological adjustment exists when the concept of the self is such that all the sensory and visceral experiences of the organism are, or may be, assimilated on a symbolic level into a consistent relationship with the concept of self.

16. Any experience that is inconsistent with the organization or structure of self may be perceived as a threat, and the more of these perceptions there are, the more rigidly the self-structure is organized to maintain itself.

17. Under certain conditions involving primarily complete absence of any threat to the self-structure, experiences that are inconsistent with it may be perceived and examined, and the structure of self may be revised to include such experiences.

18. When the individual perceives and accepts into all his or her sensory and visceral experiences one consistent and integrated system, then he or she is necessarily more understanding of others and is more accepting of others as separate individuals.

19. As the individual perceives and accepts into his or her self-structure more of his or her organic experiences, he or she finds that he or she is replacing his or her present value system—based so largely upon introjections that have been distortedly symbolized—with a continuing organismic valuing process.

As one can see, this theory relies heavily on the perceptions the individual has of the world and these perceptions play a major part in the development of one's personality. In the first five propositions stated above, it becomes clear that Rogers saw individuals developing their sense of reality from the world around them and that one strives to become actualized while having various experiences. The positive aspect of the person's behavior being goal-directed and acting according to one's reality is essential knowledge for the athletic trainer working with an individual. The athletic trainer's world view may vary greatly from the patient's because each person has created a reality based on his or her unique life experiences.

Rogers (1951) notes in proposition six that emotions come into play as individuals strive in their development. In addition, in proposition seven, he believed that the best way to understand another is from his or her internal perceptions, rather than from our perceptions of the situation, which are external to the person. Further down the list in proposition 12, he emphasizes that individuals behave based on the adaptations they have made in their lives, reflecting their beliefs about themselves. He goes on to note in proposition 16 that when one has an experience that is seen as threatening, the individual's beliefs about him- or herself become more rigid as a way to protect him- or herself from perceived harm. Consequently, the person tends to "dig in," resulting in less openness to new information and rather than being flexible and open to this information, he or she becomes rigid and closed. Rogers notes in proposition 18 that the individual can develop a better understanding of others and the information they may provide through the process of acceptance.

A question many people have is, "How does a person help another within the framework of these propositions?" Rogers addressed this very thoroughly in 1957. He noted that for change to take place in a person, there is a need for the client and the helper to be in psychological contact. The individual seeking help is seen as being in a state of incongruity, thus having an unclear picture of who he or she is, feeling vulnerable and disorganized. The helper is seen as being congruent. Rogers describes the helper as being genuine, which is one of his basic core conditions for helping. The helper has self-awareness and is able to interact with the patient without needing to present a façade of who he or she is.

The second core condition for effective change that Rogers (1957) wrote about is unconditional positive regard. This is tied directly to the ability of the helper to accept the experiences of the client. There are no conditions surrounding this acceptance, as one cares for the client in a genuine manner. Accepting another's point of view can be challenging for some individuals because they may feel uncomfortable listening to the story of another. The caring one demonstrates is a caring built out of concern for the person based on the individual's uniqueness, not the helper's need to change or control the client.

Empathy represents another core condition (Rogers, 1957). It consists of trying to experience the world of the client as if it is the helper's. Rogers notes:

> When the client's world is this clear to the therapist, and he moves about in it freely, then he can both communicate his understanding of what is clearly known to the client and can also voice meanings in the client's experience of which the client is scarcely aware. (1975, p. 99)

When experiencing empathy for another, it is important to enter the subjective world of the patient—realizing that this is not your world, but allowing yourself to experience it as if it is. In being able to achieve empathy with another, you must trust yourself and know yourself well enough that you can experience the world of another.

Lastly, Rogers (1957) addressed the client's perception of the helper. He suggests that unless the patient perceives the helper's attitudes of congruence, unconditional positive regard, and empathy, the therapeutic process will not exist. He says, "...therapist behaviors and words are perceived by the client as meaning that to some degree the therapist accepts and understands him" (p. 99).

The work of Rogers has provided a sound foundation the athletic trainer can use when working with patients. The core ingredients he presents will enhance professional relationships. Next, William Glasser's Choice Theory will be presented.

Choice Theory

In his early work in Reality Therapy, Glasser (1965) developed some new ways of examining human behavior and motivation. As his work evolved, he eventually reworked his concepts and renamed his approach Choice Theory (1998). He contends that human beings have a choice over how they respond to life events and that they actually have more control over their lives than they may believe. Glasser notes that individuals choose their happiness as well as their sadness. His ideas place great responsibility on the individual to be willing to take control of his or her life. Consequently, one must be willing to assume this responsibility rather than blaming external people, forces, and events for the way one experiences life.

Glasser (1998) notes that the first motivating factor in one's life is the need to survive. When working with an athlete, the athletic trainer often hears discussions regarding the athlete's perceptions that he or she must get through the rigors of practices to show the coach that he or she is the person who should be placed in the starting lineup. Likewise, when treating the athlete for an injury and working with him or her on rehabilitation of an injury, discussions of "just let me get through this so I can play again" are often heard. For some, adjusting to the rigors of being an athlete sends a message to the athlete that he or she is a "survivor." Knowing that one can progress through the athletic experience can be a motivation for some athletes with whom the athletic trainer may work.

The second motivating factor that influences the behavior of athletes is the need to belong and feel loved (Glasser, 1998). At the little league levels, youngsters may try out for teams in order to feel they belong to something. Who has not heard of the little league player who loves to attend practices, wear her uniform, but who could care less whether she starts every game? For her, being with her friends and wearing the team uniform helps meet the need to belong and feel cared for by others. The athletic trainer often hears athletes talk about not feeling that they belong and feeling unappreciated by their coach and teammates. Some may even reject efforts of being treated for their injuries in order to get attention from their coach, which may be a way of trying to make the coach show he or she is concerned about the athlete. Likewise, the athletic trainer may find that some athletes will not work on their rehabilitation program unless the athletic trainer is present throughout the process. This could be the athlete's way of eliciting some sense of caring from the athletic trainer.

A third motivating force for the athlete is power (Glasser, 1998). Glasser believes that humans are the only species on earth that is driven by power, and that some individuals will go to great extremes to achieve it. Athletes will often find the power they experience in their sport as both fulfilling and motivating. It ties in closely with athletes being "doers" and "achievers," rather than passive observers. Athletic trainers often hear and observe athletes expressing their sense of power. Athletic trainers also learn what the loss of the sense of power does to the athlete who experiences an injury that keeps him sidelined for a game or perhaps an entire career. When working with athletes in the rehabilitation process, the sense that he or she is regaining the power he or she lost in his or her ankle can be a strong motivating force in promoting the athlete's adhering to his or her rehabilitation plan.

Glasser (1998) has also noted that having freedom is a powerful motivating factor in selecting behavior. Athletic trainers at the collegiate level often hear of freshmen athletes getting into difficulty with their coaches because the athletes have not followed the rules of the team, consequently losing their freedom as a team member. Consider the basketball player who stays out and parties after having made the winning shot in the game, but parties too hard and misses weight training the next morning. The consequence of running the stairs in the arena after practice can take away the sense of freedom the athlete thought she had. The athlete who chooses to miss her appointment with the athletic trainer because her rehabilitation session is scheduled early in the morning may be trying to exert her sense of freedom to sleep in rather than conform to the expectations of the athletic trainer. Some athletes may appear to be uncooperative when in fact they are choosing behavior to maintain their sense of freedom to control their own behavior.

The fifth of Glasser's (1998) concepts is having fun. He contends that individuals will control their behavior to achieve a sense of fun in their lives. Athletes will talk of wanting to have fun. They often describe the fun they experience in winning games or in achieving personal goals in their lives. Little league athletes sometimes quit their sports because it is not as much fun as it used to be for them. Athletic trainers know that having some fun in the process of rehabilitation can lighten the sense of work involved in the process. Some will purposely vary their procedures to insert a fun dimension in the process of working with athletes. Fun in the athletic training process can do much to keep the athlete motivated to follow through the rehabilitation process.

In this section, various theories of counseling have been presented. The basic structure of a helping interview will be presented next.

The Basic Helping Interview

Ivey and Ivey (2003) discuss the helping interview as a process in which the helper listens to the story of the patient and attempts to get a clear picture of the strengths and weaknesses the patient expresses. The helper then suggests seeking out the positive assets of the patient and uses these to help the individual find a way to improve the situation being discussed. Building from strengths is a positive way to approach the problem solving involved in the helping relationship. As the patient develops new ways of facing the problem, he or she enters the restory phase of the helping process. After the restorying has taken place, the patient is then able to take action and develop new ways of thinking and feeling about the problem. If the patient does not move into the action mode, the helping process has not been successful.

Cavanagh and Levitov (2002) provide a six-stage model one can use in an interview. Their work was originally developed for individuals in the counseling profession, and the model has direct application for the athletic trainer in working with patients. These six steps help demystify the process and provide a workable structure that is useful to the athletic trainer. They note that it is important to establish an alliance with the person seeking help. This is the cornerstone to developing the kind of relationship in which the patient will feel comfortable to express concerns to the athletic trainer. Although it appears to be something easy to accomplish, one must be alert to factors that may influence the patient's willingness to invest in the relationship. Be aware that the patient's previous experiences with an athletic trainer may have an impact on how the individual feels about working with the athletic trainer. Issues such as trust, confidence, and the power the athletic trainer held in previous relationships can have an impact on the relationship the current athletic trainer will have with the patient. It is essential that the athletic trainer demonstrate Rogers' (1957) concepts of empathy, congruence, and unconditional positive regard cited earlier in the chapter in order to form a solid alliance.

The second stage, information gathering, is the most useful way of securing information from the patient (Cavanagh & Levitov, 2002). During this time, the use of questions will be a helpful skill (later in the chapter, these will be discussed). The athletic trainer can use this time to find out more about the situation facing the patient. Also, the athletic trainer can gather knowledge regarding the patient's previous experiences with athletic trainers and what was and what was not successful.

The third stage that Cavanagh & Levitov (2002) note is evaluation and feedback. Here is where one determines the symptoms the patient has had, their causes, their relief, the patient's readiness for help, and how well the "fit" is between the helper and the patient. The HOPS model (Prentice, 2006) wherein one takes the History of the injury, Observes various facets of the patient, Palpates boney and soft tissue structures, and then conducts Special tests is a well respected model followed by athletic trainers. The feedback aspect is important because it allows the patient to determine if the athletic trainer is the one the individual wishes to work with in the particular setting. During this stage, the athletic trainer can give the patient feedback that will allow the patient to make an informed choice regarding treatment. Feedback should be directly related to the behaviors of the patient, free of professional jargon, nonjudgmental, and include the strengths and limitations the athletic trainer sees for the patient. During this time it is most helpful for the athletic trainer to answer questions in a straightforward, direct manner. Also, it is professionally sound to continue this behavior when making recommendations for treatment, thus demonstrating respect for the patient's concerns.

Stage four is the agreement stage (Cavanagh & Levitov, 2002). During this time, the roles of the individuals are clarified and the expectations of each person are expressed. The athletic trainer needs to stipulate his or her role in the relationship with the patient and get an understanding and agreement from the patient regarding the expectations of his or her responsibility in the process. This is essential as both parties need to agree on the goals being set for the patient. These need to be realistic and within the capabilities of the patient to achieve. Goals that are set too high will frustrate the patient and those that are set too low may not provide the motivation for the patient to continue in the work with the athletic trainer. At the end of the chapter is the SPORT Goal-Setting model that can be used in this fourth stage.

At the fifth stage, the athletic trainer and the patient begin to look for changes to take place (Cavanagh & Leitov, 2002). Here is where the athletic trainer can record the progress the patient has been making and revise the treatment plan to help the patient reach the goals set previously. From here, new goals can be formulated to promote further progress for the patient.

At the final stage, termination (Cavanagh & Levitov, 2002), the athletic trainer can help the patient assess the progress made in their work together. Much of this will be based on the goals that had been set previously and their accomplishment. Athletic trainers and their patients realize that along the way to meeting the goals they had set, benchmarks of the patient's progress have been constant reminders of the success of their efforts. As termination nears, it is helpful to use feedback in the process and note how the patient has been progressing since beginning his or her work with the athletic trainer.

The six-stage model of Cavanagh and Levitov (2002) has provided a sound sequence for the athletic trainer to follow in establishing a working relationship with a patient. Next, specific helping skills presented in the intentional interviewing model of Ivey and Ivey (2003) will be discussed.

Intentional Interviewing

In the profession of counseling, a variety of models have emerged for educating beginning helpers in sound interpersonal skills for interviewing individuals they are trying to assist. Ivey and Ivey have written extensively in this arena. Allen Ivey published his first book about microcounseling in 1971 (Ivey, 1971). His intent was to examine counseling interviews and determine what specific skills good counselors were able to demonstrate with their clients. Through his research, he has identified a specific set of skills that are useful in the interviewing and helping processes. As the athletic trainer works with patients, these skills will promote a positive relationship and be useful in setting goals with the athlete.

Attending behaviors are the first skills noted by Ivey and Ivey (2003). These involve the ability to maintain eye contact with the patient, the tone of voice presented by the athletic trainer, verbally tracking what the person is saying, and the body language of the athletic trainer. Positive eye contact involves looking directly at the person one is speaking with and staying focused on him or her. It is a skill that lets the patient know the athletic trainer is interested in what is being said. The athletic trainer needs to be culturally sensitive in using eye contact because some athletes of Latin or Native American decent may not reciprocate, as in their cultures eye contact with someone in a position of authority may actually be a sign of disrespect.

The tone of voice of the athletic trainer communicates much about the professional's feelings toward the patient. The pitch, volume, and tempo of one's voice can promote the establishment of a positive relationship. Remember, the patient's response to your voice may have been something learned when he or she was a child, so be sensitive to how you speak and consider how this may sound to the patient.

Verbal tracking involves staying on the topic the person is presenting to you. If she is talking about her disappointment with how her injury is healing, do not introduce some other topic, such as how the team is performing without her in the lineup. This skill lets the patient know you are interested in what is being said and challenges the athletic trainer to "tune in" to what is being said. Staying with the person's conversation indicates a great deal about the respect you are showing to the person, whereas changing the topic of conversation may be indicating that you are not interested in what the patient is saying, that you cannot deal with what is being said, or that the individual is not important enough to you to engage in conversation with him or her about a concern.

Finally, the last of the attending behaviors is the body posture the athletic trainer takes when conversing with the athlete. According to Ivey and Ivey (2003) one should sit or stand within a reasonable distance from the individual. Again, consider that in some cultures, standing at arm's length is the norm, whereas patients from other cultures may almost stand toe to toe with you. Also, it is helpful to sit or stand squarely in front of the person you are speaking with along with placing one's arms and hands in an open position versus a closed one. The typical closed position is when one crosses his or her arms over the chest when speaking or shifting sideways in one's chair when talking. Another barrier to good body posture is having a desk or table physically between the athletic trainer and the patient. Such an authority position may inhibit good communication with the person.

In summary, the attending behaviors are quite subtle, yet powerful skills in establishing positive relations with patients. Remember to attend to each person from the first time you meet throughout the individual's experiences with you. These skills will do much to promote a positive relationship that will enhance your work with the patient.

The components of attending behaviors are instrumental in helping develop the sense of empathy. Brems (2001) has presented a Five-Phase Cycle of Empathic Skillfullness that begins with the patient stating his or her situation and communicating both verbally and nonverbally. The athletic trainer's best strategy in this initial phase is to calmly listen to the patient and pay attention to the manner in which the individual expresses him- or herself. According to Welch (1998), "people do not use the words they use by accident" (p. 37). Thus, listening involves active participation on the part of the athletic trainer.

In phase two of the empathy model (Brems, 2001), the athletic trainer can focus on the DCT representations of the patient and try to "hear, see, and sense what the client is attempting to communicate" (p. 187). During this time, the athletic trainer must attempt to sift through the material presented to pinpoint the principal issues of the patient. Listening skills play a big part in gaining this understanding, while at the same time one must disregard preconceived ideas formed about the patient prior to taking time to listen to the individual. It is important to remain psychologically open to the person and not identify with his or her problem or show sympathy toward him or her.

The third phase of empathy (Brems, 2001) involves the athletic trainer gaining an understanding of what the patient is saying within the context of the patient's experiences. Depending on which of the theories of counseling one may use, during this phase the athletic trainer can develop a framework for the problem and begin to consider if a behavioral, cognitive, person-centered, or choice theory approach may be most beneficial to the patient. The development of this framework depends on the patient's life experiences and their impact on the patient's current level of functioning.

In the fourth phase of the empathy cycle (Brems, 2001), the athletic trainer demonstrates the understanding and caring for the patient as discussed by Rogers (1951). The responses to the patient need to include both affective and cognitive components. It is helpful to adapt one's responses to the verbalization style of the patient. Brems (2001, p. 191) indicates the need to be aware of the following:

- Using the client's native language whenever possible
- Using a volume sufficient to be heard
- Using the same phrases and vocabulary as the client does (as appropriate; e.g., racist language would be avoided even if used by the client)
- Adapting to the client's preferred modality (e.g., using visual, auditory, or tactile language)
- Avoiding jargon
- Using simple phrases and easy-to-understand vocabulary
- Keeping statements brief and nontechnical

Brems (2001) also notes in this fourth phase that one must respond to the patient with caring and warmth. She suggests that the following factors be considered when the helper responds to the patient (p. 192):

- Waiting for appropriate rapport
- Waiting for the client to be in an emotional state that is receptive to clinician input
- Using a soothing voice or a voice that matches the content to be expressed
- Making appropriate eye contact
- Achieving appropriate physical proximity
- Being congruent in verbal and nonverbal expressions
- Being genuine in what is being said
- Being calm and centered during delivery
- Having more concern for the client's well-being than for the clinician's need to be right
- Paying careful attention to the client's nonverbal reactions while the clinician is speaking

In the fifth phase, Brems (2001) indicates that the cycle is not complete unless the patient receives the message from the helper. The patient needs to be able to fully understand the information presented by the athletic trainer. It is important to speak in a manner that honors the patient's style of communicating, therefore increasing the likelihood that your message will be heard.

- Some patients may be visual in their conversations with the athletic trainer, therefore, responding in the following ways will be helpful: "Tell me your views on this"; "It looks to you as if _____"; "The way you see it is _____"

- For patients who express themselves using feeling words, it is helpful for the athletic trainer to respond with phrases like "You feel _____"; "There is a lot of _____ inside you right now"; or "It really touched you when you felt _____"

- There are patients who may express themselves from an auditory framework and using terms such as "It sounds like _____ to you"; "The way you heard it was _____"; or " You heard _____"

- Finally, some of the patients may be best approached from a cognitive perspective with such phrases as "Your understanding is _____"; "You've been thinking _____ and then _____ happened"; or "In your mind it was _____"

In order to increase the probability that the message the athletic trainer is sending will be heard, it is important to consider the timing of the delivery of the message. Once the athletic trainer has developed a rapport with the patient and has knowledge of how the person processes information, the appropriate timing can be determined. A major signal that the time is on target will be the increased verbalization of the patient and a willingness to further explore the concern presented.

The following are specific roadblocks to avoid because these can compromise one's ability to listen fully to another person (Brems, 2001, p. 121):

- Inadequate listening happens when the clinician becomes preoccupied with his or her own worries.

- Evaluative listening happens when the clinician is making judgments, thus losing objectivity.

- Filtered or selective listening happens when the clinician hears only what he or she wants to hear and misses the other messages of the person.

- Rehearsing-while-listening happens when the clinician is preoccupied with formulating his or her own responses, and therefore not fully attending to the patient.

- Sympathetic listening happens when the clinician gets so involved in the story of the patient and ends up over-identifying with the patient.

Each of these contributes to a communication breakdown between the athletic trainer and the patient. With inadequate listening, the patient feels unheard; evaluative listening results in the patient feeling judged and misunderstood; selective listening also contributes to the client feeling misunderstood; rehearsing-while-listening adds to the patient feeling misunderstood and disrespected; and sympathetic listening results in the patient feeling heard but not helped (Brems, 2001, p. 121).

In the next section, the athletic trainer will be introduced to questioning skills. The use of closed and open questions will be discussed and the impact of these will be presented.

Questioning skills are seen as very valuable in the Ivey and Ivey (2003) model as they support the intentional use of questions designed for specific purposes.

Egan (1998) also addressed the appropriate use of questions and notes, saying, "when in doubt about what to say or do, novice or inept helpers tend to ask questions that add no value" (p. 101). Such a questioning style has no intention and consequently will not be helpful to the patient.

It is necessary to distinguish between the types of questions the athletic trainer can use. Closed questions are useful when one is seeking specific information from the patient. For example, one may ask, "Where does your shoulder hurt?' which will result in specific details as to the specific area where one is feeling the pain. Closed questions are very useful to the athletic trainer in pinpointing specific areas of concern. These questions often start with the words "is" as in "Is this painful?" "when" as in "When does this help?" and "where" as in "Where does this hurt?" Such questions are often given short, specific answer. An open question is one that expands the discussion with the patient. The open question, "what is hurting in your shoulder?," will probably result in a broader range of discussion about the specific injury and how it is impacting one's shoulder movements. Open questions usually start with words such as "what," as noted earlier, "how" as in "How is your rehab going?," and "could" as in "Could you explain what your goals are for this rehab plan?" If the athletic trainer asks an open question, she must be prepared to use the attending skill of verbal tracking to stay with what the athlete is saying rather than quickly jumping to another topic.

The closed questioning skills are designed to get specific information that will be useful in the diagnosis of a patient's injury. The open questions will assist the athletic trainer in promoting more discussion with the person as they work together in exploring what is concerning the individual. The athletic trainer will find both of these types of questions useful and must learn to blend them appropriately. Brems (2001, p. 145) addresses questions like those noted above and provides a clarification of their purposes, which is paraphrased below:

- "What" questions elicit facts and specific details about a situation.
- "How" questions elicit processes of sequence about a situation and may be helpful in eliciting emotions.
- "Why" questions elicit reasons and may lead to rationalizations or defensiveness.
- "When" questions elicit specific details about various time frames.
- "Where" questions elicit specific details about location(s).
- "Who" questions elicit specific details about individuals involved with the patient.

Paraphrasing represents a skill that lets the patient know the athletic trainer has really heard what the individual has said. When paraphrasing, the athletic trainer tries to respond to the content presented by the athlete. Ivey and Ivey (2003) note that this is not parroting what has been said, but represents a condensed description of what the person has said. Brems (2001) indicates three specific reasons for paraphrasing: to paraphrase content, to facilitate disclosure and communication, and to demonstrate understanding (p. 174). Hackney and Cormier (2005, p. 57) specify four steps to making a successful paraphrase:

1. Recall the patient's message to make sure you have heard it.
2. Identify the content of the message to decide what the patient is talking about.
3. Rephrase concisely the key words and concepts of the patient in order to rephrase what has been spoken in fresh or different words.
4. Include a perception check that allows the patient to agree or disagree with you.

Some patients with whom one works may tend to describe situations according to the facts and content of what is going on with them. When the athlete speaks in a concrete, specific manner, the athletic trainer will find the paraphrasing useful. For example:

> *Patient:* I was running down the field and then I saw the defensive back move toward me and then I moved to the center of the field and then the linebacker hit me and then I fell on my hip.
>
> *Athletic Trainer:* You were running, were hit, and landed on your hip. Is that correct?

Notice how in this example the person describes the event with numerous words and then the athletic trainer condenses it into a few words. In addition, the athletic trainer used the short question "Is that correct?" to check out the accuracy of the paraphrase. The use of the check-out question helps in verifying the accuracy of the paraphrase. Also notice the use of the words "and then," as these are also indicators that the patient describes events in a concrete, sequential manner. Paraphrasing can be very useful with patients who use such speaking patterns.

Some final suggestions on paraphrasing come from Young (2000, p. 102) who suggests:

- Do not paraphrase too early. Wait until you have a firm grasp of the important details, then compress them into a short paraphrase.
- Early on, use minimal encouragers and door openers liberally to encourage the client to supply essential information.
- Do not repeat the client's exact words. Give a distilled version in slightly different words.
- Do not add a moral tone to your paraphrase.
- When you can, paraphrase the client's thoughts and intentions as well as the basic facts.

Encouragers represent short statements the athletic trainer can use to keep a conversation going with a patient. Ivey and Ivey (2003) indicate that these can be both verbal and nonverbal messages. Phrases such as "go on," "tell me more," "please continue," and "uh-huh" are encouragers. Nonverbal encouragers involve a slight nod of the head; moving one's hands toward the athletic trainer as the person is speaking and smiling, when appropriate, can promote sound discussions with the individual. For example:

> *Patient:* My coach tells me that if I get this sprain better in the next 3 days, then I will be able to play on Friday night.
>
> *Athletic Trainer:* Tell me more about this discussion with your coach.

In this situation, the athletic trainer is encouraging the patient to continue with the discussion in an effort to learn more about how the athlete understands the expectations of the coach. Encouragers can be very effective in continuing the conversations the athletic trainer has with the individual. As Brems (2001) has suggested, encouragers can help to elicit more content, to encourage further disclosure, and to express interest in hearing more.

Reflecting feelings requires the athletic trainer to become aware of the main emotional words the patient may be expressing. According to Ivey and Ivey (2003), using the specific feeling words used by the individual is a sign of an effective reflection.

Hackney and Cormier (2005, p. 58) have stated:

> *Learning to reflect client feelings involves three steps. The first is to recognize the client's feelings or affected tone. The second step involves choosing the words to describe those feelings. The third step is to give your perception back to the client in a manner that is reflective rather than prescriptive.*

Some patients' main way of expressing themselves is through their feelings. Consequently, reflection of feelings can be a useful skill when working with these individuals. The athletic trainer does not want to use words that may minimize the feelings of the person, nor does he or she want to use terms that may escalate the feelings experienced by the individual. Earlier, it was noted that paraphrasing deals with the content of what the patient is saying whereas with reflection of feeling the athletic trainer is focusing on the feelings expressed by the athlete. For example:

> *Patient:* My injury has really changed my outlook about sports. Man, for years soccer was the prime thing in my life since I was 7 years old. Now you are telling me I have to sit out a year to get over this blown out knee. Man it sucks. It really makes me mad to think I have spent all this time and here I am a junior on a winning team and all I can do is sit on the bench. College soccer has been my thing, man it hurts and bums me out.
>
> *Athletic Trainer:* You are hurt and bummed out. Is that right?

Notice how the patient's story is rather long, but the reflections of the athletic trainer are concise and focused mainly on how the soccer player feels about the situation. Also, note how the athletic trainer used the exact terms of the athlete and focuses on these and then incorporates a check-out question to seek verification of the accuracy of the reflection of the athlete's feelings. Brems (2001) has written that reflection can be most useful to demonstrate deep listening, feed back overt or covert affect, feed back underlying messages, and to deepen rapport and expressed caring (p. 174).

Young (2000) has identified specific considerations when reflecting feelings. He notes that it is not wise to ask the patient "How do you feel?" since this may result in the person not being able to articulate the feeling, thus putting the patient on the defensive. Secondly, it is important to reflect feelings as close as possible when they are expressed.

Delaying a response may send the message that the athletic trainer is not comfortable dealing with the patient's feelings or that the athletic trainer is not interested in them and does not see their importance in the helping process. Young (2000) also notes that some individuals may overshoot the patient's feelings, thus expressing the reflection with more intense feelings than the patient spoke. Also, he notes that one can undershoot the feelings of the patient by using feeling terms that are considerably weaker than those expressed by the patient. It is very important that the athletic trainer seeks to reflect the feelings of the patient by staying focused on the feelings stated and responding on the same intensity level.

Summarizing is a skill that ideally combines the skills of paraphrasing and reflecting feelings (Ivey & Ivey, 2003). Whereas paraphrasing and reflecting feelings tend to be concise responses to the patient, summarizing is somewhat longer. For example in the situation presented about the soccer player, a summarization would be:

> *Athletic Trainer:* You've played soccer since you were seven. Here you are in college, injured and feeling hurt and bummed out. Right?

In this example, the athletic trainer includes both the content of the patient's statement as well as the feelings the person has expressed. In addition, the athletic trainer has checked out the summary for accuracy.

Summarizing incorporates both the thoughts and feelings of the patient and enhances the person's efforts to make sense of what he or she has been discussing. Young (2000) discusses focusing summaries (p. 131) as ways to bring a patient back to the main point of an interview when the patient's conversation has moved into areas not directly related to the issue at hand. It can help highlight themes and issues for the patient and keep the individual on target to reach the goals that have been set.

Young (2000) indicates that signal summaries (p. 131) are statements by the helper that what the patient has expressed has been digested and that it is now time to move on to discussing the next matter to be addressed. These are usually effective when the patient has come to the end of the story and pauses, not sure where to move the conversation.

Thematic summaries (Young, 2000, p. 132) encompass the content, emotions, and meanings the patient has been discussing. These are advanced as they require the athletic trainer to absorb the information on three distinct levels and then summarize these to the patient. These types of summaries will be appropriate after having sufficient time for the various themes to unfold in further interviews with the patient.

Confronting is sometimes necessary to help the patient examine the discrepancies he or she may be experiencing (Ivey & Ivey, 2003). Confrontation is often seen as a negative interaction and therefore it may help the athletic trainer to put the term *caring* in front of *confrontation*. A caring confrontation indicates that one is concerned enough about the patient to bring into the open the conflict the person may be experiencing.

Young (2000) has noted a variety of discrepancies that individuals may present. He notes to look and listen for the following (pp. 183-184):

- Incongruity between verbal and nonverbal messages
- Incongruity between beliefs and experiences
- Incongruity between values and how the client behaves
- Incongruity between what the client says and how the client behaves
- Incongruity between experiences and plans
- Incongruity between two verbal messages

Once the athletic trainer becomes aware that the patient is presenting information with one of the incongruities cited above, it is time to provide a caring confrontation to the patient. Young (2000, pp. 184-185) has developed the following four steps that will be helpful in the process:

1. First, listen carefully and make sure the relationship is well established before confronting. Be non-judgmental and make sure the timing is right.
2. Present the challenge in a way that the client will most likely accept it.
3. Observe the client's response to the confrontation.
4. Follow up the confrontation by rephrasing or retreating.

When confronting a patient, the athletic trainer can follow these four steps and not try to shock the person in dealing with the incongruity presented. However, the athletic trainer can also firmly let the patient know how he or she sees the incongruity impacting their work together, or how the incongruity may be impacting the patient's progress in another area related to the work they are doing together.

For example, a patient may be scheduled to meet with the athletic trainer for treatment of an injury but repeatedly fails to show up for treatment. When the athletic trainer sees the person in the hallways around school, the patient tells him that he hopes to be ready to play in 2 more weeks. Here is an example:

> *Athlete:* Hi. I wanted to see you but had a paper due for history, you know how that is. I want to play in 2 weeks, big game, but the elbow is still swollen. Maybe it will be ok.
>
> *Athletic Trainer:* Jim, on the one hand you tell me you want to play next week, but you have yet to get to rehab. Your plans to play and your involvement in rehab are really not in line with the training program here at school.

Notice how the athletic trainer does not blame Jim for missing rehabilitation and for taking time to work on his history paper. However, the athletic trainer does point out the conflict between what Jim is saying and what he is actually doing to treat the injured elbow. No blame is being made; however, the athletic trainer is clear about what has been going on with the athlete's behavior. Caring confrontations need to focus on the behavior of the patient and are not designed to place blame. They must stress the discrepancies presented by the athlete.

Reflection of meaning is designed to help a person explore the meaning an event or situation has for him or her (Ivey & Ivey, 2003). Athletic trainers know that participation in athletics means much for the individual patient. Glasser's (1998) concepts come into play as the athletic trainer talks with the person and begins to understand what a specific injury means as well as what the rehabilitation efforts will mean to the patient. For example, the athlete who cannot compete may be concerned about the loss of power, the loss of belonging, and the loss of fun when competition ceases. There was a high school football player whose ACL was seriously damaged in the final game of his high school career. He had hopes of going on to a Division I school and continuing his career for at least 4 more years. After months of rehabilitation, he entered college and watched football games from the stands. During his sophomore year he tried out for the team, made it, and played a year as a safety. He decided not to return to the football team his junior year and when asked why he make this choice, he replied, "I just wanted to prove to myself that I could do it, but there are other things I want to do now." Coming back to play for him had meaning and by playing he was able to experience the power and fun that he once had in his high school days.

On the other hand, consider the meaning a career-ending injury has for the professional athlete, whose self-image, fan adoration, and financial resources are now removed. For the person whose self-concept has emerged from this athletic identification, the meaning is very different. What does it mean when the athlete sees him- or herself as now being less due to the injury? What does it mean when the fans are no longer around to bolster one's self-concept? What does it mean when one has not considered what type of a career and lifestyle he or she will live once the playing is done?

As the athletic trainer works with the patient, it helps to listen to what is being communicated regarding the athlete's view of the injury and the impact he or she sees it having on him- or herself. Does he or she have a self-image that is more inclusive than that of an athlete? What will it mean to him or her to participate in the rehabilitation process? What does the progress or lack of progress in the rehabilitation process mean to him or her?

The meanings that the patient places on his or her unique situation are important to understand. The athletic trainer wants to understand this meaning and use it in the rehabilitation process with the athlete. It goes beyond rehabilitating the broken ankle and moves into treating the athlete as a person, not a joint to be repaired.

Be Aware

Learning and using the information presented thus far may result in some individuals taking on professional roles that are counterproductive to the patient. Although much of it is written about counselors and psychotherapists, athletic trainers can fall into similar roles. Welch (1998) describes a variety of roles psychotherapists may take when they have reached a stage in their professional lives that they opt to distance themselves from their clients. Each of these shows a lack of faith in the patients with which they are working and provides a buffer between the therapist and the patient.

Pundits (Welch, 1998) will listen to the stories of their patients, gather information, and analyze the information presented to them. From this they begin to offer their own opinions of what the patient should do, thus shifting the focus from the patient to themselves. The pundit is able to explain everything that is going on and remains detached from the person in an aloof, hygienic manner. In this role, the patient gains little understanding from the helper.

Wizards (Welch, 1998) use their magic to make things better. This magic involves special techniques, methods, devices, and approaches that they use to help themselves stand out as "unrecognized geniuses" (p. 89). In the field of psychotherapy, these types of individuals are look at with much disdain.

Priests (Welch, 1998) are great pontificators as to how things should be. They use psychological concepts and jargon to develop strategies by which others should live their lives. They believe individuals are unhealthy and need their form of salvation. Such helpers are arrogant, having a sense of moral superiority. They also present distortions about the therapy process, wanting patients to follow their ways of living. Such individuals prey on the vulnerabilities of their patients and use their power and influence in ways that are destructive for the patients.

Clerks (Welch, 1998) are the kind of helpers who keep comprehensive records about their patients and make it appear that they are providing professional care for them, when they are actually accomplishing very little. The clerks assess the patients and provide diagnostic labels for them but do not do anything therapeutic with the information. They end up discounting the patient by not providing the therapeutic interactions and interventions needed to help the individual progress. By remaining objective and using the diagnostic labels, they do not allow themselves to enter the subjective world of the patient, where much of the therapy must be done.

All of these styles of helping are counterproductive and allow the helper to distance him- or herself from the patient. Welch (1998) does note that many therapists today see themselves as the instrument in the helping process. He notes, "how an individual practices psychotherapy is, instead, a personal and unique process guided by research into effective psychotherapy and tempered by the therapist's individual qualities" (p. 94). In keeping with the ideas presented by Rogers (1951, 1957), it is important for the therapist to present him- or herself in a clear fashion to eliminate the patient having to second guess who the therapist is and what the therapist stands for in the helping process.

In this section of the chapter, the specific intentional interviewing skills of Ivey and Ivey (2003) have been examined. Starting with the attending behaviors, moving through the various types of questions, and following up with appropriate paraphrases, reflections and summaries will be useful tools in communicating with athletes. When one confronts with care and attempts to learn the meanings the athlete places on an injury, the athletic trainer enhances his or her understanding of the athlete with whom he or she works. In addition, nonproductive styles of working with people were presented in this section. When initially examining an athlete, it is helpful for athletic trainers to utilize common interview skills appropriate for any physical, psychological, or emotional problem. In the next section, the HOPE protocol will be introduced to assist athletic trainers during the assessment phase of a potential patient.

HOPE

Providing a thorough injury assessment of an athlete is an important role of a certified athletic trainer. The initial assessment is often done on the playing field for the purpose of ruling out life-threatening conditions. After life-threatening injuries are ruled out, a more detailed injury evaluation needs to be completed in the athletic training room or clinic. It is during this evaluation process that an athletic trainer plays a vital role in assessing, treating, managing, and possibly referring an injured athlete. This evaluation process is critical for caring for an injured athlete and has been broken down into four areas to help athletic trainers facilitate appropriate care: history, observation, palpation, and special tests (HOPS) (Prentice, 2006). All athletic trainers should be familiar with the acronym HOPS and have implemented this evaluation tool to help with assessment of an injured athlete.

Certified athletic trainers play a vital role in assessing both physical and psychosocial problems of athletes. An athletic trainer must be able to direct a thorough evaluation of an athlete suffering from a psychosocial problem as well as for an athlete suffering from a knee injury. We would like to introduce a similar acronym that is specific for athletic trainers in assessing and helping athletes with psychosocial problems. The HOPE (History, Observation, Planning, Evaluation) protocol offers a similar evaluation scheme for athletic trainers to use in the assessment of athletes suffering from a variety of psychosocial issues. It incorporates the open questions of Ivey and Ivey (2003) as a way to facilitate the helping process with an athlete suffering from psychosocial problems. The tool can be used in the same way as the HOPS acronym in assessment of musculoskeletal injuries.

History taking is essential when trying to pinpoint an issue about the patient. The following questions can be useful in the phase of the model:

- What was the event that alerted the athletic trainer that a problem exists?
- How long has the athlete been dealing with the issue?
- What types of help have been sought in the past or present?

Observations that the athletic trainer has made will help further define what has been experienced by the patient. These should be based on specific behaviors and not include hunches or speculations.

- What did the athletic trainer observe?
- What does the patient share about the situation and its impact on him or her?
- What has the coach, a friend, or colleague observed about what is going on with the patient?

Planning may involve the athletic trainer and the patient, as well as other individuals with special skills whose consultation can help in making an appropriate plan.

- What does the patient plan to do?
- What resources are needed to achieve the plan?
- What is a reasonable timeline for completing the plan?

Evaluation is essential to any intervention with the athlete. It is helpful to have specific benchmarks to look for in examining the progress of the patient's efforts to complete the plan.

- What benchmarks has the athletic trainer observed?
- What does the athlete report about the progress being made?
- What does the coach report about the progress being made?

It is essential that the athletic trainer incorporate the intentional interviewing skills and use the motivating factors cited by Glasser (1998) when using the HOPE protocol with a patient. Understanding what has been experienced by the person is crucial, but understanding alone will not help the person move toward behaviors to change the situation and choose behaviors that will better meet the needs of the individual. The athletic trainer wants to help the patient find healthy and beneficial behaviors to replace those

---

Table 2-1

The SPORT Model

- State what you want to have happen: _____
- Performance expected of you to accomplish this: _____
- Organize yourself for success by doing: _____
- Reality check (circle one): Yes, I can do this.   No, I cannot do this (try again).
- Time table for completing your goal: _____

Patient: _____   Date: _____
Athletic Trainer: _____   Date: _____

---

which have been counterproductive. In the next section, a goal-setting strategy to incorporate in the planning phase of the HOPE protocol will be presented.

SPORT

When the athletic trainer begins the process of helping the athlete deal with a specific situation, it is important to establish a plan of action. Oftentimes such efforts may not be successful due to not having a clear plan that both parties can agree to follow. The SPORT (Miller & Pappas, 2003) model, originally developed for athletic advisors, can be modified to provide a goal-setting strategy that can prove useful in helping an athlete set a goal with the athletic trainer (Table 2-1).

This model can be very useful at the outset of goal-setting and can, over time, present a helpful way to examine the progress the patient is making toward completing a goal or goals he or she has set with the athletic trainer. If, for some reason, the goal has not been achieved, there may be a need to examine the steps along the way and determine where the athlete must reconsider and make more of a commitment to completing the goal. The framework is one that athletic trainers can incorporate with a variety of interventions with patients.

Conclusion

This chapter has addressed issues of healthy personality development and has included an overview of major approaches to counseling. In it the athletic trainer has had the opportunity to learn about the needs that motivate human behavior based on the work of Glasser (1998). Some of the intentional interviewing skills of Ivey and Ivey (2003) have been presented to promote positive interaction and relationship development between the athletic trainer and the athlete. Also, the HOPE protocol for intervention analysis and preparation along with the SPORT goal-setting model have been introduced.

Chapter Exercises

1. Using Glasser's five needs of individuals, rank the order (1 = lowest to 5 = highest) of the needs you believe your patients see as most important for them. After ranking these, write statements you have heard or anticipate hearing from your patients that represent these need areas.

Rank Order	Need	Statement
_____	Survival	_____
_____	Belonging	_____
_____	Power	_____
_____	Freedom	_____
_____	Fun	_____

   Next, discuss the written statements with your classmates.

2. After discussing the statements presented above, consider how you would develop an open-ended question for one of these:

   Statement: _____.

   Open-ended question: _____?

3. Select another statement from the first practice activity and prepare a paraphrase to it, including a check-out question.

   Statement: _____.

   Paraphrase: _____.

   Check-out question: _____?

4. Now, select another statement and reflect the feelings of your patient.

   Statement: _____.

   Reflection of feelings: _____.

5. This is a role play activity using a group of three. One person will be the patient, one will be the athletic trainer, and the third will be the observer.

   a. The patient will discuss some discrepancy that is often heard by athletic trainers. Select one that demonstrates the discrepancy between what the patient is saying versus what the patient actually does.

   b. The athletic trainer will confront the patient about this discrepancy following the four steps suggested by Young (2000) in the chapter.

   c. The observer will note how the athletic trainer follows Young's (2000) model of confrontation, and at the end of the role play will describe what has been noted and observed.

   d. At the end of the role play, after the observer has discussed the observations, the patient will share how the confrontation sounded and impacted him or her.

   e. The group members will switch roles so all can participate in each role.

   f. NOTE: Please plan to use between 20 to 30 minutes to complete this activity.

6. Using the HOPE model, incorporate the three-person role play process focusing on the following patient: an 18-year-old volleyball player who has told you that

she has just learned that she has to have an operation on her shoulder that may prevent her from completing the rest of the season. Use one of the intentional interviewing skills noted in the chapter in each of the four stages of the HOPE model. Write down what you would say and then determine which of the intentional interviewing skills was used.

History:

    Event: _____.

    Time: _____.

    Help: _____.

    Intentional interviewing skill: _____.

Observation:

    Athletic trainer: _____.

    Impact on athlete: _____.

    Coach: _____.

    Intentional interviewing skill: _____.

Planning:

    Athlete: _____.

    Resources: _____.

    Time line: _____.

    Intentional interviewing skill: _____.

Evaluation:

    Benchmarks: _____.

    Athlete progress: _____.

    Coach's report: _____.

    Intentional interviewing skill: _____.

NOTE: Please plan to use 20 to 30 minutes for this activity.

7. Using the SPORT model, develop a plan for yourself for using specific intentional interviewing skills.

    State what you want to have happen: _____.

    Performance expected for you to accomplish this:_____.

    Organize yourself for success by doing: _____.

    Reality check (circle one): Yes, I can do this.   No, I can not do this.

    Time table for completing your goal: _____.

8. Below are listed some of the typical statements patients may make to the athletic trainer in the training room. Please read them and respond in the space provided. Try to classify the nature of your response based on the intentional interviewing skills described in the chapter.

"Here I am sitting in this training room. Nobody on the team cares where I am."

Response: _____.

Intentional interviewing skill: _____.

"I've been coming here for the past week and nothing seems to be getting better with this knee. This is a bummer; I want to be on the court."

Response: _____.

Intentional interviewing skill: _____.

"Move it this way you say, but each time I move my shoulder this way, it hurts. I cannot see how this is making it better."

Response: _____.

Intentional interviewing skill: _____.

"Why doesn't the coach believe I am hurt? All he says is 'Suck it up and play.'"

Response: _____.

Intentional interviewing skill: _____.

"Man, they are always pulling me out for drug tests. Let 'em get the guys who are really using on this team."

Response: _____.

Intentional interviewing skill: _____.

References

Blackham, G.J. & Silberman, A. (1980). Modification of child and adolescent behavior (3rd ed.).Belmont: CA. Thompson Learning.

Brems, C. (2001). *Basic skills in psychotherapy and counseling.* Belmont, CA: Brooks/Cole Thompson Learning.

Brickman, P., Rabinowitz, V. C., Karuza, Jr., J., Coates, D., Cohn, E., & Kidder, L. (1982). Models of helping and coping. *American Psychologist, 37,* 368-384.

Cavanagh, M. E., & Levitov, J. E. (2002). *The counseling experience: A theoretical and practical approach* (2nd ed.). Prospect Heights, IL: Waveland Press.

Cramer Roh, J. L., & Perna, F. M. (2000). Psychology/counseling: A universal competency in athletic training. *Journal of Athletic Training, 35,* 458-465.

Egan, G. (1998). *The skilled helper* (6th ed.). Pacific Grove, CA: Brooks/Cole.

Ellis, A. (1958). *Sex without guilt.* Secaucus, NJ: Lyle Stuart.

Ellis, A. (1994). *Reason and emotion in psychotherapy* (rev ed.). New York, NY: Citadel.

Ellis A. & Dryden, W. (1997). The practice of rational emotive behavior therapy (2nd ed.). New York, NY: Springer.

Glasser, W. (1965). *Reality therapy: A new approach to psychiatry.* New York, NY: Harper and Row.

Glasser, W. (1998). *Choice theory: A new psychology of personal freedom.* New York, NY: Harper Collins.

Hackney, H. L., & Cormier, L. S. (2005). *The professional counselor: A process guide to helping* (5th ed.). Boston: Pearson Allyn & Bacon.

Heath, D. H. (1980). Wanted: A comprehensive model of healthy development. *Personnel and Guidance Journal, 58,* 391- 399.

Ivey, A. E. (1971). *Microcounseling innovations in interview training.* Springfield, IL: Charles C. Thomas.

Ivey, A. E., & Ivey, M. B. (2003). *Intentional interviewing and counseling: Facilitating client development in a multicultural society* (5th ed.). Pacific Grove, CA: Thompson Brooks Cole.

Ivey, A. E., Ivey, M. B., Myers, J. E., & Sweeney, T. J. (2005). *Developmental counseling and therapy promoting wellness over the lifespan.* Boston, MA: Lahaska Press.

Krumboltz, J. D. (1966). Behavioral goals for counseling. *Journal of Counseling Psychology, 13,* 153-159.

Miller, G. M., & Pappas, J. C. (2003). Student-athletes: How do they cope? *Academic Athletic Journal, 171*), 65-72.

Moulton, M. A., Molstad, S., & Turner, A. (1997). The role of athletic trainers in counseling collegiate athletes. *Journal of Athletic Training, 32*, 148-150.

Nye, R. D. (1975). *Three views of man: Perspectives from Sigmund Freud, B.F. Skinner and Carl Rogers.* Monterey, CA: Brooks/Cole.

Prentice, W. E. (2006). *Arnheim's principles of athletic training: A competency-based approach* (12th ed.). Boston, MA: McGraw-Hill.

Rogers, C. R. (1951). *Client-centered therapy.* Boston, MA: Houghton Mifflin.

Rogers, C. R. (1957). The necessary and sufficient conditions of therapeutic personality change. *Journal of Consulting Psychology, 212*), 95-103.

Thorensen, C. E., & Mahoney, M. J. (1974). *Behavioral self-control.* New York, NY: Holt, Rineholt, & Winston.

Walen, S., DiGiuseppe, R., & Wessler, R. L. (1980). *A practioner's guide to rational-emotive therapy.* New York, NY: Oxford Press.

Welch, I. D. (1998). *The path of psychotherapy matters of the heart.* Pacific Grove, CA: Brooks Cole.

Young, M. E. (2000). *Learning the art of helping* (2nd ed.). Upper Saddle River, NJ: Merrill Prentice Hall.

Zunin, L., & Zunin, N. (1972). *Contact: The first four minutes.* New York, NY: Balantine Books.

Chapter

Systematic Referrals: Issues and Processes Related to Psychosocial Referrals for Athletic Trainers

Matthew E. Lemberger, PhD

Chapter Objectives

- ❖ Introduce issues germane to the referral process for the athletic trainer.
- ❖ Introduce a practical explanation of counseling and present two paradigms for understanding the usefulness of psychosocial services.
- ❖ Identify issues pertaining to psychosocial referral and present a series of rationales why an athletic trainer would need to refer in his or her professional practice.
- ❖ Introduce a number of the specific types of professionals to whom the athletic trainer can refer an athlete.
- ❖ Explain a model that explains what a referral is and to whom you might refer an athlete, as well as a model to demonstrate appropriate referral processes.
- ❖ Discuss a series of psychosocial special topics that might arise when working with patients/athletes.

NATA Educational Competencies

Psychosocial Intervention and Referral Domain

1. Explain the psychosocial requirements (i.e., motivation and self-confidence) of various activities that relate to the readiness of the injured or ill individual to resume participation.

2. Explain the importance of providing health care information to patients, parents/ guardians, and others regarding the psychological and emotional well-being of the patient.

3. Describe the roles and function of various community-based health care providers (to include, but not limited to, psychologists, counselors, social workers, human resources personnel) and the accepted protocols that govern the referral of patients to these professionals.

4. Describe the basic signs and symptoms of mental disorders (psychoses), emotional disorders (neuroses, depression), or personal/social conflict (family problems, academic or emotional stress, personal assault or abuse, sexual assault, sexual harassment); the contemporary personal, school, and community health service agencies, such as community-based psychological and social support services that treat these conditions; and the appropriate referral procedures for accessing these health service agencies.

5. Describe the acceptance and grieving processes that follow a catastrophic event and the need for a psychological intervention and referral plan for all parties affected by the event.

6. Explain the potential need for psychosocial intervention and referral when dealing with populations requiring special consideration (to include, but not limited to, those with exercised-induced asthma, diabetes, seizure disorders, drug allergies and interactions, unilateral organs, physical and/or mental disability).

Medical Conditions and Disabilities Domain

1. Describe and know when to refer common psychological medical disorders from drug toxicity, physical and emotional stress, and acquired disorders (e.g., substance abuse, eating disorders/disordered eating, depression, bipolar disorder, seasonal affective disorder, anxiety disorders, somatoform disorders, personality disorders, abusive disorders, and addiction).

Nutritional Aspects of Injuries and Illnesses Domain

1. Describe disordered eating and eating disorders (i.e., signs, symptoms, physical and psychological consequences, referral systems).

Acute Care of Injuries and Illnesses Domain

1. Identify information obtained during the examination to determine when to refer an injury or illness for further or immediate medical attention.

Health Care Administration Domain

1. Differentiate the roles and responsibilities of the athletic trainer from those of other medical and allied health personnel who provide care to patients involved in physical activity and describe the necessary communication skills for effectively interacting with these professionals.

2. Describe the role and functions of various community-based medical, para-medical, and other health care providers and protocols that govern the referral of patients to these professionals.

As the adage goes, athletics are about mental toughness. The mental aspects of athletics are tied to every sprint, every throw, and every leap that ultimately inspires these actions. Athletic activity has become increasingly widespread in our modern societies. The increased demand of athletics has also become increasingly competitive and so has the laurels of athletic accomplishment. The growing demand of athletics has resulted in the stressful evolutions in sport and other life stressors in the lives of athletes. In times when this stress is so intense that it becomes debilitating or distracting, athletes find that they need to seek outside assistance. In the cases of the mental duress experienced by athletes, a psychosocial referral to a mental health professional can be the first step toward optimal functioning. Read the following vignette and consider the psychosocial influence of the events in this athlete's life and how the inclusion of a mental health professional might assist in making a difference.

Jorge, Football's Fabled Folk Hero

If you ever had the opportunity to watch young Jorge play a sport, you—like everyone else—would find yourself recanting stories of a truly gifted athlete well beyond his years. As a child, his friends were often in awe of his almost innate ability to pick up every sport instantaneously. Within hours of his first exposure to the new game, Jorge effortlessly found a unique rhythm for the sport. Soon after "picking up" the nuances of the activity, Jorge excelled beyond the levels of more seasoned players. Jorge approached athletics more like an artist than a competitor. Each movement created an energy, an actual presence in every spectator's life.

Jorge was always notably larger, faster, and stronger than all other kids. As he aged, Jorge continued to develop these athletic talents and his legend ensued. Tales of Jorge's talent began to even outgrow Jorge (and even his amazing talent).

Though Jorge played each sport well, it was evident that his future was in football. In his small town football was "third only to God and family" and, hence, Jorge was perceived as an athletic savior of this otherwise fledgling community. Young and old alike rallied around Jorge and looked to him to bring pride to his township. Instinctively, Jorge fell in love with the modest celebrity that he experienced.

After excelling in high school, the natural course was for Jorge to accept a scholarship to play for the flagship school of his home state. The means to play on a larger, more visible field was set and Jorge was seemingly well on his way to the stardom that everyone was certain would be his.

In his college playing days, there was no profound tragedy, injury, or life trauma. However, there was also no profound accomplishment; at least no athletic accomplishment commensurate with the expectations that he set upon himself, that he felt from his home community, and that would be necessary to become a professional football player. For the first time in Jorge's life, his athletic ability was considered "relatively normal." Jorge was still a good player, just not a great one.

Throughout his first 3 years of college, Jorge held steadfast to the belief that "his time would come" or that "next year, that'll be my year." It was not until late into his final football season did Jorge begin to consider what his life would be like without football. He began to literally feel the pressure of his community and family weighing on his soul. Jorge considered his athletic accomplishments to this point a complete failure—he considered himself a failure in life. He feared returning home to face the unmet expectations of his family and friends. He feared the final games on the schedule and the inevitable transition in his life. For so long football and athletic success defined his life.

With this newfound awareness, Jorge began to struggle in his remaining classes, in his personal life, and even on the field. He felt that the life that he knew was spiraling out of control and that there was no reprieve in sight.

Professional Response to the Athlete

As an athletic trainer, you are charged with the task of supporting the athlete as he or she strives to reach the highest potential of his or her athletic goals and abilities. Imagine that you are one of the athletic trainers that has been working with Jorge throughout his college career. Do you believe that you could help Jorge? If so, how would you identify that he was in need of assistance and the specific issues that prompted this need? Do you believe that Jorge's current dilemmas are only athletic related or that they might be associated with other, more intrapersonal considerations? What precise actions could you take to aid Jorge and what possible obstacles would hinder your efforts? Will you be able to take on these actions by yourself or will you need additional support, guidance, and even alternative professional expertise? These and countless other questions will be relevant in your work with cases similar to Jorge's. The ultimate question will be how will you react in situations when it is a real name, a real human, and the real-life conditions that surround your work as an athletic trainer?

Modern athletic pursuits are diverse in their expression and intention. Some athletes use sport and competitive activities as a recreational departure from their everyday life, whereas other athletes' livelihood and identity are completely tied to the perfection of their sport. Similarly, outstanding athletes are also often diverse and multifaceted in that there are a wealth of variables that contribute to or obstruct from their athletic aspirations reaching the highest levels. To support these athletes, an athletic trainer should remain cognizant of the diverse forces that affect and influence these athletes and their athletic pursuits. Whereas the greater part of one's professional preparation has provided the necessary skills to account for the bodily factors in supporting athletes, this chapter shall introduce how the professional athletic trainer might support the athlete in his or her mental pursuits and influences. Specifically, this chapter shall present information to assist the athletic trainer in making psychosocial referrals.

Inevitably at some point during one's professional tenure, the athletic trainer will confront psychosocial issues that are either outside of one's professional expertise or simply not pragmatic to engage upon without the professional expertise and support of a mental health professional. In these situations, the ability to refer the athlete to the most appropriate mental health professional is vital to both parties involved. In addition to supporting the welfare of the athlete, such referrals will also protect your needs professionally and personally.

One might think that the referral process is a relatively simple and unsophisticated task. It is true that one can make referral as simple as speculating that an athlete has a "mental problem" and then thumbing through the local telephone registry for the most convenient psychotherapist. Proceeding from the genuine belief that one is acting in the "best interest of the athlete," the athletic trainer schedules an appointment with the psychotherapist's office manager, never directly speaking to the individual that will be performing the mental health services. Upon the next occasion of seeing the athlete, you inform the athlete that you have scheduled an appointment and engage in little-to-no dialogue about the considerations or actions that you have made. At this point, from the "simple referral" perspective, you have completed your task. You take credence that the athlete should be in good hands. Or so you would like to believe.

In rare situations, this "simple referral" gamble might actually prove to be beneficial to the athlete. More often, the athletic trainer will find that the referral process is a complex venture containing many variables, both evident and hidden. The situations that evoke referrals are frequently sophisticated and contain nuances that are particular to the athlete and the environment contributing to these situations. The challenge of appropriately referring the athlete to the appropriate professional is found in one's ability to consider all of these variables as they mesh with the available resources in your community.

While it is true that the referral process contains many elements to consider, you should remain assured that these features are manageable. The key to successful referral will be found chiefly in having the willingness, confidence, and capacity to be aware of distinctions relative to the particular referral situation and to match these details with the appropriate professional. The athletic trainer should reframe the complexities of the referral process into an opportunity for improved professional care. The more detailed and complex referral situation requires the athletic trainer to be more personal and proceed with more depth than would be necessary in a "simple" situation. This personal concern and action will enhance the referral situation, resulting in better athletic training services for patients.

The scope of this chapter is to introduce many of the issues germane to the referral process for the athletic trainer. The information presented will enhance one's professional development for participating in the referral of athletes. To begin, this chapter shall introduce a practical explanation of counseling and then present two paradigms, or philosophical approaches, for understanding the usefulness of psychosocial services. The two paradigms presented herein should serve as a theoretical compass for the types of situations in which psychosocial referral might be useful to athletes. These paradigms present counseling as both a process to remediate trouble spots in the psychosocial functioning of athletes and, additionally, as a potential proactive process for learning preventative skills before the psychosocial issues become unmanageable. Next, a definition of psychosocial referral is presented and then a series of rationales as to why an athletic trainer would need to refer in his or her professional practice is discussed. This chapter also introduces a number of the specific types of professionals to whom the athletic trainer can refer an athlete. In addition to having an understanding of what a referral is and to whom you might refer an athlete, a model is presented to demonstrating this procedure. Finally, this chapter closes with a series of psychosocial special topics that might arise when working with patients. These special topics can serve as a potential guidepost to ensure that the referral process leads to effective management of the patient's psychosocial issues.

Before proceeding into the contents of the chapter, the author would like to offer one additional consideration regarding your own stressors and psychosocial functioning as an athletic trainer. You might find at some point in your professional career that the best psychosocial referral that you might make is a self-referral. In working with people, there exists the implicit emotional connection with that person and entering the psychosocial aspects of his or her life. Compound this with the present issues that occur in one's own personal and professional life, the athletic trainer might find that there are times when he or she could use some assistance. The benefits of this self-awareness and self-maintenance are invaluable to one's personal well-being and even one's professional care of others.

Athletic trainers are endowed with plentiful skills that will accommodate athletes in need of psychosocial referral. As an athletic trainer, one's athletic and physiological focus necessitates a connection with the social and emotional attributes of the athletes under his or her care. There are particular skills (i.e., those mentioned in Chapter 2 of this text) such as the manner in which you interact with an athlete, the types of conversations you naturally engage upon, and the shared interests that you have with the athlete that will translate into good referral opportunities. Referral then becomes a mere extension of the activities one does to ensure the total wellbeing of the athlete. Psychosocial referral opportunities, put simply, are the opportunities to contribute to the overall training successes of athletes.

What Is Psychosocial Referral?

Psychosocial referral is a dynamic helping process in which one human service provider connects a patient to a resource that can better assist in the patient's life functioning. Psychosocial referral is a triangular process shared between the referrer, referee, and referred. The athletic trainer will take on the role of the referrer, the athlete is the referee, and the mental health professional that you connect the patient with is the referred. This shared union between the referrer, referee, and referred is only as strong as each of the individuals involved. Additionally, the athletic trainer needs to ensure that there is strength and support in the tridactic bond of the psychosocial referral.

Psychosocial referral necessitates that each of the following considerations are met to ensure the effectiveness of the referral: identification of the psychosocial need and the contributing variables (e.g., what life stresses are present); evaluating potential referral sources; preparing one's self, the patient, and the specialist; coordinating the referral; and following through with any necessary postreferral tasks. There are multiple dimensions to be considered in the referral process and each building upon previous dimensions in a line of events beginning with the initial event of the referral issue continuing through its ultimate resolution.

Psychosocial referral is the intentional process of addressing the psychosocial needs of an athlete or patient. These psychosocial needs may be overtly related to the athletic training relationship that you share with the patient or something in the individual's life beyond athletics. In either case, these psychosocial issues are implicitly connected with the athletic pursuits of the person and, therefore, are cause to consider referral.

What Is Counseling?

To recognize the value of counseling and the need for referral of patients, one must first recognize that psychosocial issues play a major role in the physical and psychological lives of individuals. Psychosocial issues are those situations, influences, and conditions that affect the manner in which a person perceives, receives, and responds mentally to life experiences (Cnaan, Blankertz, Messinger, & Gardner, 1989). Put simply, one's thoughts and feelings affect the manner in which the world is experienced and how one acts in response to these thoughts and feelings. Therefore, thoughts and feelings can impede the athlete in physical activities.

Often, events that occur in life are not perceived to be any more or less significant than any other life event. In such cases, these experiences can be managed quite simply. This balanced state of being can be understood as a type of psychological homeostasis. For the most part, this homeostasis is desirable and affords one the mental standing necessary to function optimally. Other events, outside of one's range of psychological balance, can be perceived as more arduous or uncertain and, therefore, invoking stress for the individual. There are various degrees of life stressors that can be experienced, ranging from mild discomfort to completely debilitating stressors. Additionally, different people interpret and experience the same exact occurrences in distinct ways. Thus, what might be debilitating for one person is experienced as normal or manageable for another person. The manner in which one experiences life and stress is highly personal and unique.

In terms of athletic pursuits and psychosocial issues, everyday athletes are entangled in life and athletic-specific scenarios that could potentially invoke stress. There are stressors that are specific to their athletic pursuits, such as the pressure to achieve, social and performance anxiety, and postinjury stress. Additionally, there are life and social stressors in the lives of these individuals that impact their athletic pursuits. For example, a student athlete mired in academic shortcomings can detract from one's performance and further impair the effort needed to remedy the school difficulties. In many of these stressful situations, the athletic trainer will find that the athlete feels trapped in a chronic spiral of stress that produces more complex and agonizing stress.

Counseling is the exploration of the important events in one's life; the possible psychological and social elements that are contributing to life stress; and the potential thoughts, feelings, and behaviors that can lead to a breakage from the spiral of life stress. Counseling promotes the development of safeguards to promote psychological stability. This latter facet of counseling works to ensure that the therapeutic activities that occur in the clinical session translate into the patient's everyday life outside of counseling.

The actual term *counseling* has many layers of definition within the various psychosocial helping professions. The words *counseling*, *therapy*, and *psychotherapy* will be used interchangeably and focus on the generic process of a professional helper jointly restructuring life wellness with an individual. The construct of wellness (Gladding, 2001, p. 127), or a state that emphasizes good mental and physical health, positive lifestyle patterns, and prevention, marks the shared utility between psychotherapists and athletic trainers in that both promote wellness to enhance the lives of individuals.

PSYCHOTHERAPEUTIC PRACTICES

The athletic trainer learns about the particular aspects of the profession, the issues that are relevant to patients, and the contexts under which one offers support to patients. The athletic trainer benefits from having a general familiarity with the practices of counseling and should ask for further elaboration about counseling before a referral is made. It is reasonable to assume that the athlete will ask about what he or she can anticipate regarding the processes, potential benefits, and even potential deficits and threats related to counseling. As the individual who has taken on the responsibility of connecting the athlete with the psychotherapeutic professional via the referral process, the athletic trainer has the responsibility of trying to answer these questions.

The task of clearly articulating an understanding of psychotherapeutic practices can be the most significant task in the entire therapeutic process. Counseling can be perceived by a patient as intimidating, mysterious, irrelevant, or simply not worth the effort. In fact, many individuals who consider counseling are understandably ambivalent about actually committing to attend, as most people cannot fathom the relevance and benefit of counseling to their lives. The athletic trainer can clarify the process, assisting the patient in making a commitment to participate in counseling.

In the following sections, a general portrait of the processes and procedures of counseling and the typical forms of counseling are discussed.

Processes and Procedures

In many ways, the processes and procedures of counseling are similar to the everyday interactions one shares with any trusted friend. As is the case with a friend, the bond that you share with a psychotherapist must be grounded in confidence, candor, and give-and-take. For the relationship to have any value and effectiveness insofar as psychosocial improvement, the patient must feel a degree of confidence and trust in the ally counselor. In fact, research has consistently shown that the nature of the shared relationship itself can be psychologically curative in the lives of clients (Catty, 2004). The relationship necessitates an inherent degree of disclosure and candor to have any relevant transferability back into the patient's life beyond counseling. Because each of the particular aspects and considerations are critical to the manner in which the person understands his or her world, a therapist must work with the same conditions and perceptions that make up the person's world view. Finally, there must be some degree of experienced gratification for the therapeutic relationship to account for the psychosocial needs of the athlete. The individual must experience improved satisfaction and, furthermore, be able to clearly identify life changes. Good counseling cannot simply be isolated to the quality of feeling experienced during the "therapy hour"; instead, there must be a transferable value to the patient's pursuits in life.

A factor differentiating counseling from any relationship with a trusted friend is that counseling is fashioned with an intentional curative goal. This curative goal is explored in a relationship shared between the patient and a qualified professional who employs specific approaches to meet the needs of the patient. The curative nature of counseling is sustained by the intentional exploration of the life issues and potential remedies for enhanced life functioning and wellness. Furthermore, each issue and remedy is explored by means of a safe counseling environment that protects psychological vulnerabilities without the potentially dangerous implications that may occur outside of counseling.

Counseling is a psychosocial approach to healing that explores the psychological worldview of the patient and the cultural realities of their circumstance. This psychosocial awareness is vital in accomplishing the goals of wellness. Additionally, counseling operates in a four-prong approach to human functioning, including the cognitive (thoughts), affective (feelings), behavioral (actions), and contextual (outside culture) domains. Often one or multiple of these domains are experiencing stress. The process of counseling explores these domains and promotes the individual's reactivation to each of the domains related to life-goals, functioning, and wellness.

Counseling, as a helping profession, has theoretical and research bases, and each demonstrates the effectiveness of its practices with patients (Shadish & Baldwin, 2003; Suzuki & Ahluwalia, 2004). Though there is great variety in the theoretical orientations used by the various counseling practitioners, generally speaking, the premises of counseling are specifically grounded in the personality formation and eventual life improvement of the patients. Furthermore, research has shown success with working with a number of different populations of individuals (Fischer, Jome, & Atkinson, 1998), over a diversity of different types of psychosocial issues, which can be further applied to the specific psychosocial functioning of individuals. Because of this theoretical and research grounding, the counseling is a unique process for psychosocial change for individuals. In Chapter 2,

some basic theories of counseling were presented. Ways to apply these counseling strategies are presented next.

Forms and Approaches to Counseling

Like the populations that counseling serves, the profession itself is quite diverse. There
are literally over 200 different theoretical approaches to counseling (Day, 2004), each one
with its own belief systems and techniques. A good practice in making a referral is to
inquire, in advance, how a psychosocial professional views his or her therapeutic practice,
how people change, and his or her particular thoughts about working with your patients.
This information will assist one in understanding the other professional's practice and is
helpful in communicating the process to the athlete.

In addition to the many diverse theories of counseling, there are a number of possible
forms of counseling, such as individual or group, that can each prove to be potentially
helpful to the psychosocial needs of a person. While it will typically be the responsibility
of the psychotherapist and patient to decide which form of counseling is most applicable,
a general familiarity with the forms of counseling will aid you in the referral process.

Individual Counseling

Individual counseling is the one-on-one counseling between a counselor and a client
(Gladding, 2001, p. 62). This process will often vary between dialectic sharing and exploration, educating, problem solving, goal setting, and other wellness-focused activities.
This form of therapy positions the client to be the lone "driving force" in terms of what
occurs (e.g., the amount of disclosure, depth, and intensity) and what the focus of the
counseling will be.

Group Work

Group work describes the process of giving of help or the accomplishment of tasks in
a group setting (Gladding, 2001, p. 56). Therapeutic groups are typically formed around
a shared purpose with the members providing help to the other participating members
of the group. Group work is typically led by a trained group leader who works with the
dynamic of the group to ensure the desired outcomes are addressed and worked on in
the group. Group counseling works under the premise that people are inherently social
and, therefore, psychosocial issues can be efficiently exposed, explored, and made more
manageable via the group dynamic. Members of groups grow as much from the vicarious
learning as they do from the individual attention experienced during the group.

Two Paradigms of Psychosocial Assistance for Athletes

When people consider psychosocial issues and counseling, it is often assumed that
these psychosocial issues are simply either a personal deficit or a psychological pathology. In other words, the prevailing belief is that there is a specific "problem" that needs
to be "fixed." Associated with this manner of consideration, there is a certain taboo in our
culture linked with counseling and yet, counseling offers much more than mere corrective
and problem-focused interventions. Counseling can account for the problems and pathologies of people, and the athletic trainer will find that there is a wide range of possible
benefits to counseling and referral that are beyond simply the remediation of a problem.

The most common approach to counseling focuses on problem or pathological remediation. Remediation is the therapeutic process by which counseling procedures are implemented with the goal of correcting the problem situation (Gladding, 2001, p. 194). From this vantage point, there is an isolated issue or series of issues causing the psychosocial disturbances in the individual. Counseling from this context suggests that the therapist works in conjunction with the patient to remedy the issues regarding the psychosocial issue. Once the issue is resolved, it is assumed that the patient is able to return to a "normal" or fit level of functioning.

The second, and far too underutilized, paradigm of counseling is prevention. Prevention is the therapeutic process used to avoid, avert, or minimize potential problems before they occur (Gladding, 2001, p. 95). Prevention is proactive, reinforcing the individual's positive resiliency skills and ensuring that he or she is ready and able to confront potential issues before they occur. This proactive manner of functioning focuses on extending prevention throughout one's life.

Prevention is an especially powerful mechanism for psychosocial enhancement and promotion of optimal functioning. The counseling process is designed to enhance one's existing assets, rather than "going back" to fix a deficit that inhibits optimal functioning. It is easier to prevent the potential problem issues before they manifest. Counseling can be powerful in identifying potential strengths for psychosocial reinforcement and promoting the processes necessary to use these for preventing issues from becoming detrimental. Like counseling, athletic training also incorporates a preventative paradigm as many individuals have their own array of abilities prior to entering a professional relationship with an athletic trainer.

In terms of psychosocial referral specifically, discuss with the patients that counseling and therapeutic experiences support psychological, social, and even physical successes. For example, a sports psychologist can work with a single athlete or team in mental rehearsal and visualization techniques. Research has shown a positive effect on athletic performance and these psychosocial preparations (Harwood, Cumming, & Fletcher, 2004; Robazza, Pellizzari, & Hanin, 2004). Seasoned athletes often are cited to say that though they might not have the physical skills that they possessed in their youth, they now find that in age and experience the "game comes to them." Counseling can be a similar metacognitive (i.e., "thinking about their thoughts") way of slowing down the mental speed of the game and making it more manageable to the athlete at any age. Additionally, referral might be valuable when a patient has a major event pending and there is a high likelihood of stress. Maybe an athlete faces a transitional period in his or her life out of formal athletics and the athlete could use someone to "bounce some ideas off of." There is an endless array of preventative psychosocial opportunities for people to experience in life and there are similarly an equal number of ways that psychosocial interventions can be a supportive force in these experiences.

Psychosocial Intervention and Referral Standards

The NATA has established a series of educational competencies for psychosocial intervention and referral. These are the requisite conditions and expectations that athletic trainers must adhere to concerning potential referral situations. Though these competencies present a valuable and very pragmatic reference point for psychosocial referrals, remember that these standards only account for the minimum competencies that are expected in referral situations. These standards are a guidepost for "best practices" in a referral situation. These best practices include going beyond the minimum standards of practice and meeting the idiosyncratic needs of the athlete.

In addition to serving as a helpful guidepost, these competencies also represent a portion of one's professional identity. Being able to recall these competencies with some degree of proficiency will better assist one in communicating with others during the referral process. The NATA's (NATA, 2006) standards related to psychosocial referral are as follows:

- Explain the psychosocial requirements of various activities to the readiness of the injured or ill individual to resume participation.

- Explain the importance of providing health care information to patients, parents/guardians, athletic personnel, and others regarding the psychological and emotional well-being of physically active individuals.

- Describe the roles and function of various community-based health care providers (sports psychologists, counselors, social workers) and the accepted protocols that govern the referral of physically active individuals to these professionals.

- Describe the acceptance and grieving processes that follow a catastrophic event and the need for a psychological intervention and referral plan for all parties affected by the event.

- Explain the potential need for psychosocial intervention and referral when dealing with populations requiring special consideration (e.g., those with exercise-induced asthma, diabetes, seizure disorders, drug allergies and interactions, or unilateral organs).

These competencies delineate the minimal conditions to be met in your referral efforts with patients. By integrating the considerations and procedures discussed in this chapter, the athletic trainer will satisfy these core conditions and satisfy the specialized psychosocial needs of patients when referral is needed.

When and Why Do I Make a Psychosocial Referral?

To this point in the chapter, the case has been made that athletic trainers must support the psychosocial needs of patients by offering referral. Though the need might seem relatively evident, the precise occasions when an athletic trainer should consider referral are yet still obscure. The occasions when and why it is critical for an athletic trainer to consider psychosocial referral will now be presented. The following list of occasions should be read as a generic list of sample considerations that are relevant to psychosocial referral. In reality, the occasions that might prompt referral will not be as specific and as clearly identified, thus it is sensible for the athletic trainer to consider this list for deliberation of any potential psychosocial referral situation. By engaging in this process of exploring the why's and when's to consider referral, the athletic trainer will begin thinking in the psychosocial context of the patient and, consequently, be better prepared for the psychosocial situations as they uniquely exist in the lives of athletes.

Selected psychosocial situations that are typical to one's work as an athletic trainer will be explored in later sections. Upon reading the list, try to contextualize these considerations in terms of the athlete trainer's patients. How might these situations arise? How will you know how to identify them if and when they occur? What will you do in response to these situations? What personal strengths and difficulties do you have in each of these situations?

♦ *When there are serious threats or risks to the health, safety, or welfare of the patient, other people in the person's life, or you, the athletic trainer.*

At the foundation of all psychosocial referrals is the expectation of accountability for the basic life needs and safety of one's athlete. If the athletic trainer believes that there is any eminent or potential threat in the athlete's life or that the athlete is threatening the wellness of others, referral is critical. In such cases, it is essential that you balance timeliness and the proper considerations necessary for the referral and safety goals to be met. Additionally, in the face of potentially injurious issues, referral to law enforcement, medical professionals, and others should be considered as primary protection to the athlete and others alike. Examples of such risk include the threat of suicide, self-injury, homicide, violence, and other related forms of harm to another person. In all such cases of referral, the athletic trainer must ensure that she or he is adequately prepared and have sufficient support from one's employer.

♦ *When an athlete is dealing with psychosocial issues that are affecting him or her in such a way that they are counterproductive to the life or athletic goals; daily functioning; or general cognitions, affect, and behaviors of the athlete.*

When working with patients, there will be occasions when the psychosocial issues are so taxing and arduous that the patient's life and physical activities will begin to suffer. On some occasions, the patient will be completely aware of the correlation between his or her psychosocial struggles and his or her life and physical functioning. Based upon this awareness, some individuals may openly ask for a referral, whereas others may not. Some patients will not be aware of the influences of their current difficulties, but may be experiencing unusual difficulty in attaining their life and physical goals. In either case, referral serves as a possible catalyst for exploration and eventual resolution of the presenting psychosocial issue. Embedded in this potential psychosocial referral consideration are those occasions where there is not an existing problem, but instead an opportunity for preventative enhancement. If the athletic trainer considers the attributes and goals of the patient and believes that the patient's life and athletic performance can be enhanced by psychosocial exploration, one can have a discussion with the patient about the possible benefits of counseling.

♦ *When the athletic trainer does not have the professional expertise to account for the psychosocial needs of the patient.*

Self-awareness and humility are often essential to the prosperity of any successful relationship. In the professional relationships that one sustains with patients, this same value system is highly applicable. Being aware of one's personal and professional confidence and competence is critical in ensuring that the person receives the most optimal support. Confidence is the will and commitment to meet the needs of the patient. It also includes the professional's ability and entitlement to provide competent services. Therefore, an athletic trainer should know one's professional capacities and limits. Be aware that there are some psychosocial issues that are relevant to one's everyday work with patients and that there are other psychosocial issues that are beyond the athletic trainer's expertise. In the case of the latter, there are liability factors associated with practicing beyond one's level of skill and professional entitlement. Working in concert with other relevant professionals will ensure the athletic trainer's own professional behavior and provide the best conditions for the patient's eventual success.

- *When the athletic trainer does not have the time or resources to meet the needs of the patient.*

  Certain psychosocial issues that an individual might present could be appropriately within one's professional competence. For example, the athlete could be seeking "just someone to talk to, nothing is really going on out of the ordinary... I just need someone I can trust to kind of hear me out, someone objective." It is easy to interpret this request as something one has an obligation or responsibility to attend to. However, frequently the athletic trainer will find that multiple demands and a high caseload do not allow one to attend to such inquiries. An athletic trainer cannot allow the psychosocial issues of one patient to supersede the needs of the total caseload. Because the athletic trainer evidently possesses the trust of the patient and he or she values one's judgment, the athletic trainer serves in a unique role allowing for the opportunity of connecting the patient with a professional who can offer similar levels of trust, time, and resources to attend to the total needs of the patient.

  An additional word of caution: In demanding scenarios, an essential ingredient in the athletic trainer's care for patients is one's own self-care. Ensuring and sustaining appropriate personal and professional boundaries are critical to one's own long-term success in attending to the training needs of individuals. This philosophy might prove to be an efficient and useful way of framing a referral to an athlete, "I can see that you really need to get some of these issues out and I appreciate your trust. Part of what makes me trustworthy is that I know how and when to trust myself and who I can trust myself with. I really want to help you, but I will not do either of us any good giving you my splintered attention. I know someone that I trust in similar situations, a professional; would you be interested in connecting with him or her?" Such a statement lets the athlete know the athletic trainer cares about a given situation and is trying to connect the athlete with the appropriate trained professional.

- *When the athletic trainer has no support system or supervision to assist in the psychosocial needs of the patient.*

  Psychosocial issues are complex and can be too overwhelming for one person to handle. They can spiral into problems for the patients. The same can be said of the athletic trainers that share in these psychosocial explorations with individuals; it can be simply too much for one, or even two, people to handle. In such occasions, invite the support of a third party who has the freedom, expertise, and willingness to thoroughly engage in these issues. Also, there are those occasions when professionals shortsightedly believe they are giving sufficient care to patients. But, because one lacks adequate supervision to "reality check" one's work, the potential for oversight exists. Psychosocial referral can be a great safeguard against the blinders of one's own wisdom. At its worse, such kinds of referral can simply validate our practices and reinforce the "good stuff" we offer patients.

- *When the psychosocial interface that you share with the patient serves your, the athletic trainer's, needs more than it serves the patient seeking help.*

  Generally speaking, those individuals that work with others as a profession typically have the best interest of that individual at heart. Even with the best of intentions, there are occasions where professionals might find themselves too invested, too intense, or too biased to serve their patients. The athletic trainer will indubitably connect with the cognitive and affective sentiments of his or her patients. Though one's intention might be noble and seemingly altruistic, remember the professional's role is one of influence and power. Inadvertently, such power can become manipulative or harmful to the person. If the athletic trainer feels that the athlete is becoming too enmeshed, or powerless, in the relationship, it would be wise to consider referral to another athletic trainer and, possibly, referral to a mental health professional. In the case of the latter type of referral, an enmeshed patient could misinterpret a referral as an effort to reject or harm him or her. In cases in which the athletic trainer chooses to sustain the athletic trainer–patient relationship, outside support from a mental health professional can assist in keeping the relationship productive and professional, thus empowering all parties.

Though these mentioned considerations should help guide you in a number of referral situations that might arise as an athletic trainer, there is no "cookbook" or instinctive way to identify an individual's need or desire for psychosocial referral. Each person is different and each life situation in which he or she is engaged is different. These considerations should prompt further exploration and dialogue with the patient. While remaining sensitive and compassionate to the amount of information that the patient is willing to disclose, these considerations should better assist the athletic trainer in the process of exploring the potential needs and benefits for psychosocial referral. Neither these considerations nor the referral itself is the end to the referral process. They should stimulate an internal dialogue that one has when facing a potential referral situation.

Who Are the Relevant Persons to a Referral?

The most essential elements to any psychosocial referral situation are the people involved. Behind every referral is the human element. The patient possesses a range of personal experiences, emotions, and sentiments that are far more authentic than are the mere stories that are often whimsically brought to light in a referral context. Respecting the humanity and emotionality of the psychosocial referral is an imperative that transcends the athletic trainer's own investment and, when appropriately conducted, there is an awareness that the athletic trainer has promoted the well-being of the patient.

This section highlights the various psychosocial professionals to whom a referral can be made. The information is grounded in a systemic way of applying psychosocial referrals and challenges the athletic trainer to consider the complexity of the human dynamics inherent in any referral. Most referrals are born out of the social lives of patients, thus it is sensible to assume that these referrals should account for the social lives that patients will return to everyday.

WHO IS REFERRED?

The NATA states that athletic trainers are to potentially work with all types of individuals participating in an athletic-related activity (NATA, 2006). Thus any person engaged in a physical activity who enters into a fiduciary athletic trainer–patient relationship is a potential psychosocial referral. The athletic trainer has a professional obligation to support and enhance the total well-being of a patient, including their psychosocial functioning.

In terms of the psychosocial needs of patients that could provoke a potential referral situation, one will find a wide range of behaviors, moods, thought processes, and influencing variables. Patients will come with situational disturbances that are merely affecting an isolated part of their life (e.g., trouble balancing their academics and their athletic schedule). On the other end of the continuum, there will be individuals who are plagued by chronic and intense distress that affects the entirety of their life (e.g., patterns of hostility and violence both on the athletic field and at home). Each of these types of psychosocial concerns for patients, and each of the psychosocial issues between these two extremes, deserves the attention and professional care through a referral.

Psychosocial referrals are relevant to any patient who wants to enhance his or her present life functioning. At some time in the past, we have all experienced the type of stress, anxiety, or confusion that could be assisted by a caring professional. Patients of athletic trainers, especially given the demanding nature of their lives and physical pursuits, are no different.

There are a wide variety of potential psychosocial issues that could benefit from psychotherapeutic assistance and, therefore, are grounds for a possible referral. While it is not within the scope of this chapter to explicate the various psychosocial issues, it is important to recognize that athletes will customarily be confounded by such issues. A more detailed discussion of these psychosocial issues can be found in Chapters 4 through 11 of this text. For example, student athletes will have the dual stressors of athletic and academic pressures and expectations (Fletcher, Benshoff, & Richburg, 2003). Athletes of all sorts face the complexities of training and over-training (Kirk, Singh, & Getz, 2001), the perceived need for perfectionism (Anshel & Eom, 2003; Hopkinson & Lock, 2004), and social pressure for success (Burgess & Martin, 2004). Athletes have also been shown to have psychosocial issues related to diet, eating disorders (Murphy & Gutekunst, 1997; Petrie & Rogers, 2001), and alcohol and drug usage (Damm, 1991). Another potentially problematic issue for athletes is the transition out of professional, collegiate, or formal athletic competition (Stankovich, Meeker, & Henderson, 2001) and transcending an athletic injury (Brewer, Jeffers, Petipas, & Van Raalte, 1994; Williams & Andersen, 1998). In that athletics are always tied to the personal lives of athletes, potential psychosocial referrals for patients might result with their struggles with family (Côté, 1999), friends, fellow athletes, coaches, and even gender and cultural variables (Killeya, 2001; Martin, Akers, & Jackson, 2001). This is by no means a comprehensive list of the psychosocial issues that confront a patient on a daily basis. The athletic trainer must always be cognizant of the potential stressors that are both specific to athletes, but also those mitigating life influences that inevitably enter the sporting venue.

To Whom Do We Refer?

Upon considering a psychosocial referral for a patient, the athletic trainer must take into consideration the important decision of who might be the appropriate professional to recommend to the athlete. There exist a wide variety of differing types of mental health professionals, each with their own particular training programs, professional expertise, and standards of practice. To further muddy the decision process regarding who to refer to, much shared professional territory exists between the various disciplines of mental health care. Thus, for an athletic trainer, making sense of these professional disciplines can seem arbitrary and even artificial.

Embedded within the diversity of different professional disciplines is the additional diversity between the various theoretical orientations, styles, techniques and practices, education, and personalities of the particular practitioners. It is recommended that the athletic trainer engages in an exploratory conversation with each of the various mental health professionals being considered before he or she presents these names to a patient. In conversation, ask about his or her training and education, personal style and orientation, and practical considerations (e.g., scheduling, costs, and insurance issues).

To clarify some possibly ambiguity, this section discusses some of the basic identifying elements of psychiatrists, psychologists, social workers, counselors and marriage and family therapists, and sports psychologists. While there are other types of mental health professionals that can assist patients needing psychosocial help (e.g., psychiatric nurses, self-help groups), these selected professions will probably meet most of the athletic trainer's referral needs. This section shall include the education and training, professional practice and psychosocial usefulness for patients, and affiliated professional organizations for each of these disciplines. These brief introductions provide an orientation, a starting place, for more comprehensive exploration into psychosocial professionals.

Psychiatrists
(American Psychiatric Association, n.d.; U.S. Department of Labor, n.d.)

Education and Training

Psychiatrists are medical doctors who have graduated from a medical school and have further been degreed with a specialization in the area of psychiatry. During their first 2 years of medical school, psychiatry students take the typical courses of a medical student (e.g., chemistry, biochemistry, physiology) in addition to specialized courses in psychiatry, behavioral science, and neuroscience. After their second year of education, medical students take on "clerkships," or medical specialty areas, where they study and work with physicians in at least five different medical specialties. In the case of psychiatry students, a psychiatry clerkship typically entails working with patients deemed to have a "mental illnesses" in a hospital or in an outpatient setting. After graduation from medical school, a new psychiatric physician will take state-offered written examinations for his or her given specialty area. The psychiatrist-in-training will then spend at least 3 additional years in a psychiatric residency learning the diagnosis and treatment of mental illnesses. After completing their residency, many psychiatrists opt to take a voluntary examination given by the American Board of Psychiatry and Neurology to become a "board certified" psychiatrist. Many psychiatrists continue training beyond the initial 4 years, including training in psychoanalysis.

Professional Practice and Psychosocial Usefulness for Patients

A psychiatrist is a medical doctor that specializes in the diagnosis, treatment, and prevention of mental illnesses and related emotional disturbances. Psychiatry is grounded in a medical model approach to psychosocial helping, namely identifying a problem and working toward implementation of the appropriate remedy. Psychiatrists generally have training in psychotherapy (based upon additional training outside of their formal education) as well as knowledge of the medicines that are understood to be curative for mental illnesses. A psychiatrist can therefore perform any combination of psychotherapy or psychotropic (i.e., the prescription of psychiatric medication) treatment. Generally speaking, psychiatrists work with clients who suffer from chronic and debilitating psychological distress (e.g., depression, manic-depression, panic disorder, anxiety disorders, obsessive-compulsive disorder, and schizophrenia). Psychiatrists use medications when thorough evaluation of a patient suggests that medication may correct imbalances in brain chemistry that are thought to be involved in some mental disorders.

The patients of athletic trainers, like other members of the general population, are susceptible to the psychosocial symptoms that psychiatrists have been trained to work with. These psychosocial issues tend to be more long-term and pervasive in their duration.

Affiliated Professional Organization:

American Psychiatric Association
1000 Wilson Boulevard, Suite 1825
Arlington, VA 22209-3901
(703) 907-7300
www.psych.org

Psychologists

(American Psychological Association, n.d.; U.S. Department of Labor, n.d.)

Education and Training

Psychologists are trained academically in psychotherapy and related subjects (as opposed to psychiatrists who are trained medically with a possible subspecialty in psychotherapy). The term *psychologist* is regulated by individual state licensing boards and covers people who have completed a PhD or PsyD in clinical or counseling psychology from an American Psychological Association (APA)-accredited program. PhD psychologists have approximately 5 years of graduate training in psychology in addition to whatever continuing education and specialization that they endeavor. PsyD psychologists have almost as much training but with less emphasis on the scientific and research aspects of the field. In order to obtain the license as a "psychologist," most states require a further 1 year or 2 years of postgraduate supervised experience in the field. Psychologists have completed a 1-year internship in their specialty, a specific number of hours of pre- and postdoctoral supervised clinical work, and a state-mandated licensing exam.

Professional Practice and Psychosocial Usefulness for Patients

There are many different types of professional psychologists, but for the purposes of psychosocial referral, only clinical and counseling psychologists will be investigated. Generally speaking, the work of psychologists is denoted by their training and usage of standardized psychosocial tests (e.g., intelligence, performance, personality, and aptitude tests). Additionally, these two types of psychologists typically treat the diagnostic needs of clients and often perform or consult on the psychotherapeutic remediations based upon this diagnosis. Clinical psychologists most often work in counseling centers, independent or group practices, hospitals, or clinics to assist mentally and emotionally disturbed clients adjust (Society of Clinical Psychology, n.d.). Other psychologists work with clients confounded by personal crisis (e.g., grief, depression). Clinical psychologists often interview patients and give diagnostic tests. They may provide individual, family, or group psychotherapy and design and implement behavior modification programs. Some clinical psychologists collaborate with physicians and other specialists to develop and implement treatment and intervention programs that patients can understand and comply with (selected areas of specialization relevant to athletes include health psychology, neuropsychology, and geropsychology). Counseling psychologists work with individuals in the areas of "personal and interpersonal functioning across the lifespan with a focus on emotional, social, vocational, educational, health-related, developmental, and organizational concerns" (Society of Counseling Psychology, n.d.). Counseling psychologists work to improve the well-being, alleviate distress and maladjustment, resolve crises, and increase in a diverse range of patient populations across the entire lifespan. Counseling psychologists are distinct from other APA divisions in that they serve patients both with normal developmental issues and those problems associated with physical, emotional, and mental disorders. Counseling psychologists use various techniques, including interviewing and testing, to advise people on how to deal with problems of everyday living. They work in settings such as university counseling centers, hospitals, and individual or group practices and emphasize on psychotherapy.

Affiliated Professional Organization

American Psychological Association
750 First Street, NE
Washington, DC 20002-4242
(800) 374-2721 or (202) 336-5500
www.apa.org

Society of Clinical Psychology, Division 12
www.apa.org/divisions/div12/homepage.html

Society of Counseling Psychology, Division 17
www.div17.org

Social Workers

(National Association of Social Workers, n.d.; U.S. Department of Labor, n.d.)

Education and Training

Social work students can earn degrees at the bachelors, masters, and doctoral levels, each with their own particular areas of professional knowledge and competencies. A licensed clinical social worker (LCSW) typically has 2 years of graduate schooling with an emphasis on psychotherapy, an internship emphasizing psychotherapy (approximately 900 hours of supervised field instruction), and 1 year or 2 years of supervised postgraduate work before obtaining the license. Coursework for aspiring social workers includes social work values and ethics, dealing with a culturally diverse clientele, at-risk populations, promotion of social and economic justice, human behavior and the social environment, social welfare policy and services, social work practice, social research methods, and field education. Additionally, master's degree programs continue to refine the skills required to perform clinical assessments, manage large caseloads, work in leadership roles, and develop novel ways to work with clients. Additionally, the National Association of Social Workers (NASW) offers voluntary credentials. Social workers with a Masters in Social Work (MSW) degree may be eligible for the Academy of Certified Social Workers (ACSW), the Qualified Clinical Social Worker (QCSW), or the Diplomate in Clinical Social Work (DCSW) credential based on their professional experience. Credentials are particularly important for those in private practice.

Professional Practice and Psychosocial Usefulness for Patients

A licensed clinical social worker is trained in psychotherapy and helps individuals function effectively. Typical clients of a social worker possess either a mental health or environmental disturbance that hinders their life functioning. What distinguishes social work as a profession is its devotion to helping people function within the parameters of troubling social and personal environments. To confront these environmental obstacles, social workers work with clients either therapeutically (i.e., personal change within the environmental system) or in tandem with other resources in the lives of clients to improve their social conditions (i.e., change the environment to improve psychosocial functioning). Social workers assist clients in their manner of dealing with environments and what things the clients can do to make tangible changes therein. Additionally, social workers help people function within their family, friend, and community relationships. Typical issues that social workers confront may include inadequate housing, unemployment, serious illness, disability, domestic abuse, neglect, or substance abuse. A licensed independent clinical social worker is a social worker who has the appropriate training, supervision, and state credentials to work in private or clinical practice with individuals. Licensed independent social work practice includes the diagnosis and treatment of mental and emotional disorders in individuals, families, and groups.

Affiliated Professional Organization

National Association of Social Workers
750 First Street, NE, Suite 700
Washington, DC 20002-4241
(202) 408-6800
www.naswdc.org

Counselors and Marriage and Family Therapists
(American Counseling Association, n.d.; U.S. Department of Labor, n.d.)

Education and Training

Professional counselors, as defined by the American Counseling Association, have a number of diverse specialization areas that can be relevant to the psychosocial needs of athletes, namely career, community, gerontological, mental health, school, student affairs, rehabilitation, and marriage and family counseling. For the purposes of psychosocial referral, this section shall limit the discussion to counselors and marriage and family counselors. The training for both specialty areas generally involves a 2-year master's program, followed by supervised clinical experience, and a comprehensive state licensing examination. Many counselors elect to be nationally certified by the National Board for Certified Counselors, Inc. (NBCC), which grants the designation "National Certified Counselor." Training of counselors typically includes coursework in psychotherapy and helping skills, human growth and development, social and cultural foundations, group and individual practice, appraisal, consultation, career development, research, and professional orientation. The scope of a professional counselor's therapeutic practice is conferred by the individual state legislatures, typically in the form of licensure (i.e., Licensed Professional Counselor [LPC] or, less often, through certification legislation with the title Certified Professional Counselor [CPC]). Licensure grants a professional counselor the legal right to practice through law, while restricting this right to only those persons who hold a license or the appropriate certification. It is important to note that state laws vary and therefore an athletic trainer should have familiarity with the requirements of one's particular state.

Professional Practice and Psychosocial Usefulness for Patients

Professional counselors practice in a variety of settings, including independent practice, community agencies, managed behavioral health care organizations, integrated delivery systems, hospitals, employee assistance programs and substance abuse treatment centers. Furthermore, counselors are trained to provide a full range of psychosocial services, including assessment, diagnosis, psychotherapy, and consultation. To address the cognitive, emotional, behavioral, and contextual needs of clients, counselors work from a "wellness" model, or belief that each individual possesses a wealth of innate skill that simply needs to be encouraged to flourish. To accomplish this maxim of wellness, counselors work with a variety of client types, including individuals, families, and groups to address and treat mental and emotional needs of the clients. Professional counselors are academically and clinically trained in a variety of therapeutic techniques used to address a wide range of psychosocial issues (e.g., depression; addiction and substance abuse; suicidal impulses; stress management; problems with self-esteem; issues associated with aging; job and career concerns; educational decisions; issues related to mental and emotional health; and family, parenting, and marital or other relationship problems).

Marriage and family counselors, in particular, apply these same wellness principles and therapeutic techniques to individuals, family groups, or couples for the purpose of resolving emotional conflicts in relationships, parenting and marital enhancement, crisis and abuse, and death and loss (International Association of Marriage and Family Counselors, n.d.). Marriage and family counselors work in a variety of settings, including independent practice, community mental health agencies, and managed care organizations or hospitals. Marriage and family counselors enhance client's family relationship skills by promoting effective family communication, conflict resolution, confidence, and prioritization.

Like marriage and family counselors, counselors practice in a wide range of settings (e.g., private practice, hospitals, schools, and community agencies) and promote the psychosocial wellness of the clients that they serve. The psychotherapeutic work of mental health counselors includes, but is not limited to, the following: assessment and diagnosis of psychosocial functioning, psychotherapy, treatment planning, brief and solution-focused therapy, substance abuse, psychoeducational and prevention programs, and crisis management (American Counseling Association, n.d.).

Affiliated Professional Organization

American Counseling Association
5999 Stevenson Ave.
Alexandria, VA 22304-3300
(800) 347-6647
www.counseling.org

Sports Psychologists

(American Psychological Association, Division 47,
Exercise and Sport Psychology, n.d.; Weinberg & Gould, 1999)

Education and Training

Sports psychologists are trained in programs accredited by the APA through specialized programs that employ a sports- and psychological-related curriculum. Doctoral level programs in sport psychology exist within sport science and kinesiology programs, but few sports psychologists have graduated from such programs and instead posses variant undergraduate or masters degrees. Sport psychologists may or may not be trained in programs affiliated with the APA (many sports psychologists not affiliated with APA seek certification as consultants with the Association for Advancement of Applied Sports Psychology [AAASP]). It is prudent to check on the credentialing and professional qualifications of individuals calling themselves sports psychologists, given the specialization of this area of professional practice. Certified members of AAASP work with individuals in the areas of health psychology (i.e., primarily concerned with the relationship between mental and physical health), performance enhancement, and social psychology (i.e., focuses on individual and group processes in sport and exercise settings for athletes, coaches, and spectators) (Association for Advancement of Applied Sports Psychology, n.d.).

Professional Practice and Psychosocial Usefulness for Athletes

Sport psychologists are trained to work with athletes to optimize performance and bridge their psychological functioning to their participation in sport, exercise, and physical activity. Unlike each of the aforementioned areas of psychotherapy, sports psychologists are not specifically trained or licensed to work with the psychosocial troubles that an athlete might be having outside of the sport itself. Sports psychologists work with other athletic professionals for the performance enhancement of athletes (i.e., once on the field) but not in the psychosocial therapeutic aspects in the athletes' total life (i.e., those psychosocial issues that the athlete enters the field with from their outside environment and returns to once the game or practice is over). Sports psychologists work to enhance the athlete's performance by teaching mental strategies, confronting athletic- and competition-related pressures, and treating selected psychological difficulties related to athletic injury (Murphy, 1995). Additionally, sports psychologists work with athletes to increase athletic motivation, relaxation, and the removal of psychological obstacles in performance. Sports psychologists consult directly with the athletes in a one-to-one format, with a group of athletes together, or in conjunction with the coach. Generally, it is not appropriate for sports psychologists to engage in the areas of clinical psychology or counseling psychology without further training and achieving the appropriate credentials.

Affiliated Professional Organization

American Psychological Association, Division 47, Exercise and Sport Psychology
750 First St, NE
Washington, DC 20002-4242
www.apa.org/divisions/div47

Association for Applied Sports Psychology
2810 Crossroads Dr, Ste 3800
Madison, WI
www.aaasponline.org/index.php

The North American Society for the Psychology of Sport and Physical Activity
www.naspspa.org

The preceding list of disciplines is by no means exhaustive nor is it comprehensive in its descriptions of the various specialty areas. To make an appropriate psychosocial referral, the athletic trainer must take this foundational information and learn more about the nuances of each discipline and how it applies to the needs of the patient specifically.

WHO ELSE MIGHT REFERRAL AFFECT AND WHO ELSE MIGHT WE NEED TO CONSIDER?

Every patient will have family, friends, peer athletes, and coaches that are concerned with the wellbeing of the individual. In terms of the athletic trainer's obligations in a psychosocial referral situation, one's professional scope of influence is directly rooted to the assistance of the athlete. Because of the personal and legal implications of psychosocial issues, it is wise to keep as much of the psychosocial referral information confidential. A general rule is that the patient "owns" the information. In certain circumstances, the individual may want the athletic trainer to talk with their loved ones or the athletic trainer might need to procure additional information from someone else. In these rare and carefully handled occasions, a good manner of practice is to disclose only the minimum amount of person-relevant information.

How to Refer Athletes

This chapter has offered the case that the psychosocial referral process is vital to the work of the athletic trainer. Psychosocial referral has been explored, why accounting for the psychosocial needs of athletes is inherent to the role as of athletic trainer and the enhancement of athletic pursuits, when psychosocial referrals should be considered, and to whom one might refer an athlete. It has also been mentioned that the process of referral itself is a very complex and yet achievable venture. In this section, the process will be discussed, including the how an athletic trainer appropriately refers the patient, to the what, when, why, and who in an effort to support psychosocial and athletic success.

In this section, general ingredients that are necessary for any successful psychosocial referral will be presented. Next, a specific model applied especially to the psychosocial referral needs of athletic trainers and patients will be explored. Finally, a series of helpful guidelines will be discussed to ensure that the safeguard of the athletic trainer and the needs of the referred patient are met.

THE INGREDIENTS OF A SUCCESSFUL PSYCHOSOCIAL REFERRAL

Psychosocial referrals for patients should reflect the diverse needs of the patient. Just as the individual is the sum of many distinct and personal attributes, psychosocial referrals must account for the diverse and personal demands of each of these attributes. In addition to the interpersonal ingredients particular to the person, there are numerous external forces that are active and influential in the psychosocial functioning of the individual and the potential referral situation. As such, the psychosocial referral should be considerate of this complex dynamic and strategize accordingly.

Figure 3-1 presents a graphic display of the ecological and interactive nature of psychosocial referral for patients. Referral is an ecological process because of the social contexts and influences that the athletic trainer must always be aware of during the referral process. Effective referral assumes that the athletic trainer consider and account for each of these contexts and influences in one's efforts to support the patient. Referral is interactive in that each of the context and influence forces work in relation to adjoined forces throughout the referral process. The athletic trainer must always remain aware of the dynamic elements that affect referral. As much as possible, the psychosocial referrals should work in concert with these influences, ensuring that each factor effectively contributes to the patient's psychosocial functioning.

Figure 3-1 displays adjoining circles, each representing the various elements to consider during the referral process. At the center is a core where each of these elements converge, representing the rationale behind the referral decisions. To ensure that this core aims toward the highest degree of effectiveness in the referral process, the following sections detail the *core considerations* (i.e., descriptions of the relevant elements in the life of the patient) and *core conditions* (i.e., representing the approach taken in the referral).

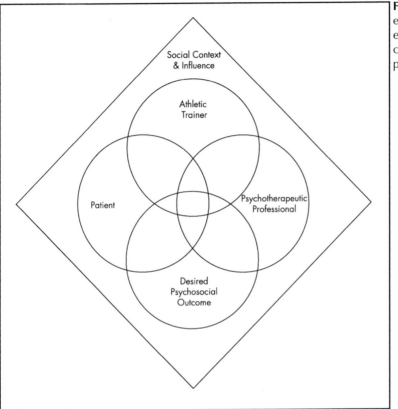

Figure 3-1. Interacting elements of consideration for the psychosocial referral of patients.

Core Considerations for Successful Psychosocial Referral

Knowledge of Self and Influence

Knowledge of how one affects the psychosocial referral process should be considered on at least three separate fronts. First, the athletic trainer must be aware of how one is viewed by the patient and, also, how the athletic trainer views the patient. In many ways, these two perceptions will form a third perception that represents the shared relationship between the athletic trainer and the patient. The total of these three perceptions will guide the professional relationship with the patient and the considerations the athletic trainer will make in a potential referral situation.

The athletic trainer must be acutely aware of the personal attributes, beliefs, mannerisms, and values influencing his or her actions. These influences cannot be disregarded in the referral process. Effective psychosocial referral relies on the athletic trainer considering and acting on objective information. The athletic trainer needs to have an awareness of the influence and power that he or she has in the athletic trainer–patient relationship. Patients value the relationship that is shared with the athletic trainer and, therefore, they will place credence in the recommendations and viewpoints offered. Consciousness of this fact will assist the athletic trainer in acting with sensitivity when evaluating the patient's needs and recommending a referral to a mental health professional.

Knowledge of self also includes an awareness of one's role as an athletic trainer and the professional, ethical, and legal standards governing one's practice as an athletic trainer. Working within the parameters of NATA's professional standards for psychosocial referral and abiding by the legal mandates of the relevant governing bodies protects the athletic trainer and the patient alike.

Knowledge of the Athlete

In many ways, one's perception is all that one possesses. The subjective manner in which the athletic trainer interprets events and people will guide the thoughts, feelings, and actions of the professional. In the process of engaging in the subjective psychosocial vantage point of the patient, one always runs the risk of misperception and assumption. It is critical that the athletic trainer respects the complexity of the individual, his or her contexts and influences, personal history, goals, and value system. To secure an authentic portrait of the patient's frame of reference, a trusting and meaningful bond must be established. This trust will enhance the athletic trainer's ability to garner the necessary information to make an appropriate referral, along with offering the patient an option, demonstrating concern, significance, and relevance.

Knowledge of the patient also includes the psychosocial and economic abilities and attributes particular to the individual. Connecting a patient with a particular psychotherapist means that the athletic trainer has a certainty that this particular patient can reasonably afford the psychological and financial costs of a psychotherapist's services.

Knowledge of the Mental Health Profession and the Local Resources

It is imperative that the athletic trainer has a practical and conversational familiarity with the processes and outcomes associated with the mental health profession. One's ability to clearly and accurately articulate the nature of psychosocial services and the proceedings associated with counseling will contribute to the experience of the patient and the overall success for the referral. In addition to a general knowledge, it is vital to have a collected list of mental health professionals whose work one knows and with whom one shares a rapport. The athletic trainer should make certain that the list of potential referral sources is large enough to cater to each of the prospective issues of his or her patients and yet is focused enough that one can sustain a sound relationship with each mental health professional.

Knowledge of the Social Context and Influences

Equally as critical to the effectiveness of a psychosocial referral is the awareness of the surrounding social context for the patient. Each element in the outside environment influences the patient and filters how he or she perceives his or her life. In the context of psychosocial referral, the person may have been born into a family system that places a very low premium on mental health services. While it might not be reasonable to completely forego a referral to this individual, it is essential that the referral be introduced in a manner that is pertinent to the patient's particular background. Keep in mind that the patient's life history and influences outside of the athletic trainer–patient relationship will influence the proceedings of the potential referral.

As illustrated in Figure 3-1, the social context and influences associated with each person are always present and literally touch every element of one's psychosocial functioning. Some of the influences that should be considered include, but are not limited to, the following: family and friends, economic and socioeconomic status, cultural and ethnic influences, gender and sexual identity issues, age and ability influences, social taboos, as well as other sociocultural variables.

A second, and equally important, aspect of social context knowledge and influence is one's awareness of the life variables on the patient as they contribute to the psychosocial issues that invoke the potential referral situation. When referring a person to another professional, the background and contextual information that one has can add further depth, insight, and transferable content that will contribute to the effectiveness of the referral and to the eventual psychosocial services to be provided. Consequently, there is no need for the athletic trainer to dig for any additional psychosocial information, leaving this task to the mental health professional. The lone expectation of the athletic trainer is to ensure that disclosures during the entire referral process are germane to the particular needs of the athlete. Remember, the patient ultimately owns his or her personal information, and the athletic trainer is ethically bound to seek the patient's permission in the referral process.

Core Conditions for Psychosocial Referral

The core conditions for psychosocial referral are those critical terms that must be met with an athlete in need of referral. More specifically, the core conditions are those personal characteristics that the athletic trainer must emanate in the shared relationship with the athlete. They represent those fundamental deliberations that must be made to ensure the appropriateness and security of the eventual psychosocial referral.

Personal Characteristics and Rapport

As a general rule, it is appropriate to treat others with the utmost respect, interest, and warmth. In cases where a psychosocial referral is potentially helpful to a person, be aware that these personal characteristics are both maintained and felt by the patient. The following is a list of personal characteristics and mannerisms that will contribute to successful psychosocial referral with a patient.

- *Honesty and candor.* Avoid insignificant pretenses as they can compromise the integrity of the relationship shared with the patient. Keep the lines of communication thoroughly clean and clear of any ambiguity, misconception, and deceit.

- *Open, accepting, and receptive.* In addition to being honest, it is critical that one remains open to the disclosures of the patient (even when these disclosures seem to be contrary to your beliefs or what you would do in a similar situation). Remember, the psychosocial issue has a specific and personal meaning to the patient. Evaluative responses to these disclosures will not likely shift the meaning that these things have to the patient and can compromise the trust that the individual has in you to further disclose. When attending to the psychosocial needs of patients, demonstrating a genuine interest and concern for the individual's well-being is essential. Also, it is vital to be receptive to these disclosures without becoming too investigative into the vulnerabilities of these issues (the mental health professional is best trained for such situations). Finally, be cognizant that certain cultural variables might exist that impact the psychosocial referral process. The athletic trainer should respond to these possibilities with heightened awareness and sensitivity.

- *Affirming and encouraging.* Some of the psychosocial issues that a patient will recant are experienced as painful. It takes an abundance of personal strength to divulge such intimate details of one's life. When entering the patient's psychosocial reality, the athletic trainer must affirm the strength and encourage the patient's psychosocial assets. These assets are critical for the patient and they will aid the patient in managing psychosocial issues until psychotherapy is to begin. Affirming includes verbally recognizing the issues that the athlete tells to the athletic trainer. Affirming can be as simple as repeating back the same words in a compassionate tone (i.e., using the "paraphrasing" skills described in Chapter 2). It can also be as complex as illustrating direct empathy with their current plight. Encouragement entails identifying the courage of the person to endure these traumatic life events and yet still find the bravery to seek help and progress.

• *Committal- and action-orientated.* The issues that a patient discloses do not cease once the conversation has come to a close or even after they have left one's athletic training facility. It is likely that the patient's time with the athletic trainer is his or her reprieve from the felt danger of the psychosocial issues that motivated the consideration for referral. One must remain dedicated to the patient as he or she proceeds with the referral—through triumphs and letdowns alike. Furthermore, as a helper, it is prudent to do more than merely attend to the verbal needs of the patient. A psychosocial referral precludes that the athletic trainer live up to the commitments he or she made (e.g., offering the contact information of a trusted psychotherapist).

These characteristics should assist the athletic trainer in sustaining meaningful rapport with the athlete as he or she confronts prior psychosocial functioning. At no time should this rapport be taken for granted—even when it is not said or even understood. The rapport and support that is offered to the patient is the precise ingredient that supports the referral, promoting the psychosocial wellness desired.

Identification of the Three Levels of Referral

There are three levels of referral that should be considered from the outset of any presenting situation. The athletic trainer's role is to analyze and respond to the particular issues related to the patient based on one of these three psychosocial levels of referral.

The fundamental consideration of any potential referral is to protect the welfare and best interests of the patient. This protective obligation means that one must ensure that the athlete is receiving adequate care and protection, even when these safeguards are in opposition with the articulated desires of the patient. While it is always prudent to work in cooperation with the patient, there might be circumstances in which the patient expresses something that could be injurious to him- or herself or others. The athletic trainer has a primary obligation to safeguard one's self, the patient, and others. Utilize the following three levels in Table 3-1, in conjunction with the other considerations presented in this chapter, to guide referral decisions.

While it is vital to consider the psychosocial referral situation in terms of its intensity and urgency, it is equally important that the athletic trainer does not devalue the seemingly less intense and urgent issues. These less intense and urgent issues are often the best occasions to refer the patient for help. As mentioned previously, taking a developmental and preventative approach to psychosocial functioning will more likely yield a sustaining, meaningful, and life-altering change in the patient's life. To work with a psychosocial issue when it has become a "problem" poses the challenge of both accounting for the problem (its history, current presence, and future) and eventually moving toward optimal functioning.

Also, it is highly likely that a person can exhibit any number of the characteristics attributed to the various levels of psychosocial referral. For example, the patient may fluctuate between level 1 and level 2 on differing times of the day. Be aware that these levels are neither fixed nor are authentic to our subjective judgment. In reality, the athlete will have very complex issues active and therefore a referral should be a very flexible and accommodating process. A more detailed discussion of the behaviors exhibited by patients can be found in Chapter 7.

Table 3-1

Levels Guiding Referral Decisions

Level 1

A level 1 potential psychosocial referral situation is when the patient is not actively confronted by an identifiable psychosocial disturbance but could benefit from working with a mental health professional. These issues are typically less intense long-term issues that are an active part of the personal or social fiber of the athlete. They are not necessarily causing a problem, but if addressed may improve the wellness of the patient. Examples of these include, but are not limited to, the following:

- Wanting to improve interpersonal relationships or sportsmanship
- Relaxation and anxiety-lessening skills
- Career and vocational guidance
- Overall social skills enhancement

These referral situations do not demand immediate attention yet should not be taken lightly. It is always easier to build a strong psychosocial wellness before troubles emerge. In so doing, the patient will be better able to confront and transcend issues if they develop. Counselors have a strong relevancy for this level of referral and therefore can be the appropriate referral source for a person wanting to improve his or her overall psychosocial functioning. This level of referral is a proactive and preventative referral.

Level 2

A level 2 referral situation is denoted by the emergence of a psychosocial problem or malady in the life of the patient. Some example characteristics the patient might exhibit are any markedly different patterns in behavior and/or mood (e.g., doing things that are "out of character"), heightened anxiety, excessively solitary behaviors, persistently tired or irritable, and decreasing personal hygiene. The patient might be resorting to alcohol or other mood-altering substances. These issues are distinctly more intense and potentially detrimental than are level 1 referral situations.

Psychosocial referrals in the case of level 2 are both increasingly urgent and, yet, increasingly troublesome for the individual performing the referral. Often the patient will either be consciously unwilling or unaware of the problematic nature of the presenting psychosocial issues. As much as possible, the athletic trainer will need to work closely with the athlete to secure his or her commitment to seeking help. Level 2 referrals are potentially life altering and therefore extreme sensitivity and commitment must be enacted by all parties. It is important that the athletic trainer refers the patient to a professional with the appropriate training, competence, and legal scope of practice at this level of referral.

Level 3

A level 3 psychosocial referral situation is one that can be categorized as an emergency situation. The patient is confronted by immediate and volatile issues that are potentially harmful to one's self or others. Some of the example behaviors might include a highly agitated manner, disruptive and aggressive behavior, loss of contact with reality, inability to communicate, suicidal or homicidal discussion, and impulsivity.

A categorical imperative for all level 3 situations is "be protective." The athletic trainer must be protective of the patient, of the people with which the patient will interact, and also one's self. The latter mode of protection is most essential, in that the athletic trainer cannot ultimately help the patient if his or her own safety is compromised. Once safeguarded, a level 3 referral must be attended to immediately. In most highly volatile situations, it is most helpful to everyone involved, even the patient, to call the proper law and heath care providers. Most athletic facilities have an institutional procedure in place for patients exhibiting level 3 behaviors.

ATHLETIC TRAINER ROLES IN REFERRAL

The athletic trainer's role in the psychosocial referral process can be likened to that of a conduit. The athletic trainer is a necessary bridge from the current manner of functioning to a whole new way of behaving. One may introduce a new awareness to the patient (e.g., maybe he or she had not taken the time or energy to consider how recent life events have affected his or her life). In other referral situations, the athletic trainer may supply the energy and initiative that the patient could not otherwise commit to without support and assurance. Within each of these potential roles, the athletic trainer serves as a valuable resource, consultant, and medium between the worlds of patients and psychosocial exploration and enhancement.

As a consultant between the patient and the mental health professional, the athletic trainer will be utilized as a unique resource person, equipped with special knowledge from both worlds, who assists patients in resolving difficulties they have not been able to resolve on their own (Gladding, 2001, p. 30). The athletic trainer's specialized knowledge will be formulated in the investigatory processes mentioned previously. This should, in turn, ensure that one has referred the patient to the most appropriate professional caregiver. In this process, the athletic trainer will be able to work within the parameters necessary to ensure that the patient is able to strive toward the desired psychosocial wellness.

As a consultant between the patient and the mental health professional, the amount of information and the type of information one is privy to is limited. For example, do not anticipate having access to the details of treatment or the patient's psychosocial records. In fact, a general rule of practice should be that you remain open and receptive to what the person chooses to disclose. Therapy is a highly personal process and often much that occurs in psychotherapy is of a sensitive and potentially vulnerable nature. The patient is able to "try on" newfound thoughts, feelings, and behaviors in therapy and thus might not be willing to initially detail the nuances of their experiences and progress. Remain respectful of this choice.

In the case that the patient does choose to openly disclose information, it is equally wise to allow him or her to choose the degree and extent of his or her disclosure. Asking personal questions can demonstrate that the athletic trainer is receptive, but asking probing questions can venture into uncomfortable realms. Additionally, whatever information the athlete shares with athletic trainer should be protected with the utmost confidentiality (of course, in-so-far as the information is not a threat to self or others).

A MODEL FOR PSYCHOSOCIAL REFERRAL OF PATIENTS

Though the psychosocial issues that a patient might bring to the athletic trainer may seem complex and demanding, the psychosocial referral process can be rather comfortable to the athletic trainer who is prepared in the process. Establishing a usable and pragmatic system of referral will enable the athletic trainer to better handle even the most intimidating scenarios as they arise. The model described below introduces many of the elements that the athletic trainer should consider in the referral preplanning process.

Gladding (2001, p. 102) defines referral as the transfer of a client to another counselor. For an athletic trainer, this transfer does not remove him or her from the professional relationship with the patient; instead, rather than transferring the individual to the total care of another professional, the athletic trainer solicits the conjoined assistance from someone with more fitting expertise. The athletic trainer should use the following model to guide the professional considerations and subsequent actions in the psychosocial referral process:

- *Pre-preparation.* It is critical to have an established list of mental health professionals on hand and ready to be used when a psychosocial referral situation arises. This list should include a large number of specialists who cover the diversity of issues that patients possess. In addition to having a list, it will prove invaluable that one has a rapport established along with a conversational understanding of the professional expertise, education, and style of these professionals.

- *Assessment.* The assessment process of a psychosocial referral challenges the athletic trainer to step into the subjective view of the patient, gauge the psychosocial issues present, and then calculate a potential fit for referral. This process of assessment is similar to the manner in which most elementary school students are first taught how to write: who, what, when, where, why, and how (athletic trainers often compile this information in Subjective, Objective, Assessment, Plan [SOAP] notes-style annotation). Who is the patient and which mental health service provider can best serve this individual? What is the psychosocial issue? What personal and environmental influences are contributing to the patient's psychosocial functioning? When and where did these issues manifest? Why are these psychosocial issues causing a problem in the life of the patient or others? How might the athletic trainer go about connecting this individual with the appropriate professional?

- *Pre-action.* The preparation process includes advanced contact with the mental health practitioner to discuss some of the general issues involved. Consider mentally rehearsing the planned conversation for suggesting the referral to the patient. Anticipating the likely events promotes preparation for the referral process and might ease some anxieties about the referral. Though psychosocial referral is nothing to fear, the athletic trainer wants to ensure sufficient private time, space, and opportunities to talk with the patient.

- *Action.* At this point, the athletic trainer is ready to introduce the psychosocial referral to the patient. A good standard for referral is to offer the patient a variety of choices in-so-far as what specific mental health professional he or she will choose to contact. Offer the patient three referral sources to ensure that the personal needs are met in the referral, which reinforces that seeking psychosocial help is the athlete's choice, and involve personal commitment. It is important to articulate in a manner that is caring, concerned, and forthright.

  For example, "Leslie, I have a feeling that you are becoming quite frustrated with all of the personal things in your life, they do seem to be overwhelming. Have you ever considered talking with a trained counselor that might be able to offer you an objective voice to sort through all of these things?"

  Action also includes committing to the offer. The athletic trainer might have to be the one who finds the counselor's phone number. In some cases, the athlete might ask the athletic trainer to even be the one to make the initial call; however, it is beneficial and contributes to the athlete's commitment level if he or she makes the call.

- *Evaluation.* The evaluation stage of a psychosocial referral does not pertain to the athletic trainer evaluating the patient or his or her progress. Instead, it is always wise to evaluate how one went about the referral process and the effect that it had. The athletic trainer should ask the patient these questions:
  - "How did that go?"
  - "Did I clearly articulate the possible benefits of counseling?"
  - "Did I help dispel any myths or misconceptions?"

Table 3-2

Lessons in Guiding Professional Considerations and Subsequent Actions in the Psychosocial Referral Process

Do's	Don'ts
• Listen to the story and be supportive	• Ignore the problem and hope it will go away or that it will be handled elsewhere in the athlete's life
• Protect self, others, and the patient	
• Express your concern for the patient's welfare and optimal well-being	• Judge, preach, or pressure the patient in the referral or therapeutic process
• Join in a collaborate brainstorming, search, and commitment for professional assistance	• Become a person's only support system—refer to a trained expert
• Assist, as requested, in the communication process with the mental health professional	• Probe or mandate into the current issues or about the process of therapy
• Continue to be supportive to the patient throughout the duration and after the conclusion of the psychotherapeutic process	• Breach confidentiality; remember, the information disclosed by the patient is still his or hers

---

  ❋   "Did I attend to your personal and cultural attributes?"

  ❋   "Was I thorough?"

  ❋   "Was I genuinely interested in you as an individual and did I act concerned?"

  ❋   "What can I do to build off of this referral for the next possible situation?"

• *Follow-up.* As mentioned, it is not the athletic trainer's role to check up on the athlete's progress. The push toward wellness can be a long and difficult road for a patient. The athletic trainer should remain supportive, be open to the patient asking for reasonable assistance, and ensure that the most optimal conditions for wellness are present. It might also prove valuable to simply note in the athlete's professional records that a recommendation for psychosocial referral was made. The follow-up process is extra assurance that the appropriate sensitivity exists in the environments in which the athletic trainer interacts with the patient (refer to Table 3-2 for a summary of lessons in this model).

Conclusion

The purpose of this chapter was to clearly articulate the need for psychosocial support of patients, recommend the utility of the referral process in meeting this need, examine the necessary considerations implicit to a positive referral process, and present a usable model for the application of referral to the athletic trainer's professional practice. It is evident that psychosocial referrals for athletes are complex. Due to the potential harm that can occur in a haphazard referral and the potential benefit one can experience from counseling, it is prudent that the athletic trainer meet these complexities head-on with sensitivity, preparation, and commitment.

As mentioned in the outset of this chapter, an athletic trainer is endowed with the potential to serve the psychosocial referral needs of patients. This unique opportunity represents the precise ingredient to help a patient make systemic and personal change.

Chapter Exercises

1(a). Identifying the psychosocial needs of patients.

Instructions: The purpose of this activity is to examine some of the psychosocial needs for patients. In clarifying the potential needs for patients, the athletic trainer will be able to make more prudent decisions in the referral process and become more competent in introducing the referral to the patient. Look at each of the prompting statements and consider the specific psychosocial issues present in the patient.

1. Who is the patient and what psychosocial issues have I witnessed directly?

2. When did these issues begin to be evident to me? What was going on in the patient's life (on the field and in his or her personal life)?

3. Where are these psychosocial issues being demonstrated? Are there certain places where the patient seems to be struggling more so than others?

4. What elements of this patient's past am I aware of? How might these issues be affecting the patient's current psychosocial functioning?

5. Who are the additional relevant parties in the patient's life? How do these individual's affect the situation?

6. What environmental influences are affecting the patient?

7. What am I feeling in the presence of the patient? How might my own biases affect the manner in which I am viewing the patient's current psychosocial functioning?

8. Is the patient and/or others safe given the current psychosocial functioning of the patient?

9. Might a psychosocial referral help the patient given each of the said issues? If yes, then what must I begin to consider? If no, how might I assist the patient (or not)?

1(b). Identifying the psychosocial needs of patients (this answered exercise uses the case of Jorge as the context).

Instructions: The following example considers the case of Jorge, the transitioning football player introduced in the chapter. Consider how the athletic trainer responded to each of these prompts. Knowing what you do about Jorge, how might you have responded to these prompts? What would you have added? What would you have omitted?

1. Who is the patient and what psychosocial issues have I witnessed directly?

Jorge. I have seen many changes in Jorge in the recent weeks. He seems to be quite sad and uncertain about his future. His school work seems to be suffering, as has his productivity on the football field. He does not seem to be able to sustain his attention for long periods of time and he is not the jovial Jorge I have known for years.

2. When did these issues begin to be evident to me? What was going on in the patient's life (on the field and in their personal life)?

    These issues with Jorge seemed to have come on in the last few weeks, about a month before the end of the football season. I think that he is getting some pressure from home about what he is going to do after college.

3. Where are these psychosocial issues being demonstrated? Are there certain places where the patient seems to be struggling more so than others?

    Everywhere. Jorge is struggling in class, on the field, and he is isolating himself from friends.

4. What elements of this patient's past am I aware of? How might these issues be affecting the patient's current psychosocial functioning?

    I know that everyone from Jorge's family had high expectations for his football career. Given his disappointing season and how important living up to the expectations is to Jorge, I think that he is taking it rather hard. He does not want to disappoint.

5. Who are the additional relevant parties in the patient's life? How do these individual's affect the situation?

    His coaches, friends on the team, as well as family and friends back home.

6. What environmental influences are affecting the patient?

    Well, he has struggled to meet his expectations as an athlete. He had a good year, but he will not get many looks from the NFL—his lifelong dream.

7. What am I feeling in the presence of the patient? How might my own biases affect the manner in which I am viewing the patient's current psychosocial functioning?

    Well, I share Jorge's disappointment with him. I know how important football is to his life. I might be impressing my own disappointment on him and seeing something that is not there... but I doubt it. He really seems to be having a hard time.

8. Is the patient and/or others safe given the current psychosocial functioning of the patient?

    Well, I do not think that Jorge is aggressive off the field... to himself or others. He is sad but he has his faculties and some support systems in place.

9. Might a psychosocial referral help the patient given each of the said issues? If yes, then what must I begin to consider? If no, how might I assist the patient (or not)?

    Jorge could benefit from counseling. He may need to be able to talk about life after football, how to communicate with his folks and his friends, and how to find meaning and pride in all of his current and future accomplishments.

2. Finding the right psychotherapist.

    Instructions: Matching the traits particular to the patient in need of psychosocial referral to the appropriate psychotherapist is integral to the ultimate success of the counseling. Consider each of the prompts listed below and answer each as it specifically applies to the case of the patient and the various psychotherapists with which you have an established working relationship.

1. List each of the psychotherapists with which I have a working relationship.
2. What is the presenting psychosocial issue with the potentially referred patient?
3. Are there any psychotherapists from my list that specialize in this psychosocial issue?
4. How does this therapist view therapy? What are the therapist's credentials and is he or she competent in the issue particular to the patient?
5. Is there a probable personality and style match between the patient and the psychotherapist? What might be the assets of this match? What might be some obstacles? How does the psychotherapist believe that people grow and change in counseling?
6. Is this referral practical for the needs of the patient (e.g., costs, distance, time)?
7. What other considerations might I need to consider in referring the patient to this psychotherapist?
8. Do my responses to numbers 2 through 7 seem to indicate that this is a good referral match for the psychosocial needs of the patient?

3. The psychosocial referral process.

   Instructions: The chapter offered a succinct model to proceed through the potential complexities of a psychosocial referral for a patient. Read each of the prompts listed below and appropriately respond to each as it is relevant to the needs of the patient.

   1. *Pre-preparation.* List each of the psychotherapists and their credentials. Ensure that I have a sample of professionals that can meet a wide range of patient psychosocial needs. Have I an appropriate knowledge of these professionals in-so-far as their practice and their personal style?

   2. *Assessment.*

      a. Who is the patient and which mental health service provider can best serve this individual? What is the psychosocial issue?

      b. What personal and environmental influences are contributing to the patient's psychosocial functioning?

      c. When and where did these issues manifest?

      d. Why are these psychosocial issues causing a problem in the life of the patient or others?

      e. How might I go about connecting this patient with the appropriate assistance?

   3. *Pre-action.* What things do I need to do before I initiate the referral? Would it help for me to talk with the possible counselor(s)? Should I set up a specific time and place to talk with the patient? Will the place be conducive to the personal nature of this referral conversation? What things might I need to do for myself to lessen my anxiety and enhance how I present the referral and relevant information?

4. *Action.*

   a. What occurred? Was there a mutual agreement that a psychosocial issue is present that could use outside professional assistance? Did we come to a viable solution and commitment to connect with such a professional?

   b. Was a specific plan made? Who is going to initiate the contact? How is this contact going to be completed and by what time? What things are going to be said? Did I help coach or role play the initial conversation with the counselor?

5. *Evaluation.*

   a. What did I do that I found to be effective in this psychosocial referral? How might I use this again in the future with other patients?

   b. What things might I be able to improve upon in the future with either this patient or in another referral situation?

   c. What are some final words of recognition and encouragement that will help support me in future referrals?

6. *Follow-up.*

   a. Are the conditions of the site that I am working at conducive to the psychosocial needs of the patient? What things might be intimidating about his or her return to succeed here with athletic training activities?

   b. What things can I do to ensure that I am servicing the total need of the patient?

   c. How can I ensure that I am supportive and receptive to the disclosures of the patient without probing into issues that he or she might not be willing or ready to tell me?

References

American Counseling Association. (n.d.). *American Counseling Association.* Retrieved January 30, 2005, from http://www.counseling.org

American Psychiatric Association. (n.d.). *American Psychiatric Association.* Retrieved January 31, 2005, from http://www.psych.org

American Psychological Association, Division 47, Exercise and Sport Psychology (n.d.). American Psychological Association, Division 47, Exercise and Sport Psychology. Retrieved July 11, 2007, from http://www.apa.org/divisions/div47

Anshel, M. H., & Eom, H. (2003). Exploring the dimensions of perfectionism in sport. *International Journal of Sport Psychology, 34*(3), 255-271.

Association for Advancement of Applied Sports Psychology (n.d.). *Association for Advancement of Applied Sports Psychology.* Retrieved February 22, 2005, from http://www.aaasponline.org/index.php

Brewer, B. W., Jeffers, K. E., Petipas, A. J., & Van Raalte, J. L. (1994). Perceptions of psychological interventions in the context of sport injury rehabilitation. *Sport Psychologist, 8,* 176-188.

Burgess, A., & Martin, S. (2004). Inner strength: The mental dynamics of athletic performance. *Sport Psychologist, 18*(4), 469-470.

Catty, J. (2004). "The vehicle of success": Theoretical and empirical perspectives on the therapeutic alliance in psychotherapy and psychiatry. *Psychology & Psychotherapy: Theory, Research & Practice, 77*(2), 255-272.

Cnaan, R., Blankertz, L., Messinger, K., & Gardner, J. (1989). Psychosocial rehabilitation: Towards a theoretical base. *Psychosocial Rehabilitation, 13,* 33-55.

Côté, J. (1999). The influence of the family in the development of talent in sport. *Sport Psychologist, 13*(4), 395-417.

Damm, J. (1991). Drugs and the college student-athlete. In E. F. Etzel, A. P. Ferrante, & J. W. Pinkney (Eds.), *Counseling college student athletes: Issues and interventions* (pp. 151-174). Morgantown, WV: Fitness Information Technology.

Day, S. X. (2004). *Theory and design in counseling and psychotherapy.* Boston, MA: Lahaska Press.

Fischer, A. R., Jome, L. M., & Atkinson, D. R. (1998). Reconceptualizing multicultural counseling: Universal healing conditions in a culturally specific context. Counseling Psychologist, 26(4), 525-88.

Fletcher, T. B., Benshoff, J. M., & Richburg, M. J. (2003). A systems approach to understanding and counseling college student-athletes. *Journal of College Counseling, 6*(1), 35-45.

Gladding, S. T. (2001). *The counseling dictionary: Concise definitions of frequently used terms.* Upper Saddle River, NJ: Merrill Prentice Hall, Inc.

Harwood, C., Cumming, J., & Fletcher, D. (2004). Motivational profiles and psychological skills use within elite youth sport. *Journal of Applied Sport Psychology, 16*(4), 318-332.

Hopkinson, R. A., & Lock, J. (2004). Athletics, perfectionism, and disordered eating. *Eating & Weight Disorders, 9*(2), 99-106.

International Association of Marriage and Family Counselors. (n.d.). *International Association of Marriage and Family Counselors.* Retrieved February 22, 2005, from http://www.iamfc.com

Killeya, L. A. (2001). Idiosyncratic role-elaboration, academic performance, and adjustment among African-American and European-American male college student-athletes. *College Student Journal, 35*(1), 87-95.

Kirk, G., Singh, K., & Getz, H. (2001). Risk of eating disorders among female college athletes and nonathletes. Journal of College Counseling, 4(2), 133-132.

Martin, S. B., Akers, A., & Jackson, A. W. (2001). Male and female athletes' and nonathletes' expectations about sport psychology consulting. *Journal of Applied Sport Psychology, 13*(1), 18-39.

Murphy, S. (Ed.). (1995). *Sport psychology interventions.* Champaign, IL: Human Kinetics.

Murphy, S., & Gutekunst, L. (1997). *Disordered eating among athletes: The athletic trainer's role.* Washington, DC: Human Kinetics.

National Association of Social Workers. (n.d.). *National Association of Social Workers.* Retrieved January 31, 2005, from http://www.naswdc.org

National Athletic Trainers' Association Education Council (NATA) (2006). Athletic Training Educational Competencies (4th ed.). Dallas, TX: National Athletic Trainers' Association, Inc.

Petrie, T. A., & Rogers, R. (2001). Extending the discussion of eating disorders to include men and athletes. *Counseling Psychologist, 29*(5), 743-753.

Robazza, C., Pellizzari, M., & Hanin, Y. (2004). Emotion self-regulation and athletic performance: An application of the IZOF model. *Psychology of Sport & Exercise, 5*(4), 379-404.

Shadish, W. R., & Baldwin, S. A. (2003). Meta-analysis of MFT interventions. *Journal of Marital & Family Therapy, 29*(4), 547-570.

Society of Clinical Psychology. (n.d.). *American Psychological Association, Division 12, Society of Clinical Psychology.* Retrieved February 22, 2005, from http://www.apa.org/about/division/div12.html

Society of Counseling Psychology (n.d.). *American Psychological Association, Division 17, Society of Counseling Psychology.* Retrieved February 22, 2005, from http://www.div17.org

Stankovich, C. E., Meeker, D. J., & Henderson, J. L. (2001). The positive transitions model for sports retirement. Journal of College Counseling, 4(1), 81-84.

Suzuki, L. A., & Ahluwalia, M. K. (2004). Two decades of research on the Problem Solving Inventory: A call for empirical clarity. *Counseling Psychologist, 32*(3), 429-438.

U.S. Department of Labor. (n.d.). *US Department of Labor: Occupational outlook handbook.* Retrieved January 30, 2005, from http://www.bls.gov/oco/home.htm

Weinberg, R. S., & Gould, D. (1999). *Foundations of sport and exercise psychology* (2nd ed.). Champaign, IL: Human Kinetics.

Williams, J. M., & Andersen, M. B. (1998). Psychosocial antecedents of sport and injury: Review and critique of the stress and injury model. *Journal of Sport and Exercise Psychology, 10*, 5-25.

Chapter

SUBSTANCE ABUSE ISSUES FOR ATHLETIC TRAINERS

Laura J. Veach, PhD, LPC, LCAS, CCS, NCC

Chapter Objectives

- ❖ Identify commonly abused substances by athletes and physically active individuals.
- ❖ Identify the signs and symptoms of drug abuse and addiction.
- ❖ Discuss societal influences toward substance abuse as related to athletes and physically active individuals.
- ❖ Discuss intervention strategies for athletic trainers when dealing with drug abuse and addiction by athletes.
- ❖ Provide an overview of the role athletic trainers play with substance abuse by athletes and physically active individuals.

NATA Educational Competencies

Psychosocial Intervention and Referral Domain

1. Identify and describe the sociological, biological, and psychological influences toward substance abuse, addictive personality traits, commonly abused substances, the signs and symptoms associated with the abuse of these substances, and their impact on an individual's health and physical performance.

Medical Conditions and Disabilities Domain

1. Identify and refer as appropriate common and significant psychological medical disorders from drug toxicity, physical emotional stress, and acquired disorders.

Acute Care of Injuries and Illnesses Domain

1. Identify the signs and symptoms of toxic drug overdose.

Pathology of Injuries and Illnesses Domain

1. Identify the normal acute and chronic physiological responses (e.g., inflammation, immune response, recovery, healing, and/or repair) of the human body to trauma, hypoxia, microbiological agents, genetic derangements, nutritional deficiencies, chemicals, drugs, and aging to the musculoskeletal system and other organ systems.

Estimates indicate the pervasiveness of substance use disorders, with the exclusion of tobacco, involve approximately 32 million Americans (James & Gilliland, 2005). Every aspect of athleticism is influenced by substance abuse and addiction issues. When compared to ancient warriors who "fortified themselves with alcohol before battle to boost their courage and decrease sensitivity to pain; many professional athletes today follow in this tradition: baseball players chew tobacco; football and basketball players often take amphetamines and cocaine" (Weil & Rosen, 1983, p. 20). Many athletic training professionals can easily recall a promising or professional athlete for whom substance problems caused major career-ending consequences. The popular media is rife with accounts of major problems facing various athletic organizations and sanctioning bodies stemming from illegal steroid use through chemical dependence. Much has been written and policies continue to be added to try and address the impact of drug use and abuse related to athletes. In addition, substance abuse issues can profoundly affect the athletic trainer; therefore, he or she "must be knowledgeable about substance abuse in the athletic population and should be able to recognize signs that may indicate when an athlete is engaging in substance abuse" (Prentice, 2003, p. 465). To better inform athletic trainers, this chapter provides comprehensive information about various commonly abused substances, societal influences toward substance abuse as related to athletes and physically active individuals, signs and symptoms of drug abuse and addiction, and intervention considerations for the athletic trainer.

Commonly Abused Substances

ALCOHOL

It is important for the athletic trainer to understand the most commonly abused substances that jeopardize the athlete's health and well-being. The most abused mood-altering substance used by many people, including athletes, is ethanol (e.g., ethyl alcohol, or as it is more commonly referred to, beverage alcohol). Based on 2002 data, approximately 120 million people in the United States over age 12 identify themselves as current drinkers (Substance Abuse and Mental Health Services Administration [SAMHSA], 2003). Alcohol is "humanity's oldest domesticated drug" (Siegal & Inciardi, 2004, p. 78) and athletes are not immune from its use and effects. Regarding its effects and attraction, an apt description notes alcohol as "the drink of deception: alcohol gives you power and robs you of it in equal measure" (Knapp, 1996, p. 95).

Even though it is a legal drug for those over the age of 21, some believe "alcohol has no place in sports participation" (Prentice, 2003, p. 479). Recent studies found patterns of extensive use of alcohol by athletes with slightly higher use in off season periods (National Collegiate Athletic Association [NCAA], 2001; Naylor, Gardner, & Zaichkowsky, 2001; The Higher Education Center for Alcohol and Other Drug Prevention, 2002; Watson, 2002). Several compelling studies utilizing large national sample sizes of college students and athletes at the collegiate level found that athletes consume more alcohol than other students, engage in binge drinking more frequently, and have more substance abuse-related consequences (Leichliter, Meilman, Presley, & Cashin, 1998; Nelson & Wechsler, 2001; The Higher Education Center for Alcohol and Other Drug Prevention, 2002). Binge drinking is defined for males as five or more drinks and for females as four or more drinks in any one drinking episode. The patterns of binge drinking by student athletes identified in research has prompted some to consider student athletes as a high-risk group for binge drinking and alcohol-related harms (Nelson & Wechsler, 2001; Thombs & Hamilton, 2002). The latest NCAA survey conducted in 2001 found decreasing trends of alcohol use from previous years, yet still found a large majority of those surveyed, 78.3%, 77.7%, and 82.1% in Divisions I through III, respectively, reported alcohol use within the past 12 months. The survey also indicated that the next highest percentage of use for a mood-altering substance was marijuana, averaging less than 33% of athletes surveyed. For further comparison, amphetamine use, which is viewed with much concern recently because of significant increases in prevalence, was used by 3.1%, 3.3%, and 3.6% of the athletes within the past 12 months of the survey date in the respective Divisions (NCAA, 2001).

Alcohol has certainly been evident in historical documents for centuries, although it is not clear how alcohol was first discovered. Historians generally believe it was an accidental discovery in the Neolithic age, about 10,000 years ago, after berries or fruits were forgotten and began the fermentation process, resulting in a crude version of wine (Erickson, 2001; Siegal & Inciardi, 2004). Distilling alcohol to get higher potency began around 800 ACE in the Middle East (Doweiko, 2006) in order to make a more concentrated type of alcohol that could be shipped in greater quantities (Weil & Rosen, 1983). Alcohol is classified pharmacologically as a depressant to the central nervous system (CNS). Due to its depressive nature, alcohol was often used as an anesthetic or sleep aid and often lived up to its reputation as a social lubricant due to its tendency to decrease inhibition.

To better determine potency, the term *proof* has been used to indicate the percentage of alcohol in a particular beverage. Using the standard formula, one roughly doubles the percentage of alcohol to determine potency. For example, beer is generally around 5% alcohol or 10 proof. The same is true for over-the-counter cough and cold preparations containing alcohol, such as a popular brand that helps one get to sleep and suppress coughs, which is approximately 20% alcohol or 40 proof. Conversely, to determine the percentage of ethyl alcohol in a beverage one can divide by half the designated proof. For example, 86 proof scotch is 43% alcohol.

Many addiction specialists and addiction educators emphasize that the critical ingredient of alcohol is ethanol whether the person consumes beer, wine, or distilled liquor. It is important that those working with athletes who provide information about alcohol address the common misconception that some alcoholic beverages are safer than others. Some have rationalized that since beer, for example, is only 5% ethyl alcohol it would be less harmful. What is important to understand is that "the same quantity of alcohol is consumed if someone drinks either a 12-ounce can or bottle of beer, a three-to four-ounce glass of wine, or a mixed drink made with one and one-half ounces of distilled spirits" (Siegal & Inciardi, 2004, p. 75). Although the overall sizes of the drinks vary, the amount of ethyl alcohol is equivalent in each drink in the preceding example and it is the ethyl alcohol that is the main mood-altering chemical in alcoholic beverages.

When beverage alcohol is consumed, it is readily absorbed into the bloodstream through the lining of the stomach and small intestines without a complicated digestive process. Beverage alcohol's mood-altering effects are felt usually within 20 minutes. The effect of ethanol can be moderated by food in the stomach, which slows the passage of alcohol, the weight of the person, the gender of the person, and the response to alcohol or tolerance. The body, primarily the liver, breaks down alcohol at relatively the same rate for most individuals. The term *intoxication* applies to an inebriated state because the liver, whose main job is to metabolize or excrete toxins, encounters ethanol as a toxin to the system (Doweiko, 2006). Old myths of drinking hot coffee or taking cold showers do not speed the rate of metabolizing ethanol, although one is likely to have a more wide awake drunk after adding caffeine to the person's system (van Wormer & Davis, 2003). Nothing exists that accelerates the rate of breakdown of ethanol (Siegal & Inciardi, 2004). Of particular note to the athletic trainer regarding ethanol metabolizing rates is the number of deaths each year of college students particularly who die of over-intoxication (Falkowski, 2000). Often those with little experience drinking alcohol do not understand that over-intoxication can be fatal. Since it happens infrequently, a youth's awareness is often limited. Therefore, it is important that athletic trainers and educators stress the risk one takes when consuming large quantities of alcohol. Signs and symptoms of acute ethanol poisoning resulting from rapid ingestion of alcoholic beverages include the following (Falkowski, 2000):

- Shallow breathing
- Vomiting
- Confusion
- Unconsciousness
- Convulsions/seizures
- Shock

If these symptoms are observed, alcohol poisoning can be fatal and constitutes a medical emergency. The athletic trainer is advised to enact emergency procedures by calling 911. Respiratory arrest or aspiration of vomit have been the primary cause of death in recent high-profile fatalities of inexperienced college drinkers after imbibing large quantities of alcohol in a short time period (Falkowski, 2000).

An additional important concept for the athletic trainer involves the method of measuring alcohol. To determine the amount of alcohol consumed, a blood alcohol concentration (BAC) is often measured either by a Breathalyzer or a blood sample. There are a number of portable, easy-to-use breathalyzers available on the market that can be purchased by an athletic organization that has a policy requiring Breathalyzer testing on a random or for-cause basis. For accuracy, a BAC level would need to be obtained within 12 hours of alcohol consumption, after which time the alcohol would likely eliminated from the body. The fact that the metabolization of alcohol is a relatively short process is one of the main reasons a Breathalyzer is the preferred measuring method as opposed to performing a urine drug screen (UDS). Because many liquid cough medicines contain alcohol in their formulas, a person may often explain a detectable odor of alcohol as a result of cough medication. Although a Breathalyzer cannot distinguish the origin of measurable alcohol, it can be important if a BAC reading is elevated from a person claiming cough medicine use.

Hospital emergency rooms are the most likely authority to obtain blood samples for a BAC and may only do so by court order if the drinker is suspected of a criminal offense or involved in an automobile crash while under the influence. As of October 2003, 45 states had enacted federally incentivized 0.08 BAC laws stating that any driver with a BAC at or above 0.08 would be charged with operating a motor vehicle illegally, commonly referred to as driving under the influence, or DUI (National Highway Traffic Safety Administration [NHTSA], 2004). Reports show that an average of 43% of drivers involved in automobile accidents resulting in serious injury or death are tested for BAC (NHTSA, 2004). Currently, over 50% of alcohol-impaired drivers involved in a fatal automobile accident have presented with a BAC at or above 0.16 (NHTSA, 2004). Sports and recreation programs are also affected negatively by alcohol-related costs. In the year 2000, the average cost for on-the-job motor vehicle accidents in the amusement and recreation service industry exceeded 197 million dollars (NHTSA, 2004). In addition, the total cost to employers related to automobile accidents where at least one driver was alcohol impaired is more than 9 billion dollars annually, and of that total 3.1 billion dollars is directly related to alcohol impairment on-the-job (NHTSA, 2004). With increasing numbers of athletic trainers working in business and industry, it is important for the athletic trainer to understand the scope of alcohol costs not only to the individual but to the organization as well. Since the athletic trainer is often the one person who has the most significant and personal contact with the athlete, it is important for him or her to be able to assess risks carefully and initiate appropriate action.

In summary, alcohol use, misuse, and dependency create significant problems for many people, and athletes are not excluded. The athletic trainer can benefit from increased knowledge and awareness about the most commonly abused substance, alcohol, which impacts far more athletes in a negative way than any other mood-altering chemical substance.

TOBACCO

The chief substance that is mood altering in tobacco products is nicotine, which has been classified as a mild stimulant. It is believed that the indigenous people of the Americas had used tobacco for perhaps thousands of years before the first European arrived (Doweiko, 2006). The resulting history and expansion of the use of tobacco has had profound effects on our world. In the United States in 2001, there were approximately 1.4 million new smokers daily, which represented a substantial decrease from 2.1 million in 1998 (SAMHSA, 2003). The same data indicated approximately 26% (61.1 million Americans) of the population aged 12 and older had smoked in the previous month and just over 3% (7.8 million) reported use of smokeless tobacco. Cigarette use is thought to be particularly prevalent with those addicted to other substances; it is estimated that 74% to 95% of chemically dependent people also have a cigarette dependency (Doweiko, 2002). Many athletes depend on their lungs to enhance their performance and are less inclined to smoke cigarettes. However, the use of smokeless tobacco continues to warrant attention by the athletic trainer.

In an effort to attain the effects of nicotine without the dangers associated with nicotine inhalation, some have rationalized that chew or smokeless tobacco might be less dangerous to one's health. However, evidence indicates that smokeless tobacco carries significant health risks for hypertension, coronary artery disease, oral cancer, oral lesions, and tumors (Doweiko, 2006; Prentice, 2003; The Higher Education Center for Alcohol and Other Drug Prevention, 2002).

With the decreasing trend in smokeless tobacco use among male youth (e.g., among baseball players 41% reported use in 2001 as compared to 60% in early 1990s [The Higher Education Center for Alcohol and Other Drug Prevention, 2002]), it seems prevention goals are beginning to be realized. Continued efforts by the athletic trainer to offer prevention programs are warranted due to the still higher-than-average rate of use of smokeless tobacco among athletes.

STIMULANTS

Another type of mood-altering substance includes stimulants, specifically ephedrine, amphetamines, and amphetamine-like medications (e.g., Ritalin [Novartis, East Hanover, NJ]). Unlike many other mood-altering substances that are primarily used for the euphoria produced by the drug, amphetamines are often used by athletes not only for the euphoric experience but also to enhance athletic performance, thus qualifying stimulants as an ergogenic aid. "Common ergogenic aids include stimulants, beta blockers, narcotic analgesics, diuretics, anabolic steroids, human growth hormone, and blood doping" (Prentice, 2003, p. 465). Indeed, many of the other mood-altering substances are more likely to impair short-term performance when compared to stimulants. Some historical information cites the use of performance-enhancing drugs in sports as early as 2,000 years ago when Roman gladiators used stimulants to reduce fatigue (Wadler, 1994 as cited in Doweiko, 2002). Although, as Weil and Rosen point out, "instead of automatically improving physical and mental performance, stimulants sometimes just make people do poor work faster" (1983, p. 38) with an added effect of depleting the body's natural energy reserves. Current research shows about a 3% usage rate of amphetamines with an alarming trend of greater use of stimulants by female than male athletes and greater use by athletes compared to nonathletes (The Higher Education Center for Alcohol and Other Drug Prevention, 2002).

One of the most controversial stimulants that has recently had a significant impact in athletics is ephedrine. Ancient Chinese medicine used the plants containing ephedrine over 5,000 years ago. More recent refinement for use in the United States began after 1930 to mainly treat respiratory issues, such as asthma. Ephedrine side effects often create anxiety and agitation with less euphoria than other amphetamines (Weil & Rosen, 1983). Almost 70 years ago, efforts to find a synthetic alternative to ephedrine with less side effects and better outcomes resulted in the pharmaceutical development of amphetamines. Approximately 4% of student athletes had reported use of ephedrine in 2001, and the highest rate of 12% was found with women's ice hockey athletes (The Higher Education Center for Alcohol and Other Drug Prevention, 2002). The recent ban of ephedrine in April 2004 was the result of a drug fraught with significant side effects (Hall, 2004).

Several sources note speed, a slang term for amphetamines, was used extensively by military personnel during wartime in the 1940s to improve endurance and alertness (Doweiko, 2006; Miller, 2004; Weil & Rosen, 1983). In the 1950s it was given by injection for the treatment of heroin addiction (Miller, 2004). Continued use of amphetamines in the 1960s and 1970s spiraled with "approximately 10 billion amphetamine tablets manu-factured in the United States in the year 1970" (Doweiko, 2002, p. 125). With such exten-sive amphetamine use, many of the negative side effects such as agitation with severe anxiety, cardiovascular damage, paranoia, severe depression, drug-induced psychosis, and withdrawal-induced suicidal ideation became much more prevalent. Warnings about the abuse and addiction potential of speed were commonplace in the early 1970s since "amphetamines had acquired a reputation as known killers" (Doweiko, p. 137).

Overall the use of amphetamines has been problematic, highlighted by methamphet-amine-related episodes of which a 30% increase was noted between the years 1999 to 2000 according to hospital emergency department data (National Institute on Drug Abuse [NIDA], 2004). Methamphetamine is often a preferred stimulant for abuse, and recover-ing addicts show impairment such as slowed motor skills and memory. Such effects persist even after ceasing any methamphetamine use for 9 months and researchers are further concerned that abusers may have an increased risk for neurodegenerative disease (Zickler, 2002). Initial information by the manufacturer as described in the *Physician's Desk Reference* (PDR) begins by stating "methamphetamine has a high potential for abuse... may lead to drug dependence and must be avoided" (PDR, 2002, p. 440). Particularly for athletes, amphetamines clearly are among the most abused of the ergogenic aids (Prentice, 2003). When athletes begin to use amphetamines sporadically and in lower doses, not only may they initially see enhanced athletic performance, they also experience the euphoric sense of well-being that becomes psychologically rewarding (Prentice, 2003). However, as increasing amounts of amphetamines are used, "abusers quickly become tolerant to amphetamine-induced euphoric feelings" (Doweiko, 2002, p. 130), which can lead to ever-increasing dosages or changing routes of administration (i.e., switching from oral tablets to injecting liquid amphetamine) usually occurring when addiction to amphetamines has developed. The athlete may then begin to experience impairment in cognitive function-ing and complex motor skills, irrationality, perseveration, pupil dilation abnormalities, hypertension, hyperreflexia, or overheating with no sustainable enhancement of athletic performance (Prentice, 2003).

Alternatives to pharmaceutically produced amphetamines are illegally manufactured amphetamines, specifically a smokeable form of crystal methamphetamine known as ice and more recently as another amphetamine: methcathinone, or Kat. Both Kat and ice produce stimulant effects and have many of the same risks and side effects as other amphetamines.

The other stimulants of particular focus for the athlete are amphetamine-like stimu-lants, such as Ritalin or methylphenidate, its generic name. For a number of years Ritalin has mainly been used in the treatment of attention deficit hyperactivity disorder (ADHD). Interestingly, consistent with a number of synthetically produced mood-altering drugs, Ritalin was manufactured as a nonaddicting alternative to amphetamines (Doweiko, 2006). Its main action in the brain involves blocking dopamine reuptake, which results in behavioral changes of improved concentration and tracking of information. It also has been found to have side effects that include weight and appetite loss, insomnia, nausea, hypertension, increased anxiety, anemia, or perseveration (Doweiko, 2006). There is con-siderable research being conducted to examine the long-term effects of this drug, which at present are poorly understood. Newer research indicates neurological damage, liver damage, decreasing seizure thresholds, and heart tissue damage in some individuals

(Doweiko, 2006). Unfortunately, more reports indicate Ritalin is being abused through illegal dispersion to those not prescribed the medication. There is growing concern among addiction professionals that this stimulant is being misused by many students to produce euphoria, especially when the drug is crushed and injected intravenously. Continued research into the addictive properties of this drug is needed.

Caffeine, a stimulant found in beverages such as coffee, tea, or colas, remains controversial as it pertains to the athlete. Some organizations restrict its use if amounts over a certain threshold are detected in urine testing. Because it also acts as a diuretic, it can create problems when being properly hydrated is important in competition (Prentice, 2003).

The athletic trainer can facilitate better outcomes for the athlete and team through continuing education, prevention efforts, and discouraging any use of stimulants as performance enhancers. The cost of amphetamine addiction far outweighs any benefit in short-term athletic performance and "it's very easy to fall into a pattern of using stimulants all the time in order to avoid the down feeling that follows the initial up" (Weil & Rosen, 1983, p. 39).

Cocaine is also classified as a stimulant, as well as is crack cocaine, a smokeable form of cocaine. Cocaine use has seen a steady decline since the mid-1990s, especially among athletes, possibly due to the interventions of athletic trainers to educate and help athletes in trouble with cocaine. At last report, approximately 2% of athletes surveyed reported cocaine use in the recent year as compared to a 5% usage rate in 1989—a significant decline (The Higher Education Center for Alcohol and Other Drug Prevention, 2002). Declining use can also be attributed to UDS testing in high school and college settings (Copeland, 2002; Goldberg et al., 2003).

Epidemics of cocaine abuse and addiction occurred in the late 1800s and again between 1921 and 1929, which lead to its prohibition, except for prescribed medical indications (Doweiko, 2002). By the late 1970s, "cocaine had been all but forgotten since the Harrison Narcotics Act of 1914" (Doweiko, 2002, p. 137), and many stimulant abusers and addicts were seeking a safer alternative to amphetamines, hence the rise in the use of cocaine. This time a new more powerful form of cocaine, "crack," was synthesized and its distribution was rampant in the 1980s and early 1990s. Many professional athletes were featured in media segments about their cocaine addictions while professional, collegiate, and high school associations organized to combat the deleterious consequences of cocaine abuse and dependency. At one time it was believed that cocaine users were most at risk for habituation or psychological dependence; however, it is now clear that physical dependence can occur as evidenced by tolerance and withdrawal symptomatology (APA, 2000).

MARIJUANA

Possibly one of the most controversial illegal drugs currently in the United States is in a drug class all by itself. Marijuana "is an ancient drug, used since prehistoric times in parts of the Old World" (Weil & Rosen, 1983, p. 113) and at times it acts similar to stimulants, at other times it is like a depressant, and still in other ways it resembles a mild psychedelic drug, yet it is in its own classification because of its many unique properties. For a number of years it was questionable whether one could develop a dependency on marijuana; however, even in 1983 experts in drug issues noted that tolerance, withdrawal, and dependence occurred with regular marijuana use. It became increasingly clear that the pattern of dependency is different: "at its worst—marijuana dependence consists of chain smoking, from the moment of getting up in the morning to the time of falling asleep... but dramatic withdrawal syndromes don't occur... and craving for the drug is not nearly as intense as for tobacco, alcohol, or narcotics" (p. 119). In one recent study, athletes aged 12 to 17 were found to report marijuana use at a rate of 6% during the previous month as compared with 10 % of nonathletes (SAMHSA, 2002). However, when looking at an extensive survey of athletes at the college level, the surveyors found just over 25% of the athletes surveyed reported marijuana use at least once within the year in both the 1997 and 2001 surveys, with the majority indicating first use occurred in high school (The Higher Education Center for Alcohol and Other Drug Prevention, 2002). Concern exists then for young athletes. Physical concerns the athletic trainer can address include an estimated 15% to 40% reduced lung capacity (Prentice, 2003). Other concerns for athletes include lowered testosterone levels, increased exercising pulse rates upwards of 20%, and decreased muscle strength (Prentice, 2003). Continued education and information can assist the athletic trainer with prevention efforts regarding marijuana use.

NARCOTICS

Athletes may initially take narcotics, a term from the Greek word meaning "stupor" (and origin of the word "stupid") (Weil & Rosen, 1983), because they are prescribed by a team physician to aid in the treatment of a painful injury. Opium is "the parent of all narcotic drugs" (Weil & Rosen, 1983, p. 80) and contains 20 different drugs, the primary one being morphine, which in 1803 became the first drug extracted from a plant. Heroin, more potent than morphine, was not extracted from opium until 1898. Like any other narcotic derived from opium compounds, heroin is referred to as an opiate or opioid (Weil & Rosen, 1983). OxyContin (Purdue Pharma LP, Stamford, CT) is the trade name for a narcotic that has received extensive media attention due to its addictive features. Recent information indicates in 2001 over 7.2 million prescriptions were written for OxyContin, resulting in sales of $1.45 billion, and sales of $1.59 billion were reported for 2002 (Inciardi & Goode, 2004). Many athletic trainers have been encouraged to advocate for other pain medications, such as nonsteroidal anti-inflammatory medications, that do not have the addictive potential of narcotics (Prentice, 2003). When narcotics are prescribed, it is important that the athletic trainer monitor usage and try to help the individual change to other non-narcotic medications as soon as is feasible to manage pain.

While it is important to understand the drugs often abused, it is also important to explore drug-using influences on the athlete or physically active individual.

Societal Influences Toward Substance Abuse in the Athletic and Physically Active Population

In the American culture, there is quite a bit of encouragement to change the way one feels. Be it through popular advertisements that promote fast pain relief, new and improved results, or more is better, the overarching frequent messages in our culture include some rendition of "better living through chemistry." In the field of addiction studies there are compelling and sometimes conflicting theories about the influence of society and cultural norms regarding substance use disorders. Many experts can agree that attitudes toward drug use vary widely both between and within various cultures. It is believed by many addiction specialists that the biopsychosocial theory, a combination of genetic, biological, and environmental influences, has a significant role in substance use disorders—from experimental misuse to polysubstance dependency, although the social influences are perhaps the most difficult to assess.

A number of social learning theorists propose that social influence is significant as it pertains to abuse and addiction patterns. For example, it is noted that "socially disruptive use of alcohol tends to occur almost exclusively in social settings; drunken behavior is seldom seen when alcohol is used in a religious context" (Erickson, 2001, p. 99). Further compounding the understanding of social influence are historical trends of drug use. After serious problems and complications become widely known in society, a decline in the use of the drug is observed; then years later an increase of use in the same drug that fell from popularity makes a dramatic comeback. For example, in the 1930s there was significant abuse of marijuana, then a decline in use, and a dramatic rise in use in the 1960s (Inciardi & Goode, 2004). Cocaine has a similar history since epidemics of cocaine abuse transpired in 1890s, 1920s, and the new version of cocaine (crack) was prevalent in the late 1980s with significant decline of use since 1990; these trends suggest "faddish patterns of popularity" (Erickson, 2001, p. 100). Other social factors include family-of-origin characteristics, such as higher risks for use occur in families with an alcoholic parent, families where parental attitudes are permissive of mood-altering substances, and families experiencing more chaos (Erickson, 2001). One theory combines these multiple social, family, and genetic factors to explain addiction.

The biopsychosocial theory looks at all factors contributing to abuse and addiction. This theory is further clarified with the following example from Erickson (2001) in which two monozygotic twins grow up in the same family, have a similar profile biologically for the development of alcohol problems, yet one twin experiments with alcohol early and is reinforced whereas the other twin becomes more involved in sports and academics and does not experiment with drinking. Each twin has a different addiction profile due more to social rather than biological influences.

It is clear that athletes often share many similar norming experiences and as such can develop their own particular culture with regard to substances. It is particularly striking to note the findings in one study: not only were athletes consuming more alcohol on a weekly basis and binge drinking more often than nonathletes, but team leaders, especially males, were less responsible in their drinking behaviors than other team members (Leichliter et al., 1998). For example, 14% of the male athlete team leaders were found to have taken advantage of another sexually while drinking, as compared to 7.7% of male non-athlete participants; also 48% of male team leaders reported driving under the influence, as compared to 38.5% of male nonathletes; with 5% of the male athlete team leaders noting arrest for DWI/DUI, as compared to 2.1% of the male nonathletes (Leichliter et al., 1998). Because team leaders and athletes are important for establishing what is acceptable behavior in a particular group, this study and others indicating negative social behaviors, such as more sexual aggression by male athletes (The Higher Education Center for Alcohol and Other Drug Prevention, 2002), support the emphasis by the athletic trainer of specialized prevention and intervention resources, particularly for student athletes.

Another important study by Thombs and Hamilton (2002) focused on the impact of social norm feedback campaigns and alcohol use by collegiate-level Division I athletes. Briefly, social norm theory involves providing more accurate data pertaining to college students on their own campuses about drinking patterns in order to reduce pressure to drink more, correct false beliefs of overindulgence, and create more healthy drinking patterns (Berkowitz, 2004). Although the findings indicated a more realistic view of campus-wide alcohol use and resulted in less alcohol use than previously perceived, the campaign showed no lessening of alcohol use among the student athletes. Although student athletes learned, for example, that a campus norm was moderate drinking, the student athlete's patterns of consumption did not decrease as a result of showing them evidence that most students drink in moderation. The researchers aptly pointed out "because of the special status often given to athletes, they may have a social mobility that exposes them to a range of campus drinking norms" (Thombs & Hamilton, 2002, p. 241). A larger question for further study might also examine the role that student athletes have in setting drinking norms among various groups because of their leadership and social status. Student athletes also have greater difficulty adapting to social challenges since they often have much less time to develop hobbies and other leisure skills (Watson, 2002).

Another social influence regarding substance abuse involves the pressure in our society to win at all costs. Athletes consider the use of drugs, especially if it enhances athletic performance. It is clear certain drugs do have the desired effect of short-term performance enhancement. However, the complications from the use relate to the drug's undesired side effects such as addiction. Many athletes who use performance-enhancing drugs become more willing to gamble with their own long-term health when faced with immediate needs to excel. Athletic excellence is often met with society's response of overwhelming approval and tremendous pressure to win and achieve dominance. Young children competing in organized sporting events learn at an early age the importance of winning and excelling in their chosen field. Sportsmanship, so often stressed by the athletic trainer, becomes a secondary focus when the stakes for winning involve financial gain, status, prestige, media focus, and greater social privilege. Thus, societal pressures to win may unduly influence athletes and physically active individuals to consider substances to aid their performance. Finally, further complicating the issues are aspects of physical activity involving injury.

For the injured athlete or physically active individual, the pressure to rehabilitate and resume his or her physical activity is often pronounced. The physical complications from the injury are challenging enough and the psychological turmoil from an injury can perhaps be the most damaging related to not being able to compete or remain physically active (Watson, 2002). Injured athletes can experience isolation and alienation for which they can never adequately prepare. As a result, the athletic trainer has a much larger role than merely helping the athlete recover physically, often operating "…in numerous daily situations in which close interpersonal relationships are important… requiring appropriate counseling skills to confront an athlete's fears, frustrations, and daily crises." (Prentice, 2003, p. 285). These psychological issues can place the injured athlete at greater risk for complications with mood-altering substances. Pain medications may be prescribed to help treat the symptoms associated with an injury, which can put the person at risk of a downward spiral into unplanned addiction. The athletic trainer is urged to closely monitor any individual being treated with prescribed medication that has a significant addictive potential. This involves (1) checking the reported daily pattern of intake of medications, (2) tracking the number of prescriptions in possession of the individual, (3) cautioning about the use of other chemicals that may potentiate the effect of the prescribed medication, such as stimulants combined with narcotics or alcohol combined with narcotics, (4) replacing medications with high addiction potential with medications without mood-altering properties for pain management, and (5) having close coordination with team physicians to discuss dosage and rehabilitation plans. Addiction specialists urge greater awareness regarding the addictive potential of prescribed medications because of the increased incidence of addiction triggered accidentally by unmonitored use of prescribed medications. For example, OxyContin, a relatively newer prescribed narcotic, has been shown to have a significant addiction potential in as little as 2 weeks when taking the drug as prescribed. When in doubt about the addiction potential of a medication, the athletic trainer can consult a licensed pharmacist. In addition, Table 4-1 provides information regarding three of the most frequently prescribed prescription medications.

Continuing research is being conducted to ascertain the unique aspects of the societal influences related to substance abuse and addiction. When abuse or addiction patterns

Table 4-1

Medication Examples

Product Name Generic Name	OxyContin, oxycodone	Desoxyn[*] methamphetamine	Xanax[†] alprazolam
Indications for use with athletes	Usually prescribed for short-term pain management related to injury or postsurgery.	No known accepted medical use for athletic performance; may be prescribed for obesity, narcolepsy, or ADHD.	Most commonly prescribed as anti-anxiety agent, especially to manage panic attacks.
Abuse potential	Significant—Schedule II, tightest regulation of medical drug.	Significant—Schedule II, powerfully addictive (NIDA, 2004).	Moderate—Schedule IV, Steinberg estimated 1 in 10 Xanax users develop addiction (Breggin, 1991).
Withdrawal issues	Similar to heroin; not life-threatening, can be assisted medically, but medical intervention not required. Symptoms: nausea, constipation, runny nose, dysphoria, muscle and bone pain, intense cravings (Erickson, 2001).	Some similarity to cocaine. Often protracted over weeks, rarely life threatening. Symptoms: sleep disturbances, abnormal EEG readings, fatigue, increased panic attacks, depression, or persistent reduced cerebral blood flow (Doweiko, 2002).	Withdrawal symptoms seen after as few as 8 to 12 weeks of use at recommended dose levels (Breggin, 1991; PDR, 2002). Symptoms: can be severe due to seizure risks, requires medical monitoring and intervention.
U.S. prevalence	OxyContin is third in illegal drug diversion cases (Inciardi & Goode, 2004). A 2002 survey estimated 1.9 million people reported nonmedical use at least once (SAMHSA, 2003).	Increasing again since late 1990s; estimated almost 1 million monthly users (Stevens & Smith, 2001).	Estimated 15 million individuals using Xanax each year; 1.5 million are addicted (NIDA, 2004). Dependence can develop within 1 to 2 months of use due to high potency of Xanax as compared with other benzodiazepines (Longo & Johnson, 2000). Recent study found Xanax ranked fourth in illegal drug diversion cases (Inciardi & Goode, 2004).

[*] Desoxyn, Ovation Pharmaceuticals, Inc, Deerfield, IL
[†] Xanax, Pfizer, Inc, New York, NY

emerge in an athlete, the athletic trainer can provide significant help by recognizing the signs and symptoms of substance use disorders.

Signs and Symptoms of Substance Use Disorders

A problematic pattern of using substances is often defined as substance abuse. Substance abuse is not the same as substance addiction. In fact, the *Diagnostic and Statistical Manual of Mental Disorders* (DSM-IV-TR) (APA, 2000) outlines specific criteria in order to recognize and diagnose substance abuse and outlines different criteria for addiction. The athletic trainer should be familiar with the following DSM-IV-TR criteria for substance abuse (APA, 2000, p. 199):

- A maladaptive pattern of substance use leading to clinically significant impairment or distress, as manifested by one (or more) of the following, occurring within a 12-month work period:

  * Recurrent substance use resulting in a failure to fulfill major role obligations at work, school, or home (e.g., repeated absences or poor work performance related to substance use; substance-related absences, suspensions, or expulsions from school; neglect of children or household)

  * Recurrent substance use in situations in which it is physically hazardous (e.g., driving an automobile or operating a machine when impaired by substance use)

  * Recurrent substance-related legal problems (e.g., arrests for substance-related disorderly conduct)

  * Continued substance use despite having persistent or recurrent social or inter-personal problems caused or exacerbated by the effects of the substance (e.g., arguments with spouse about consequences of intoxications, physical fights)

- The symptoms have never met the criteria for substance dependence for this class of substance.

It is important to note that a clinical diagnosis of substance abuse does not indicate a person will develop addiction (e.g., with the majority of alcohol abusers, alcoholism does not occur) (Center for Substance Abuse Treatment, 2003). Abusive or binge drinking is defined for males as five or more drinks in any one drinking episode; for females abusive drinking entails drinking four or more drinks in any one drinking episode (van Wormer & Davis, 2003).

In addition, the following signs and symptoms of abuse for the physically active individual or athlete may be viewed in the following three categories:

1. *Attendance problems.* Arriving late to practice or leaving practice early.

2. *Athletic performance.* Broken plays or misreading plays, increasing mistakes through inattention or poor judgment, increasingly erratic efficiency as reflected in cumulative stats, difficulty covering assignments.

3. *General behavior.* Increasing complaints from fellow teammates or workout part-ners, overreacting to real or imagined criticism, increasing physical complaints with unknown origin or evidence of injury, bragging about frequent binge drink-ing, or participating in social activities in which excessive alcohol consumption is promoted.

In general, substance abuse may be difficult to detect in the athlete or physically active person. By understanding and reviewing signs of abuse, the athletic trainer is more likely to actively assist anyone needing help with substance abuse. Often, more complicated problems occur for the athletic trainer in recognizing signs and symptoms of addiction.

Addiction can be defined as a disease that interferes with the human's ability to function normally. The disease is characterized by compulsion, obsession, and loss of control. Loss of control occurs when a person cannot, with consistent reliability, predict whether he or she is going to have a normal or abnormal using or drinking episode (Ohlms, 1982). Addiction is a disease that is primary, chronic, progressive, and fatal (George, 1990). George (1990) points out that 34.5 of every 36 people afflicted with this disease will die from it; unfortunately, many will not have received treatment for their addiction, often because the signs and symptoms are not recognized.

As early as the 1950s, the American Medical Association concluded that alcoholism was a disease, yet less than 30 patients in 1980 were referred by physicians for chemical dependency treatment in a large, urban Midwest hospital (Kubes, 1990). In 1989, with the establishment of a specialized intervention nursing team, those physician referrals increased to 500 patients per year (Kubes, 1990). Another example involves persons with disabilities who are noted to have significant substance abuse problems, yet are rarely referred (Helwig & Holicky, 1994). It is hoped that better recognition and diagnostic procedures will improve the addicted athlete or physically active individual's chances of receiving treatment with the help of the athletic trainer.

According to the DSM-IV-TR (APA, 2000, p. 197) in diagnosing addiction, one must meet any three (or more) of the following specific criteria that occur within a 1-year time period:

1. Tolerance, as defined by either of the following:
    a. A need for markedly increased amounts of the substance to achieve intoxication or desired effect
    b. Markedly diminished effect with continued use of the same amount of the substance
2. Withdrawal, as manifested by either of the following:
    a. The characteristic withdrawal syndrome for the substance (refer to Criteria A and B of the criteria sets for withdrawal from the specific substances)
    b. The same (or a closely related) substance is taken to relieve or avoid withdrawal symptoms
3. The substance is often taken in larger amounts or over a longer period than was intended.
4. There is a persistent desire or unsuccessful effort to cut down or control substance use.
5. A great deal of time is spent in activities necessary to obtain the substance (e.g., visiting multiple doctors or driving long distances), use the substance (e.g., chain-smoking), or recover from its effects.
6. Important social, occupational, or recreational activities are given up or reduced because of substance use.
7. The substance use is continued despite knowledge of having a persistent or recurrent physical or psychological problem that is likely to have been caused or exacerbated by the substance (e.g., current cocaine use despite recognition of cocaine-induced depression, or continued drinking despite recognition that an ulcer was made worse by alcohol consumption).

In addition, the following signs and symptoms of addiction for the physically active individual or athlete may be viewed in the following three categories:

1. *Attendance problems.* Absences for vague ailments of implausible reasons and sporadic attendance.

2. *Athletic performance.* General deterioration of performance, spasmodic work pace, wandering attention, lack of concentration, increased "off" days, and performance far below expected level.

3. *General behavior.* Increase in excuses; athlete's statements become undependable; begins to avoid teammates and coaches away from performance area; borrows money from teammates, trainers, or coaches; exaggerates accomplishments; repeated minor injuries on and off the field and court; unreasonable resentments; increasing difficulty with assignments; poor performance reports; increasing infraction with university, job, or team; grandiose, aggressive, or belligerent behavior; apparent loss of ethical values; money problems; malingering injuries; refuses to discuss problems; and legal problems (DWI, possession, etc.).

Various screening instruments are available to assist helping professionals validate their diagnosis. These instruments range from simple question-and-answer interviews to sophisticated, computer-scored instruments. Kinney and Leaton (1991) recommend that all helping professionals utilize some sort of screening instrument in combination with a drug-use history. Once a diagnosis is formulated, questions of how to inform the athlete arise and will be discussed in the section on intervention. In addition to recognizing signs and symptoms of addiction, it is also important to determine if an ingestive or process addiction is present. An ingestive addiction refers to the ingesting of mood-altering chemicals whereas process addictions encompass behavior patterns (e.g., gambling or sexual addictions). One particular process addiction, gambling, is included in this section because of its troubling impact in sports.

Compulsive gambling is problematic for athletes in that it puts the person and their eligibility at risk. Two categories describe problematic gambling behavior. First, problem gambling involves minor problems in family, work, or financial areas related to gambling but the behavior does not meet any diagnostic criteria (van Wormer & Davis, 2003). Second, to meet diagnostic criteria for pathological (compulsive) gambling, which is included in the DSM-IV-TR as an impulse control disorder rather than a substance use disorder, at least five or more criteria should be met (APA, 2000). Some of the criteria for pathological gambling include many of the same elements in an addiction, such as preoccupation, increasing amounts of money spent, multiple efforts to quit or control the behavior, and euphoria (APA, 2000). Men appear at higher risk for gambling-related problems, although surveys indicate one-third of compulsive gamblers are female and the trends show an increasing number of women involved in gambling (Bacon & Russell, 2004; van Wormer & Davis, 2003). Two primary resources developed out of increasing concern about gambling addiction, The National Center for Responsible Gaming (NCRC) and a National Council on Problem Gaming (Miller, 2005).

More research has recently been conducted regarding athletes and gambling problems, with mixed findings. Rockey, Beason, and Gilbert (2002) compared gambling activity of college athletes with nonathletes and found that 81% and 81.3% of the respective groups gambled. The researchers indicated concern due to high prevalence rates of pathological gambling by male athletes, which was twice that of the next highest group, male nonathletes (Rockey et al., 2002). The NCAA strictly prohibits any gambling by college athletes, and sanctions involve permanent loss of eligibility when sport gambling influences outcomes, win/loss margins, or bets involving their own institution (University of Alabama, 2002). The study further noted that 30.4% of the male athletes participated in sport gambling (Rockey et al., 2002), which highlights significant areas of concern for the athletic trainer. Further, of five addictive behaviors studied in college athletes by Bacon and Russell (2004), pathological gambling showed the highest frequency, 15.1%, meeting diagnostic criteria surpassing alcohol use disorders, other drug use disorders, eating disorders, and exercise addiction. The research conclusions reiterate the need for more comprehensive interventions that involve more than primarily educational programs regarding gambling behaviors among athletes and physically active individuals. Much more research is also needed to understand the risk and protective factors involved in preventing and treating gambling addiction in the athletic community. Many other factors, such as genetic and environmental, are involved in helping those with either process or ingestive addictions.

Most current research and treatment approaches point to the multiple genetic and environmental factors in attempting to better understand addiction (Center for Substance Abuse Treatment [CSAT], 2003). Although promising genetic research into addiction has increased in the previous decade, no single biological marker has been defined as the key link to diagnosing addiction (Doweiko, 2006; White, 1998). Addiction specialists rarely debate that addiction is a disease, but many others continue to challenge the nature of addiction with questions about psychological and physical dependency.

PSYCHOLOGICAL DEPENDENCE

An athlete who repeatedly uses mood-altering substances in the belief that the drug helps him or her perform better in school, sports, relationships, sexually, or other key areas in his or her life may be developing a psychological dependence on the drug. This can lead to a psychological belief that his or her performance can only be enhanced while under the influence in any of the previous areas of functioning. A surprising number of collegiate athletes surveyed reported using alcohol (2.2%) or marijuana or hashish (12.9%) before practice or competition (NCAA, 2001). These chemicals are not commonly believed to have athletic performance-enhancing effects, thus raising questions about the psychological perception of the need for such chemicals. Often psychological dependence involves the use of the chemical as a "crutch" (Doweiko, 2006). One who experiences psychological dependence may also meet the clinical criteria for the medical condition of substance abuse.

PHYSICAL DEPENDENCE

The person whose body does not function normally without the use of the mood-altering chemical is often experiencing physical dependence. When any drug is suddenly no longer available to the body and the body experiences difficulty adjusting without the chemical, this is frequently defined as physical dependence (Doweiko, 2006). The basic guideline to determine physical dependency is to assess the presence of a withdrawal syndrome when the drug use ceases; in the absence of a withdrawal syndrome, there is no physical dependency. As with other chemical dependencies, according to the CSAT, alcohol dependence (also referred to as alcoholism) is classified as a disease with distinct and observable symptoms and is chronic (2003).

TOLERANCE AND WITHDRAWAL SYNDROMES

It is important that issues regarding tolerance to mood-altering substances and withdrawal syndromes are available to athletic trainers. Misunderstandings exist about these two important issues when working with athletes. The first issue of tolerance has been misunderstood, especially related to alcohol. Often many drinkers, including athletes who binge drink, mistakenly believe that they are somehow less at risk of substance use complications if they demonstrate greater tolerance of the particular substance or drug combinations. For example, heavy drinkers may brag about their high tolerance for alcohol by explaining how they "can drink others under the table" and show few signs of visible impairment. In fact, studies indicate that a high metabolic and pharmacodynamic tolerance to alcohol yields a greater risk for alcohol dependency—the body is already doing something different in the metabolizing of a toxin than the normal sensitivity one should experience when alcohol is consumed (van Wormer & Davis, 2003). When the body becomes more efficient in eliminating a mood-altering substance, the term *metabolic tolerance* is accurate; when the central nervous system is less affected by the drug, the accurate term is *pharmacodynamic tolerance* (Doweiko, 2002). In fact, 44% of those surveyed in collegiate sports reported usually drinking six or more drinks at any one time and 13.5% of that number indicated 10 or more drinks at one sitting (NCAA, 2001). Thus, athletes who drink heavily are at higher risk for developing substance use disorders and display pharmacodynamic tolerance. Tolerance is one of the first signs of dependency (Doweiko, 2002), and the athletic trainer is well advised to address binge drinking or drug using patterns earlier rather than later in the athlete's career (see also the Intervention section on p. 120). Tolerance patterns help explain why approximately 11% of the drinking population consumes over 50% of the beverage alcohol in this country (Knapp, 1996; van Wormer & Davis, 2003). It takes more of the drug to achieve the desired effect when tolerance develops.

Other drug-use tolerance patterns are similarly of concern to the risk of dependency. Some estimate that an even larger percentage of users of cocaine or heroin, as compared with alcohol users, develop dependency due to a rapid progression of increased tolerance to these drugs; in other words, it takes more of the drug to achieve the desired effect in a relatively short period of time (van Wormer & Davis, 2003). Where the average progression to the end stages of some types of alcoholism involve 30 years, heroin or cocaine addiction can progress to late stages within months or a few years.

Emphasizing the importance of tolerance is important when providing education sessions to athletes in all age ranges. When an athlete, for example a swimmer, begins drinking alcohol, he or she may feel euphoric effects after one drink. With continued drinking, perhaps drinking every weekend, the swimmer may notice after 3 months that she can drink four drinks and experience minimal euphoria, so she increases her intake until there is the desired effect. In that example, the athlete could find that drinking five or six drinks in any one drinking episode is not unusual for her; yet for a female, four or more drinks per drinking episode is defined as abusive drinking. With continued drinking over multiple years, she could see her tolerance increase. It is noted that heavy alcohol use in women increases the chances of osteoporosis (National Institute on Alcohol Abuse and Alcoholism [NIAAA], 2004), a major condition for the physically active individual. The athletic trainer also needs to understand that recent research indicates that women have a greater incidence of complications from alcohol use and experience more physical damage with less alcohol in a shorter time frame than males (NIAAA, 2004). Even with some studies showing cardiovascular benefits with no more than one drink daily, for women, there is also evidence that such daily consumption may increase breast cancer risks (NIAAA, 2004). Therefore, it is critical for the athletic trainer to ascertain when and if tolerance patterns emerge in athletes since tolerance can indicate a major risk factor associated with addiction. Another critical risk factor pertains to substance withdrawal.

Substance withdrawal refers to the physical changes that occur when a substance leaves the body. These changes provide evidence that pharmacodynamic tolerance is present. Most withdrawal symptoms, which are usually the opposite of the drug effects, begin within 4 to 24 hours of last use and continue for varying lengths of time depending on the substance, degree of physical dependence, genetic factors, and overall health of the person (Doweiko, 2006). At its most benign, a hangover after an episode of heavy alcohol intake is one example of withdrawal.

In its more complicated progression, drug withdrawal can manifest in mild to extreme hand, tongue, eyelid, or body tremors; nausea and vomiting; pronounced anxiety, depressed mood, and irritability; anhedonia; delusions, headaches, sleep disturbance, mild to severe seizures; delirium tremens involving visual, auditory, or tactile hallucinations; diarrhea; goose bumps; fever or rhinitis; runny nose; elevated blood pressure and pulse and cardiac arrhythmias (Doweiko, 2006; van Wormer & Davis, 2003). Alcohol withdrawal can involve serious life-threatening conditions. Approximately 15% of alcohol dependent individuals have withdrawal seizures if not medically detoxified and as such should be evaluated by addiction specialists in a medical setting.

Intervention

When athletic trainers work with individuals whose situations are further complicated by alcohol or other drug problems, it is increasingly important to intervene in a responsible manner to address the physically active person's health. As awareness increases in recognizing addictive disorders, certified athletic trainers can learn strategies to successfully intervene in the addictive process of troubled athletes and physically active individuals. Intervening with those impacted by substance use disorders is within the parameters of an athletic trainer's work, "a unique health care provider dedicated to meeting the needs of physically active individuals" (Winterstein, 2003, p. 3). Brief interventions can be effective when working with some individuals. The first step toward determining which type of intervention to utilize often involves one or more screening instruments. Health care professionals are well advised to conduct some type of substance use screening on a regular basis with every individual provided care. There are a range of tools involving brief self-report questionnaires which may be obtained from various Web sites or substance use helping organizations, often at no charge (CSAT, 2003).

Increasing awareness directed toward drug abuse has challenged more health care providers to screen and therapeutically address troubled individuals. These helping professionals include counselors, nurses, psychologists, psychiatrists, teachers, primary care physicians, therapists, athletic trainers, and other professionals in a helping capacity. Interventions range from brief sessions combining counseling and education to the more formal intervention conducted with significant people in the addict's life facilitated by a trained addiction intervention specialist. Because a significant number of certified athletic trainers work in environments other than educational settings, such as sports medicine clinics, hospitals, or industry (Winterstein, 2003), resources within those organizations may include addiction specialists who can assist with appropriate policy development, selection of screening instruments, brief intervention techniques, and referral options. Frequently, specialists in the area of addictive disease are consulted *before* intervening to help clarify specific aspects of intervening and treating those struggling with more complex addiction issues. If at all possible, involve the Employee Assistance Program (EAP) staff in intervention issues. Most business and industry settings and some collegiate and professional teams have EAP contracts for counseling services that can help the athletic trainer in a variety of different ways, such as providing recommendations for treatment centers and monitoring the athlete's aftercare and follow-up.

Brief interventions are effective ways to reduce problems associated with substances (CSAT, 2003; NIAAA, 2003). Continued education in brief intervention techniques with

Table 4-2

Brief Screening With CAGE

Letter	Accompanying question
C	Have you ever felt that you should cut down on your drinking?
A	Have people annoyed you by criticizing your drinking?
G	Have you ever felt bad or guilty about your drinking?
E	Have you ever had a drink first thing in the morning to steady your nerves or get rid of a hangover (eye-opener)?

With one positive response to any of the four questions, investigate whether any of the positive responses occurred within the previous year, if so, then:
- One or two positive responses indicates a current alcohol-related problem needing assessment, preferably by an addiction specialist.
- Three or four positive responses indicates possible alcohol dependence and requires further assessment, preferably by an addiction specialist (Ewing, 1984 as cited in NIAAA, 2003).

individuals experiencing mild or moderate substance use problems can be obtained through workshops if no addiction specialist is available. NIAAA (2003) is one resource for training in brief intervention models and is quite involved in working with college settings to provide brief intervention trainings as well as reduce the incidence of binge drinking (Saltz & DeJong, 2002). The athletic trainer and other members of the sports medicine team can incorporate a Four-Step Model as outlined by NIAAA and are advised: "You can significantly reduce problem drinking in your patients—and its medical consequences—by conducting brief interventions" (2003, p. 3). The recommended first step includes inquiries about patterns and consequences of alcohol use, including a brief 4-item screening tool called CAGE (Table 4-2).

If the person is not referred to an addiction specialist, the next two steps involve assessment and advising by the health practitioner to either abstain if dependence is indicated or cut down on the alcohol use if alcohol-related problems are indicated (NIAAA, 2003). Examples of advising include a statement of concern about the drinking, the athletic trainer's recommendation, and determining readiness for change by the individual. Sample advising when problem drinking is indicated might include, "I am concerned about what you've shared about your drinking. I believe it is best for you to cut back. How ready are you to try to cut back drinking at this time?" If there is mutual agreement between the health practitioner and the patient to decrease alcohol use, in this case the athletic trainer and athlete, then help the athlete set a reasonable goal "to further lessen other risks, including injuries or impaired driving, the daily limit may be reduced to less than two drinks for men and less than one drink for women" (NIAAA, 2003, p. 7). Further, it is suggested that the individual examine pros and cons of drinking, situations that might foster heavier drinking, and alternatives that promote healthier consumption patterns. A major aspect of the advising stage involves providing various educational materials (see Glossary and Internet Resources on p. 303). Finally, inquire about the athlete's feelings toward this plan of action, and then in step 4 arrange how this plan will be monitored in the same way the athletic trainer monitors any other rehabilitation plan (NIAAA, 2003).

Brief interventions are not indicated if the need for specialized care for a more complicated substance use disorder is established (CSAT, 2003). The athletic trainer needs to have a clear and definite plan for referring the athlete to specialized addictive disease services.

In more complicated cases in which addiction is suspected, it can be quite challenging when an individual meets with the athletic trainer to discuss concerns. If the recommendations for treatment are shared with the athlete or physically active person, an athletic trainer may find themselves faced with strong resistance to comply. Often, denial is the hallmark of the disease of addiction; therefore, refusal to receive help for addiction is not uncommon. Working with a person in a therapeutic relationship while he or she is refusing help for active addiction complicates progress the person may be trying to make toward other goals (Johnson, 1980). The helping professional is encouraged to develop skills concerning more formal interventions with the chemically dependent person with the help of a trained addiction intervention specialist (James & Gilliland, 2005). Because of heightened sensitivity and risk management issues, it is further recommended that the athletic trainer avoid one-on-one sessions to intervene with someone with substance dependency; "individual confrontation with addicts is futile because of their superior ability to deny, threaten, cajole, plead, and otherwise subvert attempts to interfere with pursuit of their addiction" (James & Gilliland, 2005, p. 296). However, documenting any patterns of use of mood-altering chemicals or problematic behavior often provides important facts that serve as key elements in successful treatment. In addition, documentation of treatment recommendations including assessment findings is also highly recommended.

Overall, of great importance is the athletic trainer's awareness of his or her own personal attitudes toward addiction and treatment (Kinney & Leaton, 1991). Conveying genuine concern and hopefulness with empathy is particularly important (James & Gilliland, 2005; Johnson, 1980). A judgmental, moralizing attitude often gives the alcoholic/addict opportunities to be well-defended, close-minded, and untreated. Assisting the athlete to view substance-related problems as a serious medical issue, rather than a fault-finding experience, is beneficial in the intervention process (Kinney & Leaton, 1991).

When researching addiction treatment settings, it may be important for the athletic trainer to understand important aspects about treatment in the United States. Structured treatment for alcoholism began in the 1940s (Spicer, 1993; Toft, 1995). Until recently, the standard treatment for alcohol and other substance abuse was an inpatient residential approach. A belief existed that removing addicted individuals from their environment was the best approach to treating substance abuse problems utilizing a model often referred to as the Minnesota Model. It is the dominant treatment approach for addiction in the United States (James & Gilliland, 2005; Spicer, 1993). The model has been described as a multidisciplinary approach involving physicians, counselors, clergy, and recovering people caring for the individuals in treatment for substance abuse (Spicer, 1993). Two major goals of this cognitive-behavioral model are to encourage complete abstinence from all mind-altering chemicals and to "help the patient unlearn a self-destructive lifestyle" (Spicer, 1993, p. 45).

In the late 1980s intensive outpatient programs utilizing the Minnesota Model began replacing residential treatment and demonstrated equal effectiveness related to beneficial outcomes of sustained abstinence (Allen & Phillips, 1993; Washton & Stone-Washton, 1993; White, 1998). Intensive outpatient treatment had added appeal to utilization reviewers, the insurance industry, employers, family members, and clients due to reduced costs for care and flexibility of scheduling, which often allowed individuals to continue to work and live at home while receiving treatment. Overall, the efficacy of intensive outpatient treatment has been favorable and it has become the preferred treatment modality for substance use disorders (Allen & Phillips, 1993; White, 1998).

Establishing referral resources options before they are needed is vital to facilitating appropriate care. The alcoholic/addict often seeks any excuse to reject plans for treatment. A list of suggestions for developing referral resources follows:

- Make a list of treatment options, especially intensive outpatient programs, in the community. (The yellow pages often provide a comprehensive listing of agencies and counselors specializing in addictive disease cases or numerous Web sites).

- Investigate those on the list by calling and asking for written information. For example, fact sheets describing the treatment that is provided, facility license information, number of certified and licensed counselors on staff, financial requirements, referral procedures, type of client treated (alcoholics only, polysubstance dependencies, family members and/or significant others, addicts who are HIV positive, etc.).

- Select three to five treatment programs and visit them if possible. Develop relationships with clinicians, as they may consult on difficult cases.

- Follow-up with references and check to make sure that treatment specialists are recommended by other clinicians.

- Keep information with written descriptions of service providers to offer in an easy-to-access file.

- Obtain necessary consents for release of information.

- Be prepared for the athlete to refuse any counseling services.

Many providers offer evaluations or second opinions at no charge and can assist with admission to outpatient or inpatient programs. Again, alcoholics/addicts can readily fall through the cracks when given the opportunity, due to the nature of denial (Kinney & Leaton, 1991). Providing the athlete with written information regarding the referral is often useful to reduce the amount of distortion that occurs with addiction. Be prepared, with a written consent for the release of confidential information, to provide the referral site with any requested data; this data can be invaluable to the counseling staff as the athlete's denial is confronted and appropriate treatment planning is begun. A comprehensive treatment plan can make a substantial impact on beneficial treatment outcomes (Veach, Remley, Sorg, & Kippers, 2000). It is further advised that the athletic trainer specify what type of treatment updates are required from the treatment provider (e.g., monthly, bi-annually, etc.). It is also advised that the athletic trainer immediately direct the client to medical care if he or she knows of any physical complications in past withdrawal attempts or present physical distress. Since addicts/alcoholics also have a higher suicide rate than average, this should also be explored and appropriate care should be given (such as a behavioral contract) or immediate referral to a qualified mental health professional (such as a counselor or psychiatrist) (Doweiko, 2002; Erickson, 2001; George, 1990).

The athletic trainer needs to determine their comfort level regarding the possible risks of intervention. When confronted with recommendations, some individuals become hostile and agitated, especially if they perceive that a loss of job, family, team status, eligibility, or financial standing is associated with the recommendation for treatment. The stigma associated with addiction is still prevalent in the United States and this can contribute greatly to an athlete's resistance in accepting any recommendations to address substance use. There is a risk of the athlete quitting the team as a result of these issues even when the best preparation for intervening is conducted.

The family, significant other(s), friend(s), or coaching personnel may also express dissatisfaction with the athletic trainer's recommendations. This may be seen in behavior such as rescuing the athlete and refusing to support the diagnosis; minimizing the symptoms associated with addiction due to fear that the individual may lose his or her eligibility, income, and/or relationship; refusal to support treatment because of their own denial if they have an undiagnosed chemical dependency; and a variety of other nonsupportive behaviors.

There is always risk of litigation in sensitive cases and therefore the importance of strict adherence to written policies, procedures, and guidelines about confidentiality is of extreme importance with addicted individuals. If there is any illegal activity, such as selling illegal drugs, the athlete is usually increasingly suspicious and distrusting of any information being released, even for referral purposes.

Finally, the risk of a failed intervention is always a reality—the athlete may not follow through on the recommendations and a painful crisis may arise. A small percentage of those faced with intervention have walked away from school, scholarships, family, job, or home instead of accepting treatment for their addiction (Johnson, 1980). Continued assistance for the family and significant other(s) is crucial at this stage. This may involve referring loved ones to addiction specialists skilled in family addictive issues. If at all possible, preparation for this risk is well-advised before any formal intervention takes place.

INTERVENTIONS WITH ADDICTION

Perhaps one of the most utilized intervention models for confronting the newly identified chemically dependent person is the Johnson Institute Model of Intervention (Johnson, 1980). This approach involves the following critical aspects for confronting the addicted person, and obtaining the help of a trained addiction intervention specialist is highly recommended (Fisher & Harrison, 1997).

- If at all possible, significant people in the individual's life present specific facts. The presence of the athletic trainer may be critical in a formal intervention due to the important observations of behavior and valued opinion of the athletic trainer to the individual. (Two or more people are recommended; careful preparation is often advised for how these additional people share information with the client).

- Avoid generalizations, broad statements, or opinions (e.g., "You drink too much").

- Concern for the person is to be emphasized; avoid being judgmental. It is critical the athletic trainer convey concern when genuine. At no time should concern be feigned in this delicate process of intervention. However, if the athletic trainer has become over-involved with the person and is primarily experiencing anger toward the individual, an addiction specialist would advise against inclusion of the athletic trainer in the meeting since anger directed toward the athlete often increases defensive behavior and can derail the intervention.

- Relate specific facts of incidents to drinking/drug-related behavior. For example, "Over the past 3 months, I treated you for three inversion ankle sprains. I detected the odor of alcohol on your breath two of the three times I treated the injuries, and I see practice was missed on four of 12 Mondays."

- The descriptions of specific facts should include as much detail as possible, as demonstrated in the preceding example, without conclusions, generalizations, or diagnoses. An example of a statement that could follow the factual information in the preceding example and would be unhelpful might be: "So it sure looks to me that you have a bad drinking problem and you better get some help." Focus clearly on factual information that is directly observed or noted by the athletic trainer. At no time should the athletic trainer make a diagnosis; this should be done by an addiction specialist after a thorough evaluation. There are multiple reasons for the athletic trainer not to act as a diagnostician when dealing with substance use disorders. Primarily a diagnosis by the athletic trainer can jeopardize the helping relationship with the athlete or physically active person by damaging the important trust placed in the athletic trainer.

- Have the goal of intervention include conveying the facts so the person can accept help for his or her addiction.
- Present clear choices to the person. For example, "At this time, the sports medicine team supports evaluation and treatment as recommended by an addiction specialist or you will be ineligible for play this year." In addition, prepare those involved in the confrontation for possible reactions to choices presented. Discuss the course of action if the athlete storms out of the session. Designate how follow-up should occur and by whom. Many recommend that an evaluation by an addiction specialist be prearranged and transportation to the appointment be provided immediately from the intervention session.

In addition, there are some obstacles to consider (Johnson, 1980). The roadblocks to a successful intervention are as follows:

- Waiting for the alcoholic/addict to "see the light" and admit there is a problem.
- Making judgmental statements such as, "You don't care about getting better. If you did, you'd agree to get help, stop drinking, stop lying, etc."
- Broad accusations such as, "You drink all the time!"
- Getting angry with the person because he or she will not agree he or she has a problem, give excuses, blame others, etc.
- Confronting the athlete one-on-one with no leverage available (such as significant others, coaches, team physician, or family member) to help him or her get specialized chemical dependency care.
- No facts about his or her behavior related to substance abuse/dependency.
- Negative feelings about alcoholics/addicts (e.g., projection issues).
- "You" statements.
- Fear of reaction (e.g., rejection, anger, etc.).
- The person is actively under the influence of mood-altering chemicals during the intervention.
- Inadequate preparation.
- Inadequate resources for referral and/or assistance.

After considering the risks associated with confronting the alcoholic/addict about his or her disease, it is hoped that the athletic trainer can see the value to those receiving treatment for their disease of addiction. Helping professionals from various settings can make a significant difference in getting a person the care needed when faced with an addictive disease. Even when the athlete or physically active person rejects help, the family may still benefit from learning how to cope with addiction in healthier ways. This may be a catalyst for the addicted individual to accept treatment within a year rather than waiting 10 more years. The possible benefits of confrontation often outweigh the risks. In 2003, 1.9 million individuals with substance use disorders in the United States (0.8% of the total population and 8.5% of those needing specialized care) received treatment for alcohol or other drug issues. Unfortunately, approximately 20.3 million people needing specialized treatment for substance use disorders did not receive the needed care (SAMHSA, 2004). With the increased awareness of addiction and a variety of instruments to assist in identifying the alcoholic/addict, there are compelling reasons to gain skills to intervene with the troubled athlete. Roadblocks and risks associated with intervening are present, but with increasing acknowledgment and preparation these negative influences can be reduced by the athletic trainer. Until addiction is successfully addressed, progress is limited in other areas of a person's life and often sabotaged by active addiction. As Knapp recounts, "I had always thought: *I drink because I'm unhappy... Maybe, just maybe, I'm unhappy because I drink*" (1996, p. 240). Not every athlete will respond favorably to intervention, but for those who do, it is often the beginning of living a quality life.

The athletic trainer may also encounter those physically active individuals who are in recovery from addiction and are challenged with relapse prevention. In the case of any return to social drinking, "the odds are from 50:1 to 100:1 against his or her being able to handle it" (James & Gilliland, 2005, p. 313). A major emphasis by the athletic trainer can be on helping the individual to identify and reduce high-risk situations, or triggers, for using or drinking. A written, comprehensive rehabilitation plan, similar to plans dealing with recovery from a physical injury, can be most beneficial for the recovering athlete. The athletic trainer is encouraged to speak directly about recovery issues and challenges with the alcoholic or addict. Better yet, developing effective prevention strategies may help greatly reduce the need for formal intervention.

Much work has been done by athletic trainers to create prevention programs in athletic organizations. Often effective prevention can negate the need for formal intervention for many at-risk athletes. There is evidence suggesting that prevention efforts have resulted in lower use rates of mood-altering drugs. The largest percentage of athletes surveyed in the NCAA study indicated their drug use began in high school. There were an estimated 14 million adolescents (56%) who participated in team sports according to one national report (SAMHSA, 2002). Prevention specialists point out the need to do more prevention in elementary and middle school settings where students are already making decisions about use. Although high school is still an important time to work with young athletes who are exposed to opportunities to use mood-altering drugs, it can be too late to begin prevention efforts for the most successful outcome (Naylor et al., 2001). A national survey noted that the rates of use in a recent month of mood-altering substances for young people aged 12 to 17 was lower among those participating in team sports than those not participating in any team sports (SAMHSA, 2002). The college-age athlete is also amenable to focused efforts on prevention, as one study found athletes identified their participation in sports as an important factor for abstinence or limiting their alcohol intake (Nelson & Wechsler, 2001). Studies that show educational efforts as a single-focus approach do not have a significant effect on reducing harmful drinking or using patterns (Morgan, 2001; Nelson & Wechsler, 2001; Thombs & Hamilton, 2002) and are often rejected by the student athlete. This is possibly due to an over-emphasis on drug education in the past 10 years (Naylor et al., 2001). Ordinarily, education is just one component of any formal comprehensive prevention approach.

Considerable research into effective prevention efforts supports the idea that education alone is insufficient to reduce patterns of misuse of mood-altering chemicals. Comprehensive approaches include multiple levels of intervention, multiple populations (diverse and developmentally oriented), various strategies (information, effective areas, environment), collaboration with resources, various drug effects with consequences, and a long-term commitment grounded in ongoing outcome evaluation (Morgan, 2001, p. 307). In addition, some of the most recent prevention research focuses on identifying risk as well as protective factors and incorporating that information into the prevention programs. Even though involvement in sports is often seen as a protective factor in youth, research is pointing to a complicated pattern of harmful use of some drugs. For example, increased alcohol use by athletes occurs in greater frequency than nonathletes (Leichliter et al.,, 1998; Nelson & Wechsler, 2001; The Higher Education Center for Alcohol and Other Drug Prevention, 2002). Other studies found the importance of identifying the emotional factors that may influence drinking behavior of college athletes. In one study, researchers found that coping strategies and not social reasons were the most significant factors in predicting drinking patterns of female athletes, whereas male athletes were more influenced by social reasons in their drinking patterns (Wilson, Pritchard, & Schaffer, 2004). Gender differences and other diversity influences should be factored in when designing prevention efforts. Another study found significant correlations between psychiatric symptoms, especially depression, and higher rates of alcohol abuse patterns (Miller, Miller, Verhegge, Linville, & Pumariega, 2002). Continued research will help the athletic trainer by providing information such as risk factors that may lead athletes to seek environments where binge drinking is the norm (Wilson et al., 2004). The athletic trainer is best served by consulting with certified prevention specialists as programs are developed in the athletic trainer's areas of responsibility. The following areas are suggestions as the athletic trainer considers a comprehensive prevention program:

- Organize community service activities with athletes or physically active individuals, especially in organizations serving people with addiction or abuse issues, such as in a local treatment center. For example, one treatment center previously organized and marketed an annual "Sober Bowl Party" in the community to highlight having fun without mood-altering substances during the Super Bowl (B. Williams, personal communication, January 28, 2004).

- Plan activities during the off-season and school breaks that engage the athlete in focused drug-free workouts and team-building activities.

- Encourage substance-free residential options for athletes in college or professional team settings.

- Develop a yearly plan for educating student faculty, team management, and administrators about substance use issues pertaining specifically to athletes.

- Schedule individual time with every athlete to discuss and assess lifestyle risks including substance use patterns; local certified or licensed addiction specialists may offer their assistance at no charge.

- Team up with local resources in alcohol and drug enforcement, prevention, and professional substance abuse counseling services, such as an EAP to develop a working advisory board to help with policy development, monitoring, and implementation.

- Meet with local alcohol distributors, bar owners, and servers to develop strategies that emphasize moderation and responsible use with decreased marketing targeting athletes.

- Conduct ongoing outcome evaluation to determine efficacy of prevention efforts.

- Implement random drug testing and screening programs with appropriate policies and procedures.

- Provide regular training regarding the nearly 5,000 banned medications and substances as listed by NCAA and USOC (Prentice, 2003).

- Utilize resources with various Web sites listed in Glossary and Internet Resources on pp. 303 (The Higher Education Center for Alcohol and Other Drug Prevention, 2002).

Continuing efforts toward prevention and intervention can assist the athletic trainer and athletic organization toward helping people achieve healthier living. Ongoing training and collaboration with addiction specialists can assist the athletic trainer in reaching these goals.

Conclusion

This chapter contains information and suggestions in an effort to provide athletic trainers with comprehensive information about various commonly abused substances, societal influences toward substance abuse related to athletes and the physically active, signs and symptoms of substance abuse and addiction, and intervention considerations for the athletic trainer. Hopefully, this information will be a useful resource as athletic trainers work with athletes and physically active individuals whose lives have been negatively impacted by substance abuse and addiction.

Chapter Exercises

1. Engage in an assignment where you attempt to abstain from a cherished substance, behavior, or activity for 1 month. Make journal entries at least twice a week about your experience and self-awareness. How do you think this might affect your work with someone struggling with substance issues? Turn in your journal at the end of the month you selected. Write a 4-page reflection paper on what you learned and how you would utilize this in athletic training.

2. Attend at least one *open* Alcoholics Anonymous (AA) meeting in your local area. Write up your account as follows: Write a 1-page summary of what you learned about your feelings and attitudes. Include feelings about the meeting. Also, describe any feelings, issues, or resistance you experienced before attending the meetings. Did you go alone? Why? Why not? What stood out for you? How will you use this experience in your work with athletes and physically active individuals?

   Do not use any names (anonymity is essential), and remember to go to OPEN meetings for AA groups. Speaker meetings are recommended. For those who may have attended AA on a regular basis, it is recommended that they attend other types of 12-step groups for this assignment.

3. On 3 x 5 notecards, create a version of "Substance Abuse Jeopardy." On one card, write select questions from the chapter and on the next card write the accompanying answer. Test yourself by trying to match the correct answer with the correct question. For example, one answer might read, ".08 BAC," then review the questions to find the matching question, "What is the legal blood alcohol concentration limit in 45 states that constitutes DUI?"

4. Interview an addiction specialist in your local area. Prepare a list of 5 questions to ask. Write up your experience, highlighting what learned. Place all notecards in a basket and have the speaker draw out as many questions as time allows.

5. Brainstorm about a comprehensive prevention program for various work settings. List unique considerations to your ideal work setting relevant to your work as an athletic trainer. For example, you might develop a prevention program for a business setting if you imagine you will be working in a corporate environment. Report on important considerations for each particular setting and ways to address the unique issues.

6. Arrange for a phone call with at least two different treatment programs specializing in the treatment of substance use disorders. Utilize the same questions for both as they describe their referral, treatment, and aftercare services. After the phone

calls, rank your order of the centers and list the similarities and differences. Note any concerns or beneficial features that make one center your top referral choice. List ways to develop referral options for athletes and physically active individuals that the athletic trainer may be assisting. Start a file folder labeled "referral resources" and include the material you obtained from your phone interviews.

References

Allen, M. G., & Phillips, K. L. (1993). Utilization review of treatment for chemical dependence. *Hospital and Community Psychiatry, 44,* 752-756.

American Psychiatric Association. (2000). *Diagnostic and statistical manual of mental disorders* (4th ed., text revision). Washington, DC: Author.

Bacon, V. L., & Russell, P. J. (2004). Addiction and the college athlete: The Multiple Addictive Behaviors Questionnaire (MABQ) with college athletes. *The Sport Journal, 7,* 2. Retrieved February 17, 2005, from http://www.thesportjournal.org/2004Journal/Vol7-No2/BaconRussell

Berkowitz, A. D. (2004). *The social norms approach: Theory, research and annotated bibliography.* The Higher Education Center for Alcohol and Other Drug Prevention. Retrieved February 10, 2005, from http://www.edc.org/hec/socialnorms/theory

Breggin, P. R. (1991). *Toxic psychiatry.* New York: St. Martin's Press.

Center for Substance Abuse Treatment. (2003). What you should know about alcohol problems. *Substance Abuse in Brief, 2*(1), 1-6.

Copeland, J. L. (2002). *Withstanding the test of time: NCAA drug-testing program has been more than effective deterrent for substance abuse.* Retrieved January 27, 2005 from http://www.ncaa.org/news/2002/20020930/active/3920n24.html

Doweiko, H. E. (2002). *Concepts of chemical dependency* (5th ed.). Pacific Grove, CA: Brooks/Cole.

Doweiko, H. E. (2006). *Concepts of chemical dependency* (6th ed.). Belmont, CA: Brooks/Cole.

Erickson, S. (2001). Etiological theories of substance abuse. In P. Stevens & R. L. Smith (Eds.), *Substance abuse counseling: Theory and practice* (2nd ed., pp. 77-112). Upper Saddle River, NJ: Prentice-Hall.

Falkowski, C. L. (2000). *Dangerous drugs: An easy-to-use reference for parents and professionals.* Center City, MN: Hazelden.

Fisher, G. L., & Harrison, T. C. (1997). *Substance abuse: Information for school counselors, social workers, therapists, and counselors.* Needham Heights, MA: Allyn & Bacon.

George, R. L. (1990). *Counseling the chemically dependent: Theory and practice.* Upper Saddle River, NJ: Prentice Hall.

Goldberg, L., Elliott, D. L., MacKinnon, D. P., Moe, E., Kuehl, K. S., Nohre, L., et al. (2003). Drug testing athletes to prevent substance abuse: Background and pilot study results of the SATURN (Student athlete testing using random notification) study. *Journal of Adolescent Health, 32,* 16-25.

Hall, J. (2004). Ephedrine ban has holes. *The Free Lance-Star.* Retrieved February 13, 2005, from http://www.freelancestar.com/News/FLS/2004/052004/05182004/1360590

Helwig, A., & Holicky, R. (1994). Substance abuse in persons with disabilities: Treatment considerations. *Journal for Counseling and Development, 72,* 227-233.

Inciardi, J. A., & Goode, J. L. (2004). OxyContin: Miracle medicine or problem drug? In J. C. Inciardi & K. McElrath (Eds.), *The American drug scene* (4th ed., pp. 163-173). Los Angeles, CA: Roxbury Publishing.

James, R. K., & Gilliland, B. E. (2005). *Crisis intervention strategies.* Belmont, CA: Thomson Books/Cole.

Johnson, V. E. (1980). *I'll quit tomorrow* (revised ed.). New York, NY: Harper & Row.

Kinney, J., & Leaton, G. (Eds.). (1991). *Loosening the grip: A handbook of alcohol information* (4th ed.). Baltimore, MD: Mosby-Year Book, Inc.

Knapp, C. (1996). *Drinking: A love story.* New York, NY: Dell Publishing.

Kubes, N. (1990). Hospital intervention for the chemically dependent patient. *Professional Counselor,* 30-32.

Leichliter, J. S., Meilman, P. W., Presley, C. A., & Cashin, J. R. (1998). Alcohol use and related consequences among students with varying levels of involvement in college athletics. *Journal of American College Health, 46*(6), 257-263.

Longo, L. P., & Johnson, B. (2000). *Addiction: Part I benzodiazepines—side effects, abuse risks, and alternatives.* The American Academy of Family Physicians. Retrieved February 11, 2005, from http://www.aafp.org/afp/20000401/2121.html

Miller, B. E., Miller, M. N., Verhegge, R., Linville, H. H., & Pumariega, A. J. (2002). Alcohol misuse among college athletes: Self-medication for psychiatric symptoms? *Journal of Drug Education, 32*(1), 41-52.

Miller, G. A. (2005). *Learning the language of addiction counseling* (2nd ed.). Hoboken, NJ: John Wiley & Sons.

Miller, M. A. (2004). History and epidemiology of amphetamine abuse in the United States. In J. C. Inciardi & K. McElrath (Eds.), *The American drug scene* (4th ed., pp. 252-266). Los Angeles, CA: Roxbury Publishing.

Morgan, O. J. (2001). Prevention. In P. Stevens & R. L. Smith (Eds.), *Substance abuse counseling: Theory and practice* (2nd ed., pp. 299-320). Upper Saddle River, NJ: Prentice-Hall.

National Collegiate Athletic Association. (2001). *NCAA study of substance use habits of college student-athletes.* Indianapolis, IN: Author.

National Highway Traffic Safety Administration. (2004). *The economic burden of traffic crashes on employers,* posted January 15, 2004. U.S. Department of Transportation. Retrieved January 12, 2005, from http://www.nhtsa.dot.gov/people/injury/airbags/EconomicBurden/index.html

National Institute on Alcohol Abuse and Alcoholism. (2003). *Helping patients with alcohol problems: A health practitioner's guide.* NIH Publication No. 03-3769. Rockville, MD: NIAAA.

National Institute on Alcohol Abuse and Alcoholism. (2004). Alcohol—An important women's health issue. *Alcohol Alert, 62,* 2-6.

National Institute on Drug Abuse. (2004). *Methamphetamine abuse and addiction.* Research Report Series. Retrieved January 20, 2005 from http://ww.drugabuse.gov/ResearchReports/Methamph/methamph2

Naylor, A. H., Gardner, D., & Zaichkowsky, L. (2001) Drug use patterns among high school athletes and non-athletes. *Adolescence, 36*(144), 627-640.

Nelson, T. F., & Wechsler, H. (2001). Alcohol and college athletes. *Medicine & Science in Sports and Exercise, 33*(1), 43-47.

Ohlms, D. L. (1982). *The disease concept of alcoholism.* Belleville, IL: Gary Whiteaker Co.

Physician's Desk Reference (56th ed.). (2002). Montvale, NJ: Medical Economics Company, Inc.

Polcin, D. L. (2000). Professional counseling versus specialized programs for alcohol and drug abuse treatment. *Journal of Addictions & Offender Counseling, 21,* 2-11.

Prentice, W. E. (2003). *Arnheim's principles of athletic training: A competency-based approach* (11th ed.). New York, NY: McGraw Hill.

Rockey, D. L., Beason, K. R., & Gilbert, J. D. (2002). Gambling by college athletes: An association between problem gambling and athletes. *eGambling, 7.* Retrieved February 17, 2005, from http:// www.camh.net/egambling/issue7/research/college_gambling

Saltz, R. F., & DeJong, W. (2002). *Reducing alcohol problems on campus: A guide to planning and evaluation.* Rockville, MD: NIAAA.

Siegal, H. A., & Inciardi, J. A. (2004). A brief history of alcohol. In J. C. Inciardi & K. McElrath (Eds.), *The American drug scene* (4th ed., pp. 74-79). Los Angeles, CA: Roxbury Publishing.

Spicer, J. (1993). *The Minnesota Model: The evolution of the multi-disciplinary approach to addiction recovery.* Center City, MN: Hazelden Educational Materials.

Stevens, P., & Smith, R. L. (2001). Substance abuse counseling: Theory and practice (2nd ed.). Upper Saddle River, NJ: Prentice Hall.

Substance Abuse and Mental Health Services Administration. (2002). *Team sports participation and substance use among youths.* The National Household Survey on Drug Abuse Report. Rockville, MD: Office of Applied Studies, Substance Abuse and Mental Health Services Administration.

Substance Abuse and Mental Health Services Administration. (2003). *Overview of findings from the 2002 National Survey on Drug Use and Health.* (NHSDA Series H-21, DHHS Publication No. SMA 03-3774). Rockville, MD: Office of Applied Studies, Substance Abuse and Mental Health Services Administration.

Substance Abuse and Mental Health Services Administration. (2004). *Results from the 2003 National Survey on Drug Use and Health: National findings* (NSDUH Series H–25, DHHS Publication No. SMA 04–3964). Rockville, MD: Office of Applied Studies, Substance Abuse and Mental Health Services Administration.

The Higher Education Center for Alcohol and Other Drug Prevention. (2002). *College athletes and alcohol and other drug use.* Newton, MA: Education Development Center, Inc.

Thombs, D. L., & Hamilton, M. J. (2002). Effects of a social norm feedback campaign on the drinking norms and behavior of Division I student-athletes. *Journal of Drug Education, 32*(3), 227-244.

Toft, D. (1995). The Minnesota Model—Humane, holistic, flexible. *Hazelden News & Professional Update, 1-2,* 16.

University of Alabama. (2002). *Gambling: Consequences and penalties.* Retrieved February 17, 2005, from University of Alabama official athletic website: http://www.rolltide.com/Compliance/8496.asp

van Wormer, K., & Davis, D. R. (2003). *Addiction treatment: A strengths perspective.* Pacific Grove, CA: Brooks/Cole.

Veach, L. J., Remley, T. P., Sorg, J. D., & Kippers, S. M. (2000). Retention predictors related to intensive outpatient programs for substance use disorders. *The American Journal of Drug and Alcohol Abuse, 26*(3), 417-428.

Washton, A. M., & Stone-Washton, N. (1993). Outpatient treatment of cocaine and crack addiction: A clinical perspective. In F. M. Tims & C. G. Leukefield (Eds.), *Cocaine treatment: Research and clinical perspectives* (NIDA Research Monograph No. 135, NIH Pub No. 93-3639, pp. 15-30). Rockville, MD: National Institute on Drug Abuse.

Watson, J. C. (2002). Assessing the potential for alcohol-related issues among college student-athletes. *Athletic Insight, 4*(3). Retrieved December 2, 2004, from http://www.athleticinsight.com/Vol4Iss3/AlcoholAssessment.htm

Weil, A., & Rosen, W. (1983). *Chocolate to morphine.* Boston, MA: Houghton Mifflin.

White, W. L. (1998). *Slaying the dragon: The history of addiction treatment and recovery in America.* Bloomington, IL: Chestnut Health Systems.

Wilson, G. S., Pritchard, M. E., & Schaffer, J. (2004). Athletic status and drinking behavior in college students: The influence of gender and coping styles. *Journal of American College Health, 52*(6), 269-273.

Winterstein, A. P. (2003). *Athletic training student primer: A foundation for success.* Thorofare, NJ: SLACK Incorporated.

Zickler, P. (2002). Methamphetamine abuse linked to impaired cognitive and motor skills despite recovery of dopamine transporters. *NIDA Research Findings, 17*(1), 4-6.

Chapter

DISORDERED EATING

Teresa B. Fletcher, PhD, LPC, NCC
Mark E. Cole, MS, ATC, LAT, CSCS
Barbara B. Meyer, PhD

Chapter Objectives

❖ To provide a comprehensive overview of the continuum of disordered eating (DE), which includes clinical eating disorders (anorexia nervosa [AN], bulimia nervosa [BN], and eating disorders not otherwise specified [NOS]) and related disorders (body dysmorphic disorder [BDD], exercise dependence, and binge-eating disorder [BED]).

❖ To examine the etiology of DE and consequences of clinical eating disorders as a means of understanding the severity of the problem as well as developing an appreciation for early detection, education, and multidisciplinary treatment methods.

❖ To provide an overview of prevention strategies, including warning signs and suggestions for creating a healthy sport environment and developing multidisciplinary alliances will be offered.

❖ To describe types of treatment available and the multidisciplinary team of professionals (e.g., medical, mental health, etc.) who provide these services with the intent of providing athletic trainers with a global perspective of DE.

❖ To highlight the role of the ATC in the education, prevention, diagnosis, and treatment of DE.

NATA Educational Competencies

Risk Management and Injury Prevention Domain

1. Explain the risk factors associated with physical activity.

2. Identify and explain the risk factors associated with common congenital and acquired abnormalities, disabilities, and diseases.

3. Identify and explain the epidemiology data related to the risk of injury and illness related to participation in physical activity.

4. Identify and explain the recommended or required components of a preparticipation examination based on appropriate authorities' rules, guidelines, and/or recommendations.

5. Explain the precautions and risks associated with exercise in special populations.

Psychosocial Intervention and Referral Domain

1. Describe the roles and function of various community-based health care providers (to include, but not limited, to: psychologists, counselors, social workers, human resources personnel) and the accepted protocols that govern the referral of patients to these professionals.

2. Identify the symptoms and clinical signs of common eating disorders and the psychological and sociocultural factors associated with these disorders.

3. Describe the basic signs and symptoms of mental disorders (psychoses), emotional disorders (neuroses, depression), or personal/social conflict (family problems, academic or emotional stress, personal assault or abuse, sexual assault, sexual harassment), the contemporary personal, school, and community health service agencies, such as community-based psychological and social support services that treat these conditions and the appropriate referral procedures for accessing these health service agencies.

4. Explain the potential need for psychosocial intervention and referral when dealing with populations requiring special consideration (to include but not limited to those with exercise-induced asthma, diabetes, seizure disorders, drug allergies and interactions, unilateral organs, physical and/or mental disability)

5. Demonstrate the ability to conduct an intervention and make the appropriate referral of an individual with a suspected substance abuse or other mental health problem. Effective lines of communication should be established to elicit and convey information about the patient's status. While maintaining patient confidentiality, all aspects of the intervention and referral should be documented using standardized recordkeeping methods.

Nutritional Aspects of Injuries and Illnesses

1. Describe common illnesses and injuries that are attributed to poor nutrition (e.g. effects of poor dietary habits on bone loss, on injury, on long-term health, and on other factors)

2. Identify and interpret pertinent scientific nutritional comments or position papers (e.g. healthy weight loss, fluid replacement, pre-event meals, and others

3. Describe disordered eating and eating disorders (i.e., signs, symptoms, physical and psychological consequences, referral systems

4. Demonstrate the ability to recognize disordered eating and eating disorders, establish a professional helping relationship with the patient, interact through support and education, and encourage vocal discussion and other support through referral to the appropriate medical professionals.

DE can be described as a continuum of behaviors ranging from mild to severe in which consequences can lead to starvation and even death. There are two types of terms used to describe these behaviors including DE and clinical eating disorders. DE can be described as an array of behaviors ranging from making consistently bad food choices to potentially harmful eating patterns. Clinical eating disorders are mental health disorders and contain criteria that must be met in order to make a diagnosis (e.g., anorexia, bulimia). Despite beliefs that only certain athletes are at risk for DE (i.e., gymnasts, figure skaters, cross country runners), athletes from all sports (i.e., basketball, tennis) across cultures and including males and females can engage in DE behaviors. Athletic trainers are on the front lines working with athletes and subsequently in a unique position to initiate the process of recognition and treatment.

Overview of Disordered Eating

The definition of what constitutes an eating disorder has evolved over time and is the product of much thought, experience, and research. According to the DSM-IV-TR, (APA, 2000), there are three types of clinical eating disorders: AN, BN, and eating disorders NOS. Diagnosis of these clinical disorders is the responsibility of qualified medical and/or mental health professionals such as counselors, social workers, psychologists, psychiatrists, and/or physicians. In addition to the three clinical disorders identified above is a range of other related disorders or conditions that can influence or be influenced by DE, including BDD, exercise dependence, and BED.

ANOREXIA NERVOSA

AN is used to describe individuals who refuse to maintain a minimum healthy or normal weight, and is characterized by an intense fear of weight gain and significant misperception of body shape, size, or image. It should be noted that fear of weight gain often increases even if actual weight decreases. In children, failure to meet expected weight gains is common. Individuals with AN typically have poor insight into DE behaviors or deny the problem exists and may be unreliable when obtaining weight history. Therefore, outside family members can be consulted to evaluate weight loss (APA, 2000).

Subtypes of AN have been identified (APA, 2000) to reflect research illustrating presentational variation within diagnostic description. AN is structured to include two subtypes: restricting and binge-eating/purging. Individuals are identified as AN-restricting type when their primary mechanisms for weight loss are caloric restriction, excessive exercise, and/or fasting. While everyone demonstrates some variety of food preference (e.g., picky eaters), AN consists of a pattern of behavior and incorrect food-based beliefs (e.g., bread makes you fat). An individual presenting with episodic binge-eating or

---

Table 5-1

Body Mass Index Ranges and Catageories

BMI is a measure of body fat based on height and weight that applies to both adult men and women. For adults over 20 years old, BMI falls into one of these categories:

BMI	Weight Status
Below 18.5	Underweight
18.5 – 24.9	Normal
25.0 – 29.9	Overweight
30.0 and above	Obese

Reprinted with permission of Centers for Disease Control at http://www.cdc.gov/nccdphp/dnpa/bmi/bmi-adult.htm.

---

purging as the primary means for caloric control is classified within the AN-binge-eating/purging type. A binge is defined as "eating in a discrete period of time an amount of food that is definitely larger than most individuals would eat under similar circumstances" (APA, 2000, p. 589). Binging is often accompanied by guilt and subsequent compensatory mechanisms (e.g., purging). Purging can occur through a variety of means, including vomiting, diuretics, enemas, or laxatives. This subtype also defines those who restrict caloric intake and use purging methods even after eating small amounts.

Guidelines for determining low weight for the purpose of diagnosing a clinical eating disorder include use of Body Mass Index (BMI) and weight charts; the most accepted is the Metropolitan Life Insurance tables or periodic growth charts for children and adolescents (Centers for Disease Control and Prevention [CDC], 2002). BMI is a measure of body fat based on height and weight that applies to both adult men and women. It is calculated by dividing weight in pounds (lbs) by height in inches (in) squared and multiplying by a conversion factor of 703 (weight (lb) / [height (in)]^2 x 703). In order to be considered underweight, the BMI must be <17.5 or total weight must be <85% what is considered normal weight as evidenced in Table 5-1 (CDC, 2005). Although concern exists regarding the accuracy of these instruments, they are used as a rough estimate and should not be taken literally nor should they be used in isolation to determine whether or not a person has a clinical eating disorder. Further, athletes have distinctive characteristics and require special consideration to matters regarding weight. Determining ideal weight and consequently what is considered underweight is an individualized process that must take into consideration body size, historical weight, activity level, and athletic performance (i.e., what is an ideal weight for optimal performance for each particular athlete). Determining ideal weight among the athlete population is covered in the Prevention section on p. 150.

Descriptive Features

Although diagnosis is made by qualified professionals, athletic trainers are often in the unique position to notice behaviors associated with DE. Behaviors specific to AN can include obsessive-compulsiveness (i.e., perfectionism), social withdrawal, depressed mood, and restrained emotional expression. Individuals can become excessively concerned about food, eating, weight, and weight-related appearance factors. They also develop a strong desire to exert control over surroundings and tend to be irritable and/or inflexible.

Figure 5-1. The cognitive model of the maintenance of BN. (Reprinted with permission from Fairburn, C. G., & Cooper, Z. [1993]. The eating disorder examinations. In C. G. Fairburn & G. T. Wilson [Eds.], *Binge eating: Nature, assessment, and treatment* [pp. 317-360]. New York, NY: Guilford Press.)

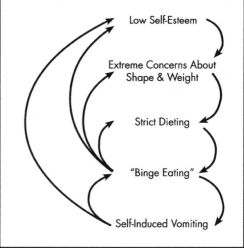

BULIMIA NERVOSA

BN is characterized by binge-eating episodes typically followed by subsequent maladaptive compensatory behaviors (i.e., self-induced vomiting; misuse of laxatives, diuretics, enemas, or other medications; fasting; and/or excessive exercise) for a period of at least 3 months. The compensatory behavior is directed at preventing weight gain following binge-eating. An eating episode is considered to be 2 hours in length and contextually specific (i.e., not inclusive of culturally specific or celebratory feasts) with a perceived lack of control over eating (APA, 2000). Foods included in the binge can vary widely, although high-calorie foods are typically present. Quantity of food consumed is typically a greater concern than the type of food consumed.

BN is a secretive illness typically resulting in guilt after a binge. To remain undetected, episodes may be planned in advance, food consumed quickly, and consumption may occur despite minor interruptions (e.g., phone ringing). However, when intrusions of greater threat occur (e.g., roommates returning home), consumption is more likely to stop. Individuals with BN demonstrate low perceived self-control, which may lead to a broader impairment in their ability to exert control over or resist impulsive (i.e., binge-eating) stimuli (Figure 5-1).

Diagnosis of BN is specified by two types: purging type and nonpurging type. The purging type includes those who regularly engage in self-induced vomiting or the misuse of laxatives, diuretics, or enemas. The nonpurging type is no less pathological but serves to identify those who use other compensatory behaviors such as fasting or excessive exercise but do not regularly engage in purging.

Descriptive Features

The difference between AN binge-eating/purging type and BN binge-eating/purging type is determined by weight. Remember that in order to be diagnosed with AN, the athlete must be underweight, at least 85% or below what is considered normal weight for him or her. Individuals with BN are typically within the normal weight range or even slightly above or below. Athletes with these disorders can also present with depressed mood and anxiety, especially in social situations (APA, 2000). They can become uncomfortable, secretive, and even paranoid around food and often spend an inordinate amount of time and energy planning, buying, and hoarding food as well as planning appropriate times to binge and purge. Substance abuse may also be a factor, particularly with use of alcohol and stimulants in order to suppress and control appetite and weight.

EATING DISORDERS NOT OTHERWISE SPECIFIED

Maladaptive eating behavior that does not meet the criteria for either AN or BN but is still considered pathological is classified as eating disorders NOS. Rationale for utilizing the NOS category is defined by the DSM-IV-TR in instances when:

- The general guidelines for a form of DE are met, but the criteria for a specific disorder and/or subtype are not met.
- Clinically significant distress is caused by a condition or behavior that only meets the general symptomatic presentation.
- Specific etiology is unclear.
- Insufficient data (or time) to make a AN or BN diagnosis.

With regard to the latter, in order for a diagnosis for AN or BN to be made, the individual must meet *all* criteria. Many individuals may meet only a few criteria or all but one criterion, and therefore cannot be diagnosed with the disorder. Yet, these individuals still have pathological DE. Therefore, this NOS category reflects the diversity of presentation possibilities across the DE spectrum.

This category has been repeatedly identified as representing the most frequently seen DE behaviors in both the general and athletic populations (Fairburn & Harrison, 2003; Franko & Omori, 1999; Lilenfeld et al., 1998; Lindeman, Stark, & Keskivaara, 2001; Tyrka, Graber, & Brooks-Gunn, 2000; Tyrka, Waldron, Graber, & Brooks-Gunn, 2002; Vervaet, Audenaert, & Van heeringen, 2003; Wade, Bulik, Sullivan, Neale, & Kendler, 2000). Inclusion of a catch-all category such as NOS is both beneficial and challenging to the identification of DE. It is beneficial because it allows for flexibility to address a serious problem without the confines of meeting specific criteria, but challenging because it is often difficult for the lay person such as an athletic trainer or coach to differentiate between a clinical eating disorder and unhealthy eating habits (Table 5-2).

As stated previously, there are three types of clinical eating disorders. However, other disorders (e.g., BDD, BED) and conditions (e.g., exercise dependence/addiction) exist. While they do not meet the criteria for clinical eating disorders, DE may be a component. Also stated previously, most athletic trainers have neither the capability nor the responsibility to differentiate among the many disorders. They can, however, provide valuable observations of day-to-day behaviors, thereby providing a more comprehensive referral to an appropriate mental health professional.

BODY DYSMORPHIC DISORDER

BDD is a preoccupation with one's appearance that goes beyond simple vanity and may result in significant distress or impairment of daily functioning. Individuals with BDD demonstrate excessive attention to personal physical features leading to detriment of life, health, and relationships (APA, 2000). It is important to note that BDD and DE often occur simultaneously. According to one study, 39% of AN patients also suffered from BDD (unrelated to weight concerns) and 81.3% considered body image their biggest or a major problem (Grant & Phillips, 2004). Further, the onset of BDD usually precedes the onset of an eating disorder (Ruffolo, Phillips, Menard, Fay, & Weisberg, 2006). Although the diagnoses can be comorbid, treatments may be different and both diagnoses should be given when appropriate (Grant & Phillips, 2004).

Table 5-2

Continuum of Disordered Eating Behaviors: Examples of Mild to Severe Cases

Behaviors	*Mild*	*Moderate*	*Severe*	*Disorder(s)*
Exercise	Has a rigid exercise schedule, but it does not interfere with other areas of functioning	Rigid exercise schedule and will miss events (work/social) to exercise	Rigid exercise schedule even when injured or sick; interferes with social/work relationships	Exercise dependence Bulimia nervosa (nonpurging type) Anorexia nervosa (both types) Body Dysmorphic Disorder
Diet restriction	Is health conscious and on occasion restricts food to maintain normal/slightly below normal weight	Is below normal weight, controls portion size, and rejects high-calorie/high-fat foods	Is well below normal weight and maintains low caloric intake for fear of weight gain	Anorexia nervosa (restricting type) Body Dysmorphic Disorder
Binging	Infrequently eats until uncomfortably full (i.e., twice a month)	More frequently eats until uncomfortably full with little control and overweight for height and body type	Uncontrollable eating until full and is obese	Binge-eating disorder Obesity
Purging	Conscious of food intake and may use natural substances such as fruit to cleanse system when feeling "full"	Frequently purges all types of food regardless of binge eating or not	Frequently purging with signs of damage to skin, teeth, esophagus, etc. and bloating/constipation	Bulimia nervosa (purging type) Anorexia nervosa (binge-eating/purging type)

A person with BDD is similar in concept to one with hypochondriasis, or a hypochondriac. For example, just like a hypochondriac will complain of pain that only psychologically exists, the individual with BDD will be preoccupied with a slight or even imagined defect. This preoccupation may include a body part (e.g., nose) or a body region (e.g., face), with an inordinate amount of time spent trying to address the problem area or area(s). Individuals with BDD may compulsively exercise in an effort to burn fat (e.g., cardiovascular activities), build muscle (e.g., lifting weights), or engage in DE to attain a desired

Figure 5-2. Body dysmorphic disorder. (© Fotolia.com.)

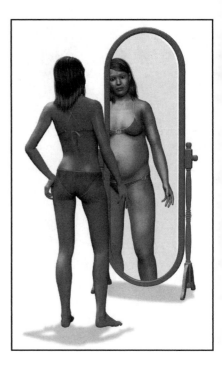

physique. Other individuals may seek more intrusive methods such as plastic surgery to change certain features (i.e., nose job). It should be noted that BDD involves an individual's *perception* of his or her body that is not necessarily consistent with reality (Figure 5-2).

The signs of BDD are similar regardless of the physical area of concern: the individual exhibits obsession and preoccupation with the body image or area and may generalize their dissatisfaction to their entire self as overt distress or general ugliness. For example, the first author once counseled a client diagnosed with BDD. She participated in fitness competitions and ate only broiled chicken, plain white rice, and lima beans for breakfast, lunch, and dinner. She would occasionally splurge on candy or cake, feel guilty, and subsequently run 5 miles to burn off the excess fat she felt. She literally pointed to her thighs to indicate where on her body the cake had settled. Although incredibly toned with a very low body fat percentage, the client believed she saw ripples of cellulite in her thighs where there clearly was none.

Related to BDD and acknowledged in the sport and exercise arena is muscle dysmorphia (MDM), the preoccupation with muscle and body size and shape or definition. The identification of MDM emerged as a result of studies examining the use of anabolic steroids among weightlifters (Pope, Katz, & Hudson, 1993). Currently, MDM is not included in the DSM-IV, although it is acknowledged as a form of BDD. As a consequence of this fixation with their body or body part(s), individuals may develop a number of defense mechanisms, including DE, to cope with their body dissatisfaction (Olivardia, Pope, Mangweth, & Hudson, 1995). Similar to anorexics perceiving their emaciated bodies as too fat, a person with MDM will view extremely muscular physiques as too small and even puny. People who suffer from MDM can engage in unhealthy behaviors (i.e., use anabolic steroids, continue to lift while injured) and are primarily concerned with underdeveloped musculature (Olivardia, 2001 ; Olivardia, Pope, & Hudson, 2000). Within the group of individuals exhibiting MDM, behaviors can include maximizing or minimizing the size of a target area. This intent may translate into the under/over consumption of certain foods, excessive exercise (especially a muscle- or muscular group-specific exercise), and numerous inquiries for validation and re-evaluation of the body image or part.

Both BDD and MDM are often associated with self-destructive behaviors that may contribute to their identification. These behaviors may include the following (Allen & Hollander, 2004):

+ DE
+ Preoccupation with exercise or workouts at significant personal expense
+ Extreme or fad diets
+ Overtraining
+ Training while injured
+ Alcohol and other drug abuse, including anabolic-androgenic steroids
+ Dietary supplement abuse
+ Low body image dissatisfaction
+ Obsessive-compulsive behaviors or rituals

EXERCISE DEPENDENCE

Although not yet considered a clinical disorder, exercise dependence is used to describe individuals who demonstrate an excessive commitment to exercise, experience withdrawal-like symptoms when away from exercise, and who choose to exercise through injury (de Coverley Veale, 1987). Exercise dependence, sometimes incorrectly labeled exercise addiction, is best operationalized through the diagnostic criteria of substance dependence. As such, we consider exercise dependence to be a "...multidimensional maladaptive pattern of exercise, leading to clinically significant impairment or distress..." (Hausenblas & Symons Downs, 2002, p. 113). This behavioral pattern is found to exist when three or more of the following conditions are met within a 12-month time frame (Veale, 1991):

+ Tolerance (i.e., the need for continually increasing amounts of exercise to achieve the desired effect or diminished effects from the same amount of exercise)
+ Withdrawal (i.e., demonstration of symptoms of concern [e.g., anxiety] when there is cessation of exercise or exercise is used to avoid symptoms)
+ Intention effects (i.e., the need to work out for longer and longer periods of time)
+ Loss of control (i.e., efforts to reduce the amount or control exercise are unsuccessful)
+ Time (i.e., an excessive amount spent exercising or with exercise-associated activities)
+ Conflict (i.e., social, occupational, and/or recreational activities are altered or terminated)
+ Continuance (i.e., when a person continues to exercise despite physical or psychological problems as a result of exercise)

The concept of exercise dependence has not received as much attention from the psychological or psychiatric community as it has in the sport and exercise domains. Therefore, it is difficult to determine the relationship between exercise dependence and DE other than to speculate comorbidity, whereby a person can meet the criteria for both at the same time. For the athletic trainer, recognizing exercise dependence is difficult because in sport, extra physical training is often viewed as a positive commitment to the sport, coach, and team (Thompson & Sherman, 1999). Until more research is conducted and objective criteria established, exercise dependence should be considered one more behavior that can be taken into consideration when evaluating the existence of DE.

BINGE-EATING DISORDER

Recurrent episodes of binge-eating without compensatory behaviors can be described as BED. This disorder is characterized by feeling impaired or out of control; consuming food without hunger and often in private; and is associated with concurrent feelings of disgust, anger, and/or guilt. Currently, one must be binging at least 2 days per week for over 6 continuous months to meet the clinical definition of BED (APA, 2000). BED is different than AN binge-eating/purging type or BN purging type because no compensatory behaviors are used to offset the binges. While this disorder can be found in the DSM-IV-TR, it remains under consideration for classification as a clinical eating disorder.

BED is associated with a variety of associated symptoms and has been found in a greater number of women than men (APA, 2000). Dysphoria, obesity, and historic yo-yo dieting with weight gain experiences are commonly seen in conjunction with this condition. The weight gains identified may preclude these individuals from high-level athletic competitions; however, individuals with BED may be more prevalent in a community fitness or outpatient clinical population. As such, the athletic trainer should remain cognizant of the signs and symptoms of BED when working with these nonelite populations.

Mental health professionals and select medical professionals are trained to be able to differentiate among unhealthy eating habits, DE, and clinical eating disorders. However, some allied health care professionals (e.g., athletic trainers, physical therapists, etc.) may find the presentation of behaviors quite confusing in terms of knowing what to look for and deciding when to step in and intervene. In attempting to provide a thorough overview of DE, it should come as little surprise that DE is not one specific thing but rather exists on a continuum.

Disordered Eating as a Continuum

The conceptualization of maladaptive eating behavior is currently under consideration, a fact which has important implications for all professionals who work closely with sport and exercise participants. Support for this revision comes from three sources: (1) the continued expansion of AN and BN diagnostic categories to include subtypes, (2) the empirical prevalence of NOS, and (3) the recognition given to related disorders. As this body of work begins to develop critical mass, more attention is directed toward acknowledging the progression of DE from mild to severe behaviors (Fairburn & Harrison, 2003; Franko & Omori, 1999; Lindeman et al., 2001; Stice, 2002).

As suggested earlier, research to date has focused mainly on AN and BN at the expense of the more prevalent and inclusive category of NOS. Focusing the empirical and clinical interest in DE on individuals with AN and/or BN serves to marginalize the many individuals who *almost* meet established diagnoses and exhibit obvious maladaptive eating behaviors (Marantz Henig, 2004). Garner, Rosen, and Barry (1998, p. 840) clarify this point in stating, "identifying DE among athletes must go beyond focusing on those who meet formal diagnoses to include those who engage in a myriad of pathogenic weight control behaviors that have clinical significance and that can severely compromise health and performance."

In an effort to promote consideration for the range of eating pathology, the terms *DE* and *clinical eating disorder* have been used throughout this chapter. The continuum is multidimensional in that it incorporates restriction (e.g., exclusion of high-calorie/high-fat foods to self-starvation), binging (e.g., infrequently eating until uncomfortably full to

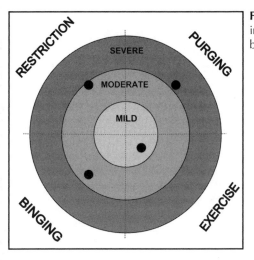

Figure 5-3. Continuum of DE behaviors (severe purging behavior, moderate restricting behavior, moderate binging behavior, mild exercise behavior).

obesity), purging (e.g., occasional use of laxatives to electrolyte imbalance and dehydration), and exercising (e.g., inflexible exercise routine of rigorous exercising despite illness or injury) (see Table 5-2). Moreover, these behaviors can range from mild to severe, and fluctuate among all four behaviors at any given point (Figure 5-3). That is, individuals can have multiple symptoms in the mild to moderate range, meet one or more criterion for several clinical eating disorders without fully meeting any, or meet the criteria for more than one disorder at the same time.

Identifying even mild DE behaviors becomes a key component because once diagnosed with clinical eating disorders, individuals already fall on the severe end of the spectrum. Currently, no tools other than the DSM categorization of "eating disorder NOS" exist to identify mild or even moderate behaviors. Reframing DE behaviors in this way may enable athletic trainers and other health professionals to place the observed behaviors (i.e., restricting, binge-eating, purging, exercising) on the continuum. The continuum can then serve as a reference point thereby guiding strategies to prevent and if necessary intervene. Athletic trainers and others would benefit from a more objective measure to inform decisions regarding when to refer athletes or clients and to whom (i.e., medical professional, nutritional counselor, mental health professional). Since this proposed system of tracking behavior is in the developmental stages, it should serve *only* as a guide to understand the progression of DE.

In addition to behavioral factors, athletic trainers should become familiar with etiology. Contributing attributes to DE behavior can include biological, psychosocial, and sociocultural. Also, short- and long-term consequences of DE are outlined below.

Etiology and Consequences

ETIOLOGY

Extensive review of the DE literature suggests that there is no single cause or influence that can predict who will exhibit mild DE behaviors or who will present with a clinical eating disorder. Although it has been suggested by some researchers (Taub & Blinde, 1992) that athletes may be at risk for the development of DE, other researchers suggest no difference in DE prevalence between college athletes and nonathletes (i.e., Ashley, Smith, Robinson, & Richardson, 1996; Davis & Strachan, 2001; Littleton & Ollendick, 2003; Madison & Ruma, 2003). This discrepancy may be the result of the conceptualization of DE or the way in which DE is identified on the continuum. These equivocal results reinforce the suggestion that there is no single risk factor to DE but rather a multitude of factors (e.g., biological, psychosocial, sociocultural, etc.) that independently or collectively contribute to DE.

Biological Factors

Researchers are attempting to identify biologically based predispositions to DE in an attempt to proactively identify individuals at risk. Research focused on neurological and hormonal imbalances is ongoing, and initial studies reveal results worthy of consideration. Also, gender and age can be contributing factors.

Imbalances

Researchers are continuously looking for biological and neurological contributors to mental disorders, and DE is no exception. Imbalances in neurotransmitters, particularly serotonin and/or hormones, may predispose individuals to DE (Goldbloom & Garfinkel, 1990; Phillips, 2004; Zhu & Walsh, 2002). Such studies reveal that serotonin activity is different between women and men and therefore may explain gender differences with respect to DE (Kaye & Weltzin, 1999). Further, these imbalances may make detection of DE more difficult because these individuals may not fit the other stereotypes associated with DE (i.e., weight-conscious, etc.).

Gender

Approximately 90% of individuals diagnosed with clinical eating disorders are female (APA, 2000). This discrepancy may be due to biological, hormonal, or evolutionary differences as well as societal expectations (see Sociocultural Factors on p. 143 for a detailed discussion) (Beals, 2004). While the majority of research and media attention is devoted to DE occurrence among women, there is a developing body of work that suggests increased prevalence of DE among men. Braun, Sunday, Huang, and Halmi (1999) indicate that while males account for only 5% to 15% of formal DE diagnoses, this percentage appears to be increasing. It is unclear whether this rise is due to increased acceptance of men admitting to DE or to an increase in the actual incidence of DE. It is also important to note that males may be less likely to meet the criteria for AN or BN but may be more at risk for other related disorders. For example, men and boys may be harboring a secret obsession about their looks (i.e., BDD) and are endangering their health by engaging in other behaviors such as excessive exercise (i.e., exercise dependence), steroid abuse, and/or overuse of nutritional and dietary supplements (Pope, Phillips, & Olivardia, 2000). The body of work on gender specificity for DE continues to evolve and has important implications for athletic trainers and other health professionals who work in the sport and exercise domain.

Age

While DE can occur at any time in a person's life, behaviors typically begin in adolescence with AN developing somewhat earlier than BN (APA, 2000). Although statistics show DE typically begins to develop first in adolescence, clinicians report admitting anorexia patients to inpatient treatment facilities as young as 8 and 9 years of age (Tyre, 2005). That said, DE is also being recognized with greater frequency in older adults. As with the men above, it is not known whether older adults are engaging in DE behaviors

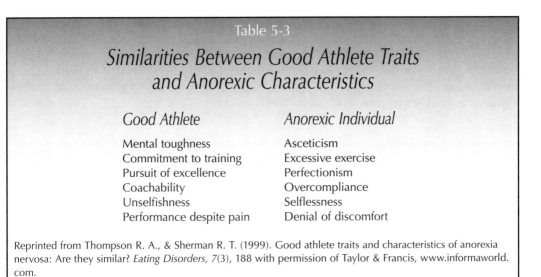

Table 5-3
Similarities Between Good Athlete Traits and Anorexic Characteristics

Good Athlete	Anorexic Individual
Mental toughness	Asceticism
Commitment to training	Excessive exercise
Pursuit of excellence	Perfectionism
Coachability	Overcompliance
Unselfishness	Selflessness
Performance despite pain	Denial of discomfort

Reprinted from Thompson R. A., & Sherman R. T. (1999). Good athlete traits and characteristics of anorexia nervosa: Are they similar? *Eating Disorders*, 7(3), 188 with permission of Taylor & Francis, www.informaworld.com.

with greater frequency or whether older adults are merely more comfortable reporting their DE behaviors. Regardless, athletic trainers often work with clients and patients across the lifespan and therefore should be aware that DE concerns may present at any age.

Psychosocial Factors

In addition to biological factors, psychosocial factors such as personality traits have also been identified as contributing factors to DE. Again, single factors cannot independently predict DE; however, it is the combination of factors that can contribute to or even exacerbate DE. The goal for athletic trainers is to be able to identify DE when behaviors are mild and prevent the downward spiral to a clinical eating disorder.

Personality Traits

There are certain individual characteristics such as personality traits that can contribute to DE. For example, perfectionism (negative or neurotic) has been linked with DE and most recently with social physique anxiety (Haase, Prapavessis, & Owens, 2002). Other personality characteristics linked to DE include but are not limited to high achievement orientation, independence, persistence, high pain tolerance, as well as high expectations and low self-esteem. Many of these traits coincide with those of competitive athletes and therefore can make DE detection among athletes more challenging (Table 5-3).

Sociocultural Factors

Family

It has been suggested that individuals at greatest risk for DE may come from dysfunctional families involving overbearing or controlling parents, parental alcoholism or substance abuse, and/or physical or sexual abuse (Brownell & Foryet, 1986; Fairburn, Welch, Doll, Davies, & O'connor, 1997). Such environments can lead to the development of low self-esteem and a struggle to gain control of anything, whereby food then becomes a source of control. This can trigger certain responses in athletes, especially when they feel out of control over recovering from injury, poor performance, or the demands of a coach. Certainly not all dysfunctional families produce children with DE and not all athletes with DE come from dysfunctional families, but family dynamics can certainly be one of many factors contributing to DE. With that in mind, technological advancements are facilitating the identification of genetic markers for DE. Preliminary data suggest that the relationships between genetics, family behavior patterns, and DE are worthy of further exploration (Bulik, Sullivan, & Kendler, 2000).

Ethnicity

Control, success, goodness, power, and beauty can be seen as equated with thinness in Western culture (Root, 1991; Silverstein & Perdup, 1988). Historically, prevalence of DE in athletes has occurred predominantly among those of Western-European descent and is lower among other ethnicities (Hsu, 1990). Although the statistics reflect a stereotype, there are extenuating circumstances that may elucidate this phenomenon. Ethnic diversity amongst athletes is low in many studies and there are greater numbers of Caucasian athletes participating in what can be considered "high risk" sports such as gymnastics, diving, and cross-country running (Beals, 2004). Researchers and clinicians also are seeing more diversity in patients with DE (Powers & Santana, 2002). There is some evidence of acculturation versus enculturation of emigrant populations, thus increasing the rate of DE in those of Asian and Latino descent. Concurrently there is a developing body of work demonstrating initially higher rates of DE in African-Americans (Mulholland & Mintz, 2001) and this may carry over to other underrepresented groups of athletes participating in all types of sports. However, some athletes may be at more of a risk than others simply by looking at the nature of the sport in which they participate.

Sport Culture

While no predictive pattern exists for the development of DE, some athletes may be at more of a risk than others by virtue of the sport in which they participate and/or the leadership style of the coach who supervises their physical development. Both of these factors will be discussed in detail in the sections following.

Sport Type

As suggested previously, some sports place more emphasis on body type than other sports, thereby increasing the possibility of athletes in those sports developing DE and at the same time creating a dilemma for athletic trainers. Health care professionals should be aware of the demands and standards of specific sports and their resultant impact on body image, yet at the same time these professionals must guard against focusing only on athletes in high-risk sports at the exclusion of endangered athletes in all sports.

While we promote an inclusive view of identifying at-risk athletes, it should be noted that sports where performance outcomes are based primarily on physical appearance or lean ideals are of particular concern (e.g., gymnastics, diving, figure skating, dance, cheerleading, ballet, synchronized swimming). DE is also a concern when optimal performance is based on leanness (e.g., swimming, cross country skiing, cross country running) or where weight classification is inherent in the activity (e.g., wrestling, boxing, rowing, weightlifting, judo, tae kwon do). It is not uncommon for athletes in these types of structured sports to participate in weight cycling (i.e., dramatic increases and decreases over short periods of time) in order to "make weight" for competition (Johnson, 1994).

Coach Influence

It has been established previously that certain aspects of the good athlete persona (e.g., achievement-oriented, independent, persistent, high pain tolerance, high expectations) may overlap with predictors of DE, thereby complicating detection of mild DE behaviors (see Table 5-3). As a result, some coaches may find themselves positively reinforcing these personality traits without the knowledge that they are indirectly influencing DE behavior. Conversely, the feedback provided by some coaches (e.g., an athlete appears to jump higher as a result of weight loss) may be misinterpreted by athletes (e.g., "If I lose more weight, I'll jump even higher"). This pressure to perform, coupled with inadequate coping skills and lack of appropriate supervision, may result in unhealthy behaviors (i.e., DE). Further risk exists when playing status or time is dependent on performance and/or the participant is highly identified as an athlete.

As stated previously, there are many factors interacting simultaneously to influence DE. As DE progresses from mild to severe, so do the consequences. In order to gain an appreciation for the consequences of DE behaviors on individuals, effects of health and athletic performance are outlined below.

CONSEQUENCES OF DISORDERED EATING

The effects of DE can range from mild to severe and in some cases of AN and BN, death can occur. Many of the side effects of DE are the same regardless of disorder and other effects are more specific. Regardless, it is important to understand the physical effects of DE as well as its impact on sport performance.

The longer a person engages in DE behavior, the greater the potential for severe and even irreversible physical damage (Warren & Stiehl, 1999). Each disorder has serious physical and psychological effects. In AN, for example, the body lacks adequate energy (i.e., calories) to function. Once energy stores are depleted, the body will begin to shut down, which may result in organ damage. The amount of time it takes for these results to occur is dependent upon an individual's genetic make-up, body type, and/or pre-existing conditions. If the body has been denied food or food intake has been restricted, the body adapts by making it difficult to digest food when it is ingested. Conversely in BN-purging type, the body becomes used to purging and will automatically continue even if the behavior is not self-induced. Unfortunately, these patterns reach a point where the athlete realizes he or she no longer has volitional control over the behaviors, and in some disorders the damage may be irreversible. The psychophysiological effects of the DE have been compared to substance abuse/addiction in that a person may be in denial and must hit bottom before the individual is ready to seek help.

Physical Effects

Many of the physical symptoms associated with DE (i.e., dry skin, brittle hair and nails, cold intolerance, lightheadedness, immunosuppression, constipation, sensation of being bloated after eating) are well documented (Johnson, 1994). Sexual and reproductive effects are also reported, including lower levels of testosterone and libido among men and higher levels of menstrual disorders (e.g., delayed menarche, amenorrhea) among women (Warren & Stiehl, 1999). Failure to maintain adequate weight over a period of time results in energy conservation, which may present as cessation of the menstrual cycle and subsequent fertility problems. Since not every athlete who presents with menstrual dysfunction is involved in DE, this condition alone should not be used to identify women with DE.

Female Athlete Triad

Menstrual disorders are only one aspect of a recognized syndrome known as the female athlete triad, an interrelated set of pathologies, DE, amenorrhea, and osteoporosis, affecting active women (Hobart & Smucker, 2000). These interconnected conditions exert far reaching impact on the health, wellness, and performance of active women, and often go unnoticed due to either their insidious nature or associated secretiveness.

In women having reached menarche, amenorrhea is the loss of menstrual periods for 3 or more consecutive months. Primary amenorrhea is characterized by an absence of the onset of menses by age 16, while secondary amenorrhea indicates the absence of menstruation for 6 months or for a length of time equivalent to at least three of the woman's previous menstrual cycle lengths. This criterion is a hallmark of AN and may actually precede it. Amenorrhea occurs as the result of a cascade of essential hormone imbalances. Research demonstrates (Zeni, 2000) that athletic participation and menstruation should and can occur simultaneously. In pre-pubescent athletes, menarche may be delayed as a consequence of AN. While there are numerous studies documenting prevalence and incidence data within the general population, the body of work within active populations is more limited in nature. Athletic trainers should discuss menstrual disorders with female athletes in order to identify changes and explore causes as a preventative measure risk of a clinical eating disorder.

Osteoporosis, the third part of the triad, is characterized by decreased bone mineral density and a deterioration of bone tissue. Adolescence is a critical time for accruing bone mass and without it, irreversible damage may result in higher incidents of stress fractures, scoliosis, and premature osteoporosis (Warren & Stiehl, 1999).

Although the lack of bone mass described above may have severe consequences for premature osteoporosis, the loss of muscle mass, especially in AN, can be devastating. Specifically, the heart muscle becomes weaker in response to exercise, thereby resulting in decreased pulse rate and blood pressure. Heart damage is usually the most common reason for hospitalization among individuals with AN and is the most common cause of death along with renal failure and suicide. If left untreated, 18% to 20% of individuals with AN will die within 20 years (Powers & Santana, 2002). This statistic puts AN at the highest mortality rate of any other psychiatric disorder.

Although individuals with BN may not present the exact outcomes as those with AN, gastrointestinal disorders can emerge within this population. Individuals who purge through induced vomiting can experience bad breath, dental problems, throat and esophageal irritation, ulcers, and eventually ruptures in the esophagus. Laxative abuse is another method of purging and can cause chronic diarrhea, severe abdominal cramping, hemorrhoids, as well as the inability of the colon to function properly. Since the body can become dependent upon the laxatives, cessation of use may result in constipation, gas, bloating, and severe abdominal cramping (Beals, 2004). Dehydration is also common among individuals with BN and may result in electrolyte imbalances such as hypokalemia or low blood potassium levels, which can lead to death.

A public health context and the connected nature of these pathologies provide the athletic trainer even greater impetus to recognize the value of early mild DE behaviors along the developmental continuum. Although some of the consequences are minor, the risks of confronting the problem far outweigh the consequences of doing nothing.

Effects on Athletic Performance

It should come as little surprise that the consequences of DE on athletic performance are primarily negative. While loss of body weight may appear beneficial at first, the consequences of continued weight loss are typically detrimental. There comes a time when performance is based on an optimal weight and going above or below that weight negatively affects performance. For example, an athlete may lose weight and as a result, performance gets better. The behavior is reinforced by the performance and often the athlete's social milieu (i.e., coach, teammates, parents) and he or she continues to try to lose additional weight. At some point performance will suffer.

Lack of energy to sustain training sessions, loss of muscle strength, increased risk of injuries, immunosuppression, as well as the psychological stress of hiding the DE behaviors can contribute to poor performance. Health care professionals cannot rely on poor performance alone to identify DE, as athletes may perform adequately or optimally for a short time while experiencing mild or even moderate DE.

Taken together, the consequences of DE can be short-lived and insignificant or long-lasting and severe. Some DE experts (Beals, 2004) claim that there is no way to predict who will succumb to the addictive qualities of DE and who will be able to maintain healthy eating behaviors regardless of the myriad of predisposing factors. When it comes to DE, it is better to be proactive than reactive. That said, athletic trainers cannot and should not bear the primary responsibility for prevention, identification, and/or treatment of DE and clinical eating disorders. Rather, these conditions are best managed through a multidisciplinary approach.

Prevention of Disordered Eating

Educational training is the first step in learning how to assess and identify DE behaviors. Experts propose a multidisciplinary systems approach, which begins with building relationships with professionals and colleagues, along with athletes, coaches, families, and other professionals who provide support for athletes. Vigilance is also a necessary component of prevention as athletic trainers must be able to identify warning signs of DE and ultimately those at risk for the development of DE behaviors. Finally, educating athletes, coaches, and family members and keeping lines of communication open between athletic staff and medical and mental health professionals may provide athletes with the best chance of averting DE altogether.

EDUCATIONAL AND PSYCHOEDUCATIONAL TRAINING

The first responsibility of the AT is to acquire both formal as well as informal information and training on DE. Training can be obtained in a number of ways, including seminars and workshops at professional conferences and keeping up with the latest research by reading professional journals. Athletic trainers can also develop and maintain referral networks of experts in the field (i.e., mental health professionals or physicians specializing in DE). Education is an ongoing process in the field of athletic training, and DE is one of many topics that may facilitate ethical and efficacious practice.

Once athletic trainers acquire information about DE, they must share it (formally or informally) with others in the athletic and health care domains (i.e., athletes, coaches, parents and family members, administrators, other athletic trainers, and members of the sports medicine staff). Communication of relevant information may occur through formal presentations or informal interactions, and must include facts about the consequences of DE and tips for developing healthy eating habits. Once again, the authors caution athletic trainers about taking full responsibility for these discussions and encourage them to call upon other health professionals (i.e., nutritionist, mental health professional) to augment the education process. This process begins with athletes themselves.

Athletes can develop intimate relationships with each other and therefore they may be privy to information and in a position to notice behaviors of teammates that few others have the opportunity to observe. As such, athletes need to know the warning signs so that they can watch out for the health and well-being of their teammates. Education can go beyond warning signs and include the contributors and the short-term and long-term consequences of the disorder, as well as what treatment entails. Finally, athletes need to know what steps to take if they suspect that a teammate is struggling with DE.

Since coaches are often implicated in precipitating or exacerbating existing DE disorders (e.g., Rosen & Hough, 1988; Ryan, 2000; Thompson, 1998), they too must be included in the educational and prevention process. According to the literature, coaches engage in both appropriate and inappropriate weight monitoring or weight management with athletes (Heffner, Ogles, Gold, Marsden, & Johnson, 2003), receive little education or training about DE (Turk, Prentice, Chappell, & Shields, 1999), and hold falsely elevated beliefs about their awareness of DE symptoms. Because coaches have power and influence over their athletes (LeUnes & Nation, 1989; Zimmerman, 1999), they can be a key component in influencing and monitoring eating behaviors. Many coaches and athletic trainers take responsibility for identifying and even treating DE, yet we recommend a team approach (as will be presented later).

Athletes' families would also benefit from DE education. Family members of athletes that are predisposed (i.e., have low self-esteem) or considered at risk (i.e., gymnasts) should definitely be included in learning about mild DE behaviors and warning signs. Parents can be invited to attend workshops or learning institutes offered through schools, universities, or the community. Parents tend to have a certain amount of influence with athletes and therefore would benefit from learning about types of DE and their warning signs. Family counseling is often included as a part of treatment and can be a big part of prevention as well.

When taking a proactive approach to DE, building relationships is a key element. This process begins with the athletes themselves. By getting to know them, the athletic trainer can discriminate among the variety of risk factors (e.g., perfectionism, low self-esteem) and warning signs (e.g., portion control, increasing amount of time exercising beyond scheduled practices) to identify which athletes may be more predisposed to DE. Also, building mutual respect and rapport with athletes leads to a sense of trust, which in turn can help athletes feel more comfortable in disclosing personal information, such as fears of gaining weight. Relationships take time and cannot be forced, but the more comfortable athletes feel, the more likely they will be to disclose honest information and the better the chance of identifying any unhealthy behaviors, particularly DE.

Coaches and athletic trainers need to have open lines of communication for many reasons such as discussing injury, recovery, and rehabilitation status as well as any factors that may be inhibiting performance. Coaches and athletic trainers work closely together and DE prevention can be readily discussed as a part of the close working relationship. Regularly addressing this issue will lead to the development of a mutual understanding of roles and responsibilities. This relationship can contribute to developing strategies for weight monitoring and nutrition-related issues among team members. This way, athletes will not feel they must participate in DE in order to be successful on the team.

Many athletic trainers have relationships with their athletes' family members and can observe interactions between parents and athletes. As alluded to earlier, family dynamics can play a part in the development of DE. The relationship between AT and parent can serve as a buffer for athletes who are under pressure to perform from family members.

Finally, relationships should be built with other professionals who work closely with athletes, such as physicians, nutritionists, strength coaches, sport psychology consultants, mental health professionals, and other athletic trainers. All supporting members can assist the AT in identifying warning signs, working cooperatively together, and developing prevention and intervention strategies when DE is suspected.

WARNING SIGNS AND EARLY DETECTION

Early detection of DE means watching for warning signs that are typical and preventing conditions from going undiagnosed. As stated previously, the earlier DE is discovered, the better the chances for consequences to be temporary and less severe. Some athletes are able to hide the signs of their DE from even their closest confidants and may appear physically normal. As such, athletic trainers cannot expect all athletes or clients with DE to look the same way (e.g., like an emaciated skeleton). By the time individuals begin to look unhealthy, the damage has already begun. In order to intervene before irreversible damage has been done, athletic trainers and other health care professionals should key into individuals who do the following:

- Begin to cut high-calorie or high-fat foods from their diets, such as red meat, dairy, carbohydrates, and sugar
- Begin to cut down on the quantity of food eaten
- Take food home to eat later when dining at restaurants
- Become preoccupied with food, calories, nutrition, and/or cooking
- Eat only "safe" foods
- Have odd rituals, such as cutting food into small pieces
- Prefer to eat in isolation to hide the amount of food actually ingested
- Spend more time playing with food than eating it
- Cook meals for others without eating
- Begin to be more conscious of what others are eating and other athlete's weights
- Become obsessed with feelings of being fat, fear of weight gain, or physical appearance
- Have difficulty sleeping
- Dress in layers to either hide weight loss or combat cold intolerance
- Reddened fingers or swollen cheeks or glands (from induced vomiting)
- Develop heartburn or bloating
- Engage in compulsive exercising or extra workouts, especially focusing on calorie-burning activities
- Take repeated trips to the bathroom, particularly after eating
- Begin to become more isolated withdrawn or secretive, depressed, or moody
- Become very secretive about food and spend a lot of time thinking about and planning the next binge
- Steal food or hoard it in strange places, such as shoe boxes or dresser drawers

In some cases, DE may be only a part of a more complex psychological problem. DE has been linked with other behaviors that are self-inflicted such as self mutilation (Favaro & Santonastaso, 2000; Lane, 2002; Reinhold, 2003). Research has shown evidence of correlation between DE and other psychological disorders such as obsessive-compulsive disorder (Yaryura-Tobias, Neziroglu, & Kaplan, 1995), dissociative disorders (Brown, Russell, Thornton, & Dunn, 1999; Demitrack, Putnam, Brewerton, Brandt, & Gold, 1990; Simeon, 2006), substance abuse (Nagata, Oshima, Wada, Yamada, & Kiriike, 2003), and borderline personality disorder (Dulit, Fyer, Leon, Brodsky, & Frances, 1994; Warren, Dolan, & Norton, 1998). Due to the complex nature of DE and severe consequences, a comprehensive assessment is crucial.

Table 5-4
Daily Food Journal

Name: Date:

Description of Food (Amount)	Calories	Fat (grams)	Protein (grams)	Other
TOTALS				

Thoughts, Observations And Feelings About Food Today:

ASSESSMENT OF DISORDERED EATING

As stated previously, DE behavior can be quite secretive, and individuals may become skilled at hiding the pathology. In order to become even more proactive, athletic trainers can initiate the use of assessment tools or instruments to determine which athletes are more at risk. Monitoring behavior can begin by using food journals that include foods consumed and thoughts and feelings regarding food (Table 5-4).

Athletic trainers can use formal questionnaires or informal interviews to access athletes' thoughts and feelings regarding food, body image, and performance (Table 5-5). Other assessments can be more formal in nature and include instrumentation targeted at measuring certain constructs, such as the Eating Disorders Inventory (EDI) (Garner & Olmstead, 1984).

The assessment process can entail a cooperative effort to determine the ideal body weight for performance and weight management. Ideal body weight in sport can be defined as height and weight or body fat percentage typical for a given sport. This discussion can take place between the athlete, athletic trainer, and coach; however, consultation with other professionals is encouraged especially if the athlete shows any signs of risk (e.g., low self-esteem, perfectionism, sport judged on leanness) or lacks knowledge of proper nutrition. The following tips for identifying the ideal body weight and body composition are taken from Manore and Thompson (2000):

- Body weight and composition that can be relatively easily maintained while consuming a healthful diet and adequate exercise
- Body weight and composition that allows adequate nutrition and calories
- Body weight and composition must be associated with optimal health as both increased and decreased weight can contribute to injury and disease
- Body weight and composition allows for optimal performance in the chosen sport
- Body weight and composition is individualized and allows consideration for genetic make-up

Be cautious, however, when entering into conversations regarding body composition as variation exists based on technique utilized. As a general rule, electrical impedance and skinfolds include greater variance than hydrostatic weighing, which has more variance than air displacement technology. Margins of error can range from 3% to 6% and be misleading. For example, an athlete who has 16% body fat actually may range in composition from 10% to 22%. Resulting preoccupation with body fat percentages and the variability of follow-up assessments can fuel DE. For example, the Canadian Academy of Sport Medicine has abandoned body composition assessment as a strategy to reduce DE among athletes (Carson & Bridges, 2001).

As stated previously throughout the chapter, prevention is extremely important in DE. However, no matter how diligent the prevention program, inevitably athletes are going to need more intense attention and some type of intervention. The referral process can be a smooth transition if mechanisms are in place (i.e., established relationships), including intervention strategies.

INTERVENTION

The standard treatment of DE is to take a multidisciplinary approach. Because of the physical, mental, and emotional nature of DE, professionals from the medical and mental health fields need to be included to assist the athlete. The role of the athletic trainer in intervention is to make a timely referral and become an active member of the treatment team by providing support for the athlete. This does not minimize the role of the athletic trainer, rather athletic DE necessitates involvement of the athletic trainer as an integral part of the treatment process. In order to understand their role, however it is helpful to understand the process of comprehensive treatment that increases the chances of success and a timely recovery.

Table 5-5

Performance Enhancement Questionnaire

Name   Date_

Date of Birth   Sport_

Height   Weight   Hightest Wt. Since 18

-

1. How long have you been at your current weight?

2. How many times has your weight fluctuated by at least 10 pounds in the last year?

3. What do you feel is your optimal weight?

4. Which of the following activities are you currently participating in?
   - ❏ Working to lose weight
   - ❏ Working to gain weight
   - ❏ Stay the same weight
   - ❏ Not doing anything about my weight

5. How many meals (i.e., breakfast, lunch, dinner) do you eat a day?
   - ❏ 1-2
   - ❏ 3-4
   - ❏ 5-6
   - ❏ 7 or more

6. How many snack times do you have each day?
   - ❏ 1-2
   - ❏ 3-4
   - ❏ 5-6
   - ❏ 7 or more

7. How often do you skip meals (#/week)?

8. Are you now or have you ever followed a special diet?

     If yes, what types?

9. Please circle any of the following foods that you avoid:

Red meat	Breads	Poultry	Pasta	Fish
Dairy	Fast foods	Vegetables	Fats/oils	Sweets
Fried foods	Fruits	Carbohydrates	Soda or Pop	Protein

Table 5-5 (continued)

Performance Enhancement Questionnaire

10. How often do you eat dairy products?
    - ☐ 0
    - ☐ 1-2 servings per DAY
    - ☐ 3-5 servings per DAY
    - ☐ 1-2 servings per WEEK
    - ☐ 3-5 servings per WEEK

11. Do you take vitamin or mineral supplements?

    If yes, what types?

12. Do you think your diet is nutritionally adequate?

13. Please rate how SATISFIED you are with the following factors:

	Very Satisfied	Somewhat Satisfied	Neutral	Somewhat Dissatisfied	Very Dissatisfied
My overall physical appearance					
My overall physical fitness					
My ability to be successful in my sport					
My body weight					
My visible muscle tone					
My cardiovascular endurance					
My muscular strength					
My body fat					
My overall athletic ability					
My body shape					

14. Do you know which dietary supplements are banned or restricted by the NCAA?

15. How easily can you maintain your current weight? (Check all that apply)
    - ☐ Very easily
    - ☐ Somewhat easily
    - ☐ Neutral
    - ☐ It is somewhat difficult
    - ☐ It is very difficult

16. What are your personal goals for body composition? (Check all that apply)
    - ☐ Gain lean body mass
    - ☐ Gain weight
    - ☐ Decrease body fat
    - ☐ Decrease weight
    - ☐ Maintain current body composition
    - ☐ Other
    - ☐ None

Table 5-5 (continued)

Performance Enhancement Questionnaire

17. Please list how many hours per day and per week do you exercise: (Include both weight training and conditioning activities)

	SUN	MON	TUES	WED	THUR	FRI	SAT
Practice/Game							
Conditioning							
Weight Training							

AVERAGE hours/day   AVERAGE hours/week

18. How many hours per day and week do you exercise
beyond what is required of you in your sport?

19. Are you or have you ever been diagnosed
or treated for an eating disorder?

20. Do you think you might have an eating disorder?

21. Please indicate the topics you would like to learn more about. (Check all that apply)
- ❏   Nutrition programs for peak performance
- ❏   Weight control
- ❏   Weight gain
- ❏   Disordered eating counseling
- ❏   Meal planning and preparation
- ❏   Tips on eating out
- ❏   Other

The following questions are for women only:

22. At what age did you have your first menstrual period?

23. How often do you have periods now?   days

24. Since your cycles began have you gone for more than
4 months without a cycle?

        If so, when?

25. How many days do your periods last?   days

26. What is the typical interval between your cycles?   days

27. How many periods have you had in the last 12 months?

28. What date did your last period start?

29. Do you ever have heavy bleeding during your periods?

Table 5-5 (continued)
Performance Enhancement Questionnaire

30. Do you ever experience cramps during your period?
If so, are they:
☐   MILD
☐   MODERATE
☐   SEVERE

31. How do you treat them?

32. Do you take birth control pills or hormones?

33. Do you have any pain or unusual discharge
during or between periods?

34. When was your last pelvic exam?

Reprinted with permission of Mark Cole and Kim Terrell.

Approach the Athlete

In cases where the athlete is attempting to hide DE behavior or is in denial, it is helpful to provide a caring and empathic environment. The athletic staff (i.e., athletic trainer, coach, administrators) must demonstrate support for comprehensive treatment and the athlete as an individual. Athletes should be part of the decision-making process so they feel more in control of the treatment process. The athlete, coach, physician, athletic trainer, and parent (especially if the athlete is a minor) should discuss whether the athlete is going to continue to practice and compete while undergoing treatment. If there is no immediate health threat, the athlete may be able to remain involved in sport as long as training and competing do not interfere with treatment. Issues of communication also need to be resolved, again with the athlete's consent. For example, what will teammates or the media be told and what are the consequences of missing practices and competitions. Remember that athletes may hide behaviors to avoid the risk of losing playing time or status and, therefore, this may be a critical point of the treatment process. Athletes must feel supported and understand that their physical and mental well-being is more important than playing time and performance.

Treatment Team

Comprehensive care begins with the inclusion of medical and mental health professions as active, empowered members of the treatment team. When establishing the treatment team, it is important to include professionals who have an understanding of and experience with DE, as well as knowledge of the athletic culture. Typical medical professionals include physicians (e.g., general practitioner, family practitioner, psychiatrist, or sports medicine) as well as a registered dietitian (RD). Due to the serious consequences of DE, a physical exam or full diagnostic evaluation with accompanying lab work and nutritional evaluation may be completed in order to determine physical condition, which will

Figure 5-4. New Life Centers Eating Disorder Treatment Facility. (Reprinted with permission of New Life Centers.)

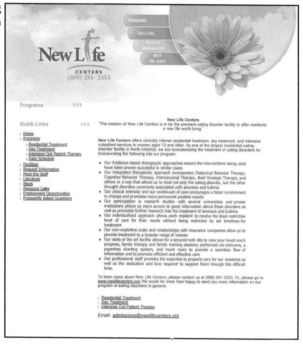

be discussed later. The second group is composed of mental health professionals. Several types of mental health professionals are qualified to provide counseling services and they include the LPC, LCSW, licensed psychologist (clinical, counseling, or sport), and/or a psychiatrist. Pre-established relationships with supportive professionals can contribute to a smooth transition for the athlete into the treatment process.

Treatment

In addition to making referrals, it is important that athletic trainers have an idea of what athletes will experience when being treated. Treatment can take many forms and consist of diverse techniques from both medical and mental health professionals. Individuals with DE often participate in individual, group, and/or family therapy as well as nutritional counseling. Individuals may be treated as an outpatient, which means they can live and operate normally and go to a facility to receive treatment. Inpatient treatment may be prescribed when the individual needs constant supervision and support as well as multidimensional counseling. This treatment involves full-time residency within a structured facility for a short amount of time (i.e., 30 to 45 days). See Figure 5-4 for an example of a treatment facility. Hospitalization may be required if the individual's health is in danger and constant supervision and support are needed.

Although different modes of treatment (i.e., individual, group, and family counseling), are used each serves a specific purpose. Individual therapy is useful in order to identify specific issues and provide more undivided attention to the client's unique circumstances. The most effective theory used in the treatment of DE is cognitive behavioral therapy or CBT. CBT is based on the notion that dysfunctional or faulty thinking (e.g., "The less I weigh, the better I will perform") causes unhealthy ways of behaving (i.e., restricting or binge-eating/purging). Therapists and individuals work on changing thoughts (e.g., "I can maintain a healthy weight and reach optimal performance") and accompanying behaviors (e.g., "I need to eat a consistently balanced diet in order to maintain a healthy weight"). During treatment, dietitians work as nutritional counselors who educate clients on all aspects of nutrition and how to maintain a healthy diet. Knowledge of healthy eating cannot be taken for granted, even among athletes.

There are two forms of treatment initiated by medical professionals, which include prescribing medication and behavioral contracting. Physicians and researchers consistently explore various types of medication for the treatment of mental disorders and DE is no exception. Certain medications have been successful in the treatment of BN (Zhu & Walsh, 2002) and BDD (Phillips, 2004), but drug trials for AN have been disappointing. Initiated by a physician, behavioral contracting can be an effective tool for motivating individuals to make changes in eating behaviors. An effective contract is based on five important principles: a collaborative physician-athlete relationship, patient involvement in setting the terms, appropriate outcome and process goals, a system for monitoring progress, and clearly defined consequences if the contract is broken (Brubaker & Leddy, 2003).

Group counseling is another mode of treatment and often incorporates CBT as well as provides a supportive and safe environment composed of others who struggle with DE. This setting permits the athlete to work on issues causing DE within the context of like-minded individuals. Group counseling supports cohesion, a shared identity, and relieves individuals of the burden of struggling alone.

Family counseling is typical when the individual is a minor; however, everyone can benefit especially when family dynamics contribute to DE. Family members can learn how interactions play a part in creating dysfunctional thinking. Most parents do not intend to pressure their children to the point of developing a DE; however, communication among family members can be misinterpreted. Either way, the family members can learn strategies to support the individual in treatment as well as to prevent relapse.

Successful recovery from a clinical eating disorder takes time, support, and commitment to the treatment process. Individuals will vary in the ability to overcome dysfunctional thoughts and behaviors and for some the struggle is a life-long process. While some athletes may be able to return to a sport after treatment, others must sacrifice playing a sport in order to live a healthy life. The role of the AT is to remain supportive and compassionate while maintaining the integrity of the sport.

Conclusion

Athletic trainers need to have a comprehensive understanding of DE. General knowledge includes familiarity with the various disorders and related behaviors, etiology, and consequences. This working knowledge can equip athletic trainers to develop effective prevention programs leading to successful treatment of DE and clinical eating disorders among all athletes.

In order to become proficient at recognizing DE, athletic trainers can conceptualize behaviors along a continuum. These restricting, binge-eating, purging, and exercising behaviors can range from mild to severe and realizing the difference between "good athlete" qualities and DE can be complex. However, identification of subtle or mild behaviors is critical to preventing DE from progressing to a clinical eating disorder with potential for long-term physical and psychological consequences.

The best strategy defense against DE is prevention. Developing and nurturing of cooperative relationships with health professionals possessing expertise and an interest in athletic populations is a worthwhile endeavor. Also, athletic trainers must keep updated on education and research in order to coordinate efforts based on the latest technology and information. Educating others and soliciting cooperation can lead to many individuals looking for warning signs of DE and increases the chances of detecting mild DE early, which in turn can potentially reduce DE as well as incidents of clinical eating disorders among athletes.

Athletic trainers can take an active role in the treatment process by developing a supportive healthy athletic environment. Communication among professionals can assist in providing comprehensive care that is based on the best interest of the athlete. Overall, the synthesis of material on DE should provide a basic understanding of DE and can serve as a resource for clinical practice.

Chapter Exercises

1. You are approached by the captains of the Women's Lacrosse team you have been working with during the last year. They voice concerns for a team mate who they feel has an eating disorder. They point to caloric restriction behavior, inappropriate emotional distress, variable performance, and fear of performance-based weight gain. Describe your responses to the team captains and outline a plan of action for investigating their claims. What resources would you utilize in your plan? Who would you discuss the conversation and plan with? Why?

2. You identify a high school wrestler at your school that is not in the lineup for the Varsity match. When you inquire as to their status the coach indicates they lost too much weight too quickly and are not feeling well. When you observe the athlete they appear drawn, pale, are dressed in layers, and are shivering. How would you respond to this situation over the remainder of the wrestling season? Also, outline and justify your approach to this situation during the off-season and next year's pre-season.

References

Allen, A., & Hollander, E. (2004). Similarities and differences between body dysmorphic disorder and other disorders. *Psychiatric Annals, 34*, 927-933.

American Psychiatric Association. (2000). *Diagnostic and statistical manual of mental disorders* (4th ed. revised). Washington, DC: Author.

Ashley, C. D., Smith, J. F., Robinson, J. B., & Richardson, M. T. (1996). Disordered eating in female collegiate athletes and collegiate females in an advanced program of study: A preliminary investigation. *International Journal of Sport Nutrition, 6*, 391-401.

Beals, K. A. (2004). *Disordered eating among athletes: A comprehensive guide for health professionals.* Champaign, IL: Human Kinetics.

Braun, D., Sunday, S., Huang, A., & Halmi, K. (1999). More males seek treatment for eating disorders. *International Journal of Eating Disorders, 25*, 415-424.

Brown, L., Russell, J., Thornton, C., & Dunn, S. (1999). Dissociation, abuse and the eating disorders: Evidence from an Australian population. *Australian and New Zealand Journal of Psychiatry, 33*, 521-528.

Brownell, K. D., & Foryet, J. P. (Eds.). (1986). *Handbook of eating disorders: Physiology, psychology, and treatment of obesity, anorexia nervosa, and bulimia nervosa.* New York, NY: Basic Books.

Brubaker, D. A., & Leddy, J. J. (2003). *Behavioral contracting in the treatment of eating disorders. Physician & Sportsmedicine, 31*, 15-18.

Bulik, C. M., Sullivan, P. F., & Kendler, K. S. (2000). An empirical study of the classification of eating disorders. *American Journal of Psychiatry, 157*, 886-895.

Carson, J. D., & Bridges, E. (2001). Abandoning routine body composition assessment: A strategy to reduce disordered eating among female athletes and dancers. *Clinical Journal of Sport Medicine, 11,* 280.

Centers for Disease Control and Prevention. (2002). *Prevalence of overweight among children and adolescents: United States, 1999-2002.* Retrieved September 9, 2005, from http://www.cdc.gov/nchs/products/pubs/pubd/hestats/overwght99.htm

Centers for Disease Control and Prevention. (2005). *Overweight and obesity: Defining overweight and obesity.* Retrieved February 19, 2006, from http://www.cdc.gov/nccdphp/dnpa/obesity/defining.htm

Davis, C., & Strachan, S. (2001). Elite female athletes with eating disorders: A study of psychopathological characteristics. *Journal of Sport and Exercise Psychology, 23,* 245-253.

de Coverley Veale, D. M. (1987). Exercise dependence. *British Journal of Addiction, 82,* 735-740.

Demitrack, M. A., Putnam, F. W., Brewerton, T. D., Brandt, H. A., & Gold, P. W. (1990). Relation of clinical variables to dissociative phenomena in eating disorders. *American Journal of Psychiatry, 147,* 1184-1188.

Dulit, R. A., Fyer, M. R., Leon, A. C., Brodsky, B. S., & Frances, A. J. (1994). Clinical correlates of self-mutilation in borderline personality disorder. *American Journal of Psychiatry, 151,* 1305-1311.

Fairburn, C., & Harrison, P. (2003). Eating disorders. *Lancet, 361,* 407-416.

Fairburn, C. G., Welch, S. L., Doll, H. A., Davies, B. A., & O'connor, M. E. (1997). Risk factors for bulimia nervosa: A community-based, case-control study. *Archives of General Psychiatry, 54,* 509-517.

Favaro, A., & Santonastaso, P. (2000). Self-injurious behavior in anorexia nervosa. *Journal of Nervous and Mental Disease, 188,* 537-542.

Franko, D., & Omori, M. (1999). Subclinical eating disorders in adolescent women: A test of the continuity hypothesis and its psychological correlates. *Journal of Adolescence, 22,* 389-396.

Garner, D. M., & Olmstead, M. P. (1984). *Manual for Eating Disorder Inventory (EDI).* Odessa, FL: Psychological Assessment Resources.

Garner, D., Rosen, L., & Barry, D. (1998). Eating disorders among athletes: Research and recommendations. Child and Adolescent Psychiatric Clinics of North America Special Issue. *Sports Psychiatry, 7,* 839-857.

Goldbloom, D. S., & Garfinkel, P. E. (1990). The serotonin hypothesis of bulimia nervosa: Theory and evidence. *Canadian Journal of Psychiatry, 35,* 741-744.

Grant, J. E., & Phillips, K. A. (2004). Is anorexia nervosa a subtype of body dysmorphic disorder? Probably not, but read on… *Harvard Review of Psychiatry, 12,* 123-126.

Haase, A. M., Prapavessis, H., & Owens, R. G. (2002). Perfectionism, social physique anxiety and disordered eating: A comparison of male and female elite athletes. *Psychology of Sport and Exercise, 3,* 209-222.

Hausenblas, H., & Symons Downs, D. (2002). Exercise dependence: A systematic review. *Psychology Sport and Exercise, 3,* 89-123.

Heffner, J. L., Ogles, B. M., Gold, E., Marsden, K., & Johnson, M. (2003). Nutrition and eating in female college athletes: A survey of coaches. *Eating Disorders: The Journal of Treatment and Prevention, 11,* 209-220.

Hobart, J. A., & Smucker, D. R. (2000). The female athlete triad. *American Family Physician, 61,* 3357-3364.

Hsu, L. K. G. (1990). *Eating disorders.* New York, NY: Guilford Press.

Johnson, M. D. (1994). Disordered eating in active and athletic women. *The Athletic Woman, 13,* 355-369.

Kaye, W. H., & Weltzin, T. E. (1999). Pharmacologic therapy for anorexia nervosa. In D. J. Goldstein (Ed.), *The management of eating disorders and obesity.* Totawa, NJ: Humana.

Lane, R. C. (2002). Anorexia, masochism, self-mutilation, and autoerotism: The spider mother. *Psychoanalytic Review, 89,* 101-124.

LeUnes, A. D., & Nation, J. R. (1989). *Sport psychology: An introduction.* Chicago, IL: Nelson Hall.

Lilenfeld, L., Kaye, W., Greeno, C., Merikangas, K., Plotnicov, K., Pollice, C., et al. (1998). A controlled family study of anorexia nervosa and bulimia nervosa: Psychiatric disorders in first-degree relatives and effects of proband comorbidity. *Archives of General Psychiatry, 55,* 603-610.

Lindeman, M., Stark, K., & Keskivaara, P. (2001). Continuum and linearity hypotheses on the relationship between psychopathology and eating disorder symptomatology. *Eating and Weight Disorders, 6,* 181-187.

Littleton, H., & Ollendick, T. (2003). Negative body image and disordered eating behavior in children and adolescents: What places youth at risk and how can these problems be prevented? *Clinical Child and Family Psychology Review, 6,* 51-66.

Madison, J., & Ruma, S. (2003). Exercise and athletic involvement as moderators of severity in adolescents with eating disorders. *Journal of Applied Sport Psychology, 15,* 213-222.

Manore, M. M., & Thompson, J. L. (2000). *Sport nutrition for health and performance.* Champaign, IL: Human Kinetics.

Marantz Henig, R. (2004). Sorry. Your eating disorder doesn't meet our criteria. *The New York Times.* Retrieved November 30, 2004, from http://www.nytimes.com/2004/11/30/health

Mulholland, A., & Mintz, L. (2001). Prevalence of eating disorders among African American women. *Journal of Counseling Psychology, 48,* 111-116.

Nagata, T., Oshima, J., Wada, A., Yamada, H., & Kiriike, N. (2003). Repetitive self-mutilation among Japanese eating disorder patients with drug use disorder: Comparison with patients with methamphetamine use disorder. *Journal of Nervous and Mental Disease, 191,* 319-323.

Olivardia, R. (2001). Mirror, mirror on the wall, who's the largest of them all? The features and phenomenology of muscle dysmorphia. *Harvard Review of Psychiatry, 9*(5), 254-259.

Olivardia, R., Pope, H., & Hudson, J. (2000). Muscle dysmorphia in male weightlifters: A case-control study. *American Journal of Psychiatry, 157,* 1291-1296.

Olivardia, R., Pope, H., Mangweth, B., & Hudson, J. (1995). Eating disorders in college men. *American Journal of Psychiatry, 152,* 1279-1285.

Phillips, K. A. (2004). Treating body dysmorphic disorder using medication. *Psychiatric Annals, 34,* 945-953.

Pope, H., Katz, D., & Hudson, J. (1993). Anorexia nervosa and "reverse anorexia" among 108 bodybuilders. *Comprehensive Psychiatry, 34*(6), 406-409.

Pope, H. G., Phillips, K. A., & Olivardia, R. (2000). *The Adonis complex: The secret crisis of male body obsession.* New York, NY: Free Press.

Powers, P. S., & Santana, C. A. (2002). Eating disorders: A guide for the primary care physician. *Primary Care: Clinics in Office Practice, 29,* 81-98.

Reinhold, S. L. (2003). Alienation and isolation from the body: A common etiology for the deliberate self-harm of eating disorders and self-mutilation? *Dissertation Abstracts International, 63,* 5534.

Root, M. P. P. (1991). Persistent, disordered eating as a gender-specific, post-traumatic stress response to sexual assault. *Psychotherapy, 28,* 96-102.

Rosen, L. W., & Hough, D. O. (1988). Pathogenic weight control behaviors of female college gymnasts. *Physician & Sportsmedicine, 16,* 141-144.

Ruffolo, J. S., Phillips, K. A., Menard, W., Fay, C., & Weisberg, R. B. (2006). Comorbidity of body dysmorphic disorder and eating disorders: Severity of psychopathology and body image disturbance. *International Journal of Eating Disorders, 39,* 11-19.

Ryan, J. (2000). *Little girls in pretty boxes: The making and breaking of elite gymnasts and figure skaters.* New York, NY: Warner Books.

Silverstein, H., & Perdup,. L. (1988). The relationship between role concern, preferences for slimness, and symptoms of eating problems among college women. *Sex Roles, 18,* 101-106.

Simeon, D. (2006). Self-injurious behaviors. In E. Hollander & D. J. Stein (Ed.), *Clinical manual of impulse-control disorders.* Washington, DC: American Psychiatric Publishing.

Stice, E. (2002). Risk and maintenance factors for eating pathology: A meta-analytic review. *Psychology Bulletin, 128,* 825-848.

Taub, D. E., & Blinde, E. M. (1992). Eating disorders among adolescent female athletes: Influence of athletic participation and sport team membership. *Adolescence, 27,* 833-848.

Thompson, R. (1998). The last word: Wrestling with death. *Eating Disorders: The Journal of Treatment and Prevention, 6,* 207-210.

Thompson, R., & Sherman, R. T. (1999). Reducing the risk of eating disorders in athletics. *Eating Disorders, 1,* 65-78.

Thompson, R. A., & Sherman, R. T. (1999). Good athlete traits and characteristics of anorexia nervosa: Are they similar? *Eating Disorders, 7*(3), 188.

Turk, J., Prentice, W., Chappell, S., & Shields, E. (1999). Collegiate coaches' knowledge of eating disorders. *Journal of Athletic Training, 34,* 19-24.

Tyre, P. (2005). Fighting anorexia: No one to blame. *Newsweek,* 51-60.

Tyrka, A., Graber, J., & Brooks-Gunn, J. (2000). *Handbook of developmental psychopathology* (2nd ed.). Dordrecht, Netherlands: Kluwer Academic.

Tyrka, A., Waldron, I., Graber, J., & Brooks-Gunn, J. (2002). Prospective predictors of the onset of anorexic and bulimic syndromes. *International Journal of Eating Disorders, 32,* 282-290.

Veale, D. M. W. (1991). Psychological aspects of staleness and dependence on exercise. *International Journal of Sports Medicine, 12,* S19-S22.

Vervaet, M., Audenaert, K., & Van heeringen, C. (2003). Cognitive and behavioral characteristics are associated with personality dimensions in patients with eating disorders. *European Eating Disorders Review, 11,* 363-378.

Wade, T., Bulik, C., Sullivan, P., Neale, M., & Kendler, K. (2000). The relation between risk factors for binge-eating and bulimia nervosa: A population-based female twin study. *Health Psychology, 19,* 115-123.

Warren, F., Dolan, B., & Norton, K. (1998). Bloodletting, bulimia nervosa and borderline personality disorder. *European Eating Disorders Review, 6,* 277-285.

Warren, M. P., & Stiehl, A. L. (1999). Exercise and female adolescents: Effects on the reproductive and skeletal systems. *Journal of the American Medical Women's Association, 54,* 115-120.

Yaryura-Tobias, J. A., Neziroglu, F. A., & Kaplan, S. (1995). Self-mutilation, anorexia, and dysmenorrheal in obsessive compulsive disorder. *International Journal of Eating Disorders, 17,* 33-38.

Zeni, A. (2000). Stress injury to the bone among women athletes. *Physical Medicine and Rehabilitation Clinics of North America, 11,* 929-947.

Zhu, A. J., & Walsh, T. (2002). Pharmacologic treatment of eating disorders. *Canadian Journal of Psychiatry, 47,* 227-234.

Zimmerman, T. S. (1999). Using family systems theory to counsel the injured athlete. In R. Ray & D. M. Wiese-Bjornstal (Eds.), *Counseling in sports medicine* (pp. 111-126). Champaign, IL: Human Kinetics.

Chapter

PSYCHOLOGICAL RESPONSE TO INJURY AND INTERVENTIONS

Eva V. Monsma, PhD

Chapter Objectives

❖ Take a NATA competency-based approach for outlining systematic cognitive, emotional, and behavioral responses to injury following a developmental framework.

❖ Specify cognitive, psychomotor, and affective competencies comprising the NATA psychosocial intervention and referral content areas.

❖ Describe life-stress and injury models for guiding athletic trainers' understanding of injury and rehabilitation processes, and pain management.

❖ Examine the importance of social support.

❖ Present motivational and anxiety theories and their various interventions.

❖ Provide case-specific examples designed to facilitate decisions surrounding interventions.

NATA Educational Competencies

Psychosocial Intervention and Referral Domain

1. Explain the psychosocial requirements (i.e., motivation and self-confidence) of various activities that relate to the readiness of the injured or ill individual to resume participation.
2. Explain the stress-response model and the psychological and emotional responses to trauma and forced inactivity.
3. Describe the motivational techniques that the athletic trainer must use during injury rehabilitation and reconditioning.
4. Describe the basic principles of mental preparation, relaxation, visualization, and desensitization techniques.
5. Describe the basic principles of general personality traits, associated trait anxiety, locus of control, and patient and social environmental interactions.
6. Describe the acceptance and grieving processes that follow a catastrophic event and the need for a psychological intervention and referral plan for all parties affected by the event.

In 1996, Larson, Starkey, and Zaichkowsky surveyed 482 ATCs and found that only 47% believed that every injured athlete suffers negative psychological effects in response to injury. The most common responses identified were stress and anxiety followed by anger, treatment compliance problems, depression, concentration problems, and exercise addiction. In a recent literature survey of psychological correlates of injury, Roh & Perna (2000) confirmed athletic injury is accompanied by significant psychological distress, which can impair rehabilitation compliance and possibly physical recovery. Psychological principles are becoming more pertinent in the athletic training room as increasing evidence indicates athletes who are better at coping with injuries can be distinguished based on their psychological characteristics and behaviors from those less able to do so (Brewer, 2003). Psychological characteristics such as a positive attitude, intrinsic motivation, and willingness to learn about the injury and rehabilitation technique are important for hastening the rehabilitation process (Wiese, Weiss, & Yukelson, 1991).

Sport scientists and allied health professionals are realizing the benefits of attending to psychological factors that improve the quality of rehabilitation and hasten and improve practice return. While elite-level athletes have access to a wide range of rehabilitation providers including sport psychologists, the majority of athletes have limited access to these professionals. In most sports settings, it is the athletic trainer who has the most frequent contact with injured athletes from the onset of injury throughout the rehabilitation process. Thus, they are in a unique position to monitor athletes' psychological states and recommend related interventions to improve rehabilitation effectiveness, compliance, and wellness. It is important for athletic trainers to understand the scope of their potential for providing psychosocial support for managing injury response and rehabilitation. To this end, athletic trainers must understand psychological concepts, models, and ways in which athletes vary in their psychological responses and abilities to use interventions. A major factor influencing individual variability is development.

Table 6-1

Progressive Reactions of Injured Athletes Based on Severity of Injury and Length of Rehabilitation

	Progressive Reactions		
Rehabilitation Length	To Injury	To Rehabilitation	To Practice Return
Short (<4 weeks)	Shock, relief	Impatience, optimism	Eagerness, anticipation
Long (>4 weeks)	Fear, anger	Loss of vigor, irrational thoughts, alienation	Acknowledgment
Chronic	Anger, frustration	Dependence or independence, apprehension	Confident or skeptical
Career-Terminating	Isolation, grief process	Loss of athletic identity	Closure and renewal

Reprinted with permission from Hedgpeth, E. G., & Gieck, J. (2004). Psychological considerations for rehabilitation of the injured athlete. In W. E. Prentice (Ed.), *Rehabilitation techniques for sports medicine and athletic training* (4th ed.). New York, NY: McGraw-Hill.

The growth of competitive sport opportunities has seen a rise in early sport specialization (participation in only one sport starting at 8 years of age) (Malina, Bouchard, & Bar-Or, 2004). The popularity of organized sport is accompanied by long intense practices, which have contributed to the rise of overuse injuries. The variability of responses extends beyond athletic ability and includes factors associated with physical and psychological development. For example, age-related variation in sport participation indicates participation intensity and sport demands reduce fun and increase perceptions of stress, a seminal injury risk factor (Wiese-Bjornstal, 2004). As employment opportunities in middle and high school settings increase (NATA, 2006), not only do athletic trainers need to be educated in psychological aspects of injury but also consider developmental differences that may impact their treatment decisions.

Progressive Reactions of Injury

Injury severity, rehabilitation length, and reactive phases of injury response are common factors among injured athletes and are considered when designing intervention strategies. The severity of injury is directly related to the length of rehabilitation. According to Hedgpeth & Gieck (2004), length of rehabilitation is categorized as short (<4 weeks), long (>4 weeks), chronic, and career termination. Regardless of rehabilitation length, injured athletes pass through three progressive, reactive phases of rehabilitation: reaction to injury, reaction to rehabilitation, and reaction to return. Typical responses to these phases by rehabilitation length are specified in Table 6-1. Factors related to length of rehabilitation and these progressive reactions should be considered when augmenting or tailoring interventions for athletes.

Hedgpeth and Gieck (2004) note that when helping athletes through short-term injuries, it is important to allow venting opportunities to enable frustrations to surface in order to help athletes see "the light at the end of the tunnel" (p. 79). Noncompliance is uncommon in short-term injuries. Keeping athletes involved in team practices, meetings, and social events can help circumvent feelings associated with losing a spot on the team or other physical aspects of performance such as loss of speed and mechanics. Maintaining sport involvement can help the athlete stay current with plays and coaching changes as well as help maintain neuromuscular connections involved in physical performance, especially if augmented by imagery.

In the case of long-term injuries, where anger is common, it is important to emphasize interventions once the athlete has come to terms with his or her anger. Exerting power to control and calm an angry athlete can exasperate the situation and diminish possibilities of determining the cause of anger. Allowing time to vent frustration is also important in long-term rehabilitation contexts. Active listening to feelings and developing a supporting relationship can help an athlete learn to trust the athletic trainer who can then help the athlete focus on the process and associated goals that lie ahead in the rehabilitation process. Negative thoughts, irrational thinking, and loss of social support are common and can potentially exasperate pain, anger, worry, fear, anxiety, and self-pity. Intervention considerations should focus on restructuring thoughts involving positive thinking, keeping things in perspective, and positive images and attitudes. Helping athletes see potential carry-over effects of psychological exercises used during intervention, especially during the latter phases by augmenting interventions with sport-specific drills, can increase motivation and confidence.

Interventions for chronic and career-ending injuries can incorporate some techniques used in short- and long-term injuries—specifically those geared at pain and anger management—but these categories of injuries require additional support. Chronic injuries are unique because rather than focusing on reactive strategies, interventions involve proactive rather than passive involvement of the athletes. Athletes with chronic injuries can become dependent on medical professionals feeling they are no longer receiving the special attention associated with the initial diagnosis. Pointing out that this is inappropriate and unnecessarily time consuming is advised. Establishing respect and trust is imperative in chronic injury cases and can be accomplished by staying current with literature; sharing information about the healing process is advised.

Career-ending injury interventions can involve psychological and career counseling as well as financial planning. Those injuries that occur at the peak of an athlete's career resulting in forced retirement are associated with poor adjustment and certainly require referral to a sport psychologist. Additionally, an abrupt withdrawal from training can also result in sudden exercise abstinence syndrome (SEAS), a condition involving both physiological and psychological symptoms. SEAS symptoms include heart palpitations, irregular heart beat, chest pain, disturbed appetite and digestion, sleep disorders, increased sweating, depression, and emotional instability (Prentice, 2006).

An athletic trainer's psychological intervention decisions should systematically correspond with the specific progressive reactions to injury, rehabilitation, and the return to practice. Additionally, aligned with the developmental approach advocated by Weiss (2003), several considerations must be made in order to develop interventions that are age-appropriate and effective for provoking behavioral change. These include progressive reactions to injury, rehabilitation, and practice return that include severity and expected length of rehabilitation time; developmental differences reflected in age periods; anxiety dimensions; motivational orientations; and self-perceptions.

Understanding Psychological Responses to Injuries

CONCEPTUAL MODELS

Psychological response to injury is a multifaceted process involving cognitions, emotions, and behaviors that are closely tied to psychological and environmental precursors of injury (Brewer, Anderson, & Van Raalte, 1999; Wiese-Bjornstal, Smith, Schaffer, & Morrey, 1998). Because managing psychological responses to athletic injuries is an inexact science, conceptual models guide responses and decision making about interventions. Conceptual models are heavily relied upon for understanding psychological characteristics associated with athletic injury. Also referred to as frameworks or theoretical models, conceptual models illustrate information garnered from both clinical and research contexts. Some models have been developed specifically for injury-related contexts while others such as life stress models and the grief model (Kubler-Ross, 1969) have been adapted to fit such contexts. The practical utility of these conceptual models are two-fold: 1) they help guide researchers toward testing proposed relationships that collectively provide the basis for theory development and 2) they provide practitioners with guidance for organizing thoughts involved in making treatment decisions. However, it is important to understand that sport psychology is whole; however, injury-related sport psychology is in its infancy where organizational models are operational but have yet to progress toward the level of theory. Understanding a variety of conceptual models is reflected in several athletic training competency requirements. Accordingly, the following sections include models illustrating the stress response, an integrated model of injury response, frameworks of motivation, and anxiety.

INJURY AND THE STRESS RESPONSE

While stress can contribute to injury occurrence, injuries themselves are stressful. In addition to dealing with pain, injured athletes must move from a familiar sport culture to the unfamiliar rehabilitation culture. This process is referred to as acculturation becomes a stressor because of conflicting messages about progress, loss of familiarity, control, confidence, and motivation. In the face of injury, the responsibility of athlete behavior shifts from the coach to sports medicine professionals who have their own rules, settings, and expectations. Additionally, rehabilitation exercises can be perceived as boring and fall short of healing progress expectations while a host of physical setbacks can further prolong the rehabilitation process. Otherwise self-confident athletes may not be able to adapt their confidence when faced with responding to an injury, especially if it is severe. Subsequently, rehabilitation can be stressful and a barrier to compliance (Hedgpeth & Gieck, 2004).

Athletic trainers are accountable for being able to explain the stress-response model and the psychological and emotional responses to trauma (NATA, 2006). Life stress can be categorized as total stress encountered from a variety of contexts, including athletic, academic, familial and social, and context-specific negative stress. Examples of the latter may include recurring psychomotor errors during a game or demands such as increasing playing time stemming from being chosen as a first string player. The stress response (Figure 6-1) can be defined as a bidirectional relationship between the athlete's perception, or cognitive appraisal, of the stressor, and physiological and attentional changes stemming from the stress-related stimuli.

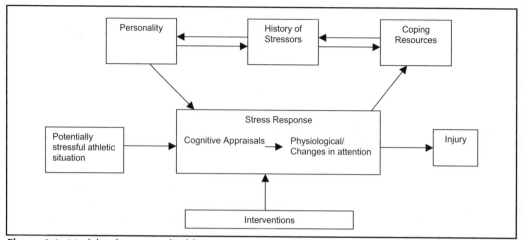

Figure 6-1. Models of stress and athletic injury. (Reprinted with permission from Williams, J. M., & Anderson, M. B. [1998]. Psychosocial antecedents of sport injury: Review and critique of the stress injury model. *Journal of Applied Sport Psychology, 10,* 5-25.)

The general premise of the relationship between life stress and injury, as depicted by Williams and Anderson's (1998) critique of the stress and injury model, is that increasing levels of stress eventually wear down an individual's ability to cope with the stressor, resulting in injury or illness. The impact on injury depends on one's personality characteristics, history of stressors, and coping resources. For example, a hockey goalie with an anxious personality (trait anxiety) and a history of previous injuries may be more susceptible to attentional disruptions. This could lead to a pulled hamstring during a vigorous practice because the two stressors diminish her coping resources, which subsequently lead to deficits in reaction time and balance (e.g., ability to shift attention and body positioning from recovering from a save to prepare for the next shot during a rapid slap shot goal targeting drill). Researchers have shown that athletes with high life stress who are placed in high-stakes scenarios experience perceptual narrowing that decreases their attention during potentially dangerous situations (see Williams, Rotella, & Scherzer, 2001 for a review). Consider a quarterback unable to focus on the open receiver, hesitating long enough to get sacked and suffers an ACL tear.

The relationship between the person's cognitive appraisal of a potentially stressful practice or competitive situation and the physiological and attentional characteristics of stress is bidirectional. Cognitive appraisals about the demands of the external situation are in terms of one's adequacy to meet those demands and the consequences of the ensuing success or failure related. It is possible to experience eustress, or "good stress," if the situation is perceived as fun, challenging, or exciting. Conversely, negative perceptions are referred to as distress, and potentially ego-threatening or anxiety-producing distress is a product of perceiving inadequate resources to meet the demands of a situation perceived as important. Cognitive appraisals may be accurate or flawed by irrational thoughts (e.g., never fully recovering from an ankle sprain). Distress subsequently leads to physiological, attentional, and perceptions of higher situation specific (state) anxiety, which in turn constantly modify cognitive appraisals.

While cognitive factors can initiate the stress response, the associated physiological changes lead to injuries. Cognitive appraisals or messages from the brain involving hormonal (e.g., cortisol) changes are sent to the muscles, which in turn shorten or contract. Because muscles are arranged in pairs, when one tightens, its opposite produces a counter tension to hold a particular body segment in place. This double pull, or bracing of the agonist and antagonist muscles, interferes with messages sent to and from the brain, reducing coordination and flexibility and increasing the likelihood of injury. Other physiological responses related to stress include shortness of breath, nausea, and increases in body temperature. After an injury has occurred, the associated pain can also be stressful because of autonomic changes including peripheral vasoconstriction, muscle spasm, and muscular bracing.

A preoccupation of these physiological symptoms, known as attending to irrelevant cues (e.g., heckling, opponent faking directional movements, and negative thoughts associated with previous performance), are involved in attentional and/or peripheral vision narrowing and blocking of adaptive responses to relevant cues such as detecting and moving away from the face of potentially dangerous situations. The stress response involves a combination of physiological, psychological, and behavioral responses, which can lead to injuries such as sprains, strains, and other musculoskeletal injuries.

Personality, history of stressors, and coping resource precursors of the stress response influence the likelihood and severity of injury. They are either directly tied to or have moderating influences on the stress response; relationships among the precursors are bidirectional. Personality characteristics such as trait anxiety, achievement motivation, locus of control, and hardiness measured specifically in athletic contexts have been shown to predispose individuals to stress or have buffering effects from these consequences (Williams, 2001). Using stress management interventions (described below) can also be an effective strategy.

A noteworthy feature of the life stress-injury model is the idea that interventions (e.g., cognitive restructuring, attentional shifting and relaxation techniques discussed later) geared at minimizing the likelihood of injury incidence occur at the level of the stress response targeting cognitive appraisals and/or physiological and attentional changes. However, one cannot assume that injured athletes have the necessary psychological skills to cope with an injury, especially in the process of acculturation to rehabilitation. In summary, where the stress response has similar characteristics as injury precursors, once injured, the process of acculturation becomes a stressor in and of itself (Hedgpeth & Gieck, 2004).

INJURY RESPONSE MODELS

In general, models that describe injury response include three interrelated dimensions: emotional, cognitive, and behavioral. Insight about emotional responses is typically gained through grief models in which the multifaceted sense of loss experienced by injured athletes is proposed to parallel other psychological losses, such as bereavement. Examples of loss experienced by athletes include loss of physical function, athletic identity, socialization opportunity, loss of income, and missed opportunities. The primary feature of cognitive models is accounting for the variability of athlete perceptions. For example, the depth of athletic identity and importance placed on social opportunities can influence an athlete's response to rehabilitation.

Grief Models

Kubler-Ross (1969) proposed that individuals experiencing bereavement-related loss sequentially pass through five stages: denial, anger, bargaining, depression, and acceptance. Applied to injury contexts, denial consists of minimizing or ignoring the significance of the injury and an unrealistic belief in rapid recovery. Anger directed at teammates, coaches, opponents, the world, themselves, and athletic trainers ensues as athletes realize the severity of their injury. This is followed by bargaining, where the athlete rationalizes or makes promises contingent on quick recovery and then depression characterized by feelings of despair and hopelessness, withdrawal, social isolation, and crying. Acceptance replaces depression as the injury is treated and the athlete realizes that recovery is possible and the focus shifts to more proactive steps toward recovery.

Although Evans & Hardy's (1995) extensive literature review has dispelled stage theory as a reaction to injury, several variations of the Kubler-Ross (1969) model reflecting different numbers of stages and different descriptions of stages have been advanced for athletic injuries. McDonald & Hardy (1990) found a two-stage process described initially as shock, panic, disorganization, and helplessness followed by a task-focused approach to rehabilitation, adaptation to their limitations, and eagerness expressed about practice return. Unlike other linear models, the Affective Cycle proposed by Heil (1993) involves repetition of distress, denial, and determined coping each with their own composite of emotions. Distress is a component characterizing disorganization and disruption of emotions, including shock, anger, guilt, humiliation, bargaining, helplessness, anxiety, depression, isolation, and preoccupation. The second component is denial, which includes disbelieve and distortion of injury severity. The final component, determined coping, is marked by acceptance of the severity of injury and the impact of the athlete's long- and short-term goals. This productive part of the cycle involves using effective coping responses and efficiently working through the recovery process. Multiple shifts can occur from phase to phase and they can occur in any order with one component dominating for periods of time depending on the context. For example, attending a practice while injured may serve to shift initial distress brought on by being unable to practice into determined coping as the athlete is motivated to rejoin his teammates and realizes the rehabilitation goals necessary for practice return.

A consistent feature of grief models is the distinction between undesirable, maladaptive emotional states and those that help athletes adapt and psychologically recover from injury. The characteristics defining emotions experienced soon after the injury, such as denial, anger, and depression, are examples of maladaptive emotions; acceptance, task-focus, and determined coping are adaptive. Despite intuitive appeal, grief models have been extensively criticized for inconsistent definitions of injuries across studies, use of invalid measures of emotions, lack of theory testing, longitudinal designs, and the failure to account for individual differences in injury perception (Brewer, 1994; Evans & Hardy, 1995).

Dynamic Model of Psychological Response and Sport Injury Rehabilitation

As can be seen in Figure 6-2, the dynamic model of psychological response to injury and rehabilitation parallels many components of the stress response model and represents the interaction between personal and situation factors (Wiese-Bjornstal et al., 1998). Personal and situational factors are moderating variables, those that affect thoughts (i.e., cognitive responses), feelings (i.e., emotional responses), and behaviors of injured athletes during rehabilitation. Examples of personal variables include injury-specific variables (i.e., history, severity, type, and recovery status) and individual difference variables (i.e., age, gender, pain tolerance, motivational orientation, psychological skills, maturity status, weight gain/loss, and use of ergogenic aids). Situational variable examples include sport (i.e., type, level of competition, scholarship status), social (i.e., family dynamics, social support provisions, coach's influence), and environmental (i.e., rehabilitation environment and accessibility). The effects of personality-, history-, and coping-resource precursors of sport injury are often amplified by the injury and moderate both physical

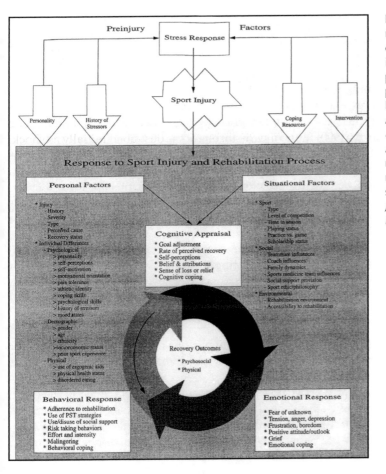

Figure 6-2. Integrated model of psychological response to the sport injury and rehabilitation process. (Reprinted with permission from Wiess-Bjornstal, D. M., Smith, A. M., Schaffer, S. M., & Morrey, M. A. (1998). An integrated model of response to sport injury: Psychological and sociological dimensions. *Journal of Applied Sport Psychology, 10,* 46-69.)

and psychological recovery outcomes (Wiese-Bjornstal, 2004). Accordingly, the athletic trainer should be prepared to discover the full gamut of an athlete's personal and situational variables so he or she can reduce his or her negative influences on interacting cognitive, emotional, and behavioral responses.

Cognitive Responses

The interaction of these responses begins with cognitive appraisal, which are thoughts occurring immediately after the injury and subsequently throughout the recovery period. Perceptions of the cause of the injury, goal of adjustment, rate of perceived recovery, attributions, ability to cope with the injury (pain and associated loss), and availability of medical and social support are examples of cognitions. Consistent with Lazarus' (1999) theory of coping, the direction of emotional and behavioral responses resulting from cognitive appraisals is based on the relationship between the demands of the injury situation and the individual's ability to meet those demands, or cope. If there is a mismatch between situational demands and individual resources, negative emotional responses will prevail. Accordingly, athletic trainers should realize their fundamental role in facilitating individual resources and how these needs reflected in personal factors may systematically differ across individuals. Systematic variation in personality factors are discussed in subsequent anxiety, motivation, and psychological skill intervention sections of this chapter.

Emotional Responses

Emotions are characterized as complex psychophysiological states that have a quick onset, short duration, and common cognitive antecedents. It is common for injured athletes to experience a wide array of emotions throughout the injury and recovery process, including anxiety and depression, which are often accompanied by a reduction in motivation. Negative emotional responses resulting form incongruent situational demands and coping perceptions can influence rehabilitation effectiveness. That is, emotions stem from injury-related thoughts and change dynamically throughout the whole injury experience. As sports medicine practitioners have typically focused on the physical rehabilitation of injuries, athletes have been left with coping with the emotional healing on their own.

Paying attention to and assessing the athlete's mood are important steps toward facilitating the emotional response and motivating the athlete to adhere to injury rehabilitation and a timely return to practice. In addition to grief-related emotions associated with loss (Evans & Hardy, 1995), the most common postinjury emotions are anxiety, tension, depression, frustration, anger, fatigue, and boredom (Wiese-Bjornstal, 2004). In contrast, some athletes respond to injury with positive emotions such as optimism, vigor, and relief—particularly if athletes perceive that the stress associated with participating in a particular sport outweighs positive outcomes.

Behavioral Responses

The utility of behavioral responses in injury contexts lies in what motivates different behaviors (e.g., rehabilitation adherence, practice return apprehension) and how to predict behaviors across a wide range of situations (e.g., game-specific apprehension, re-injury, attrition). The direction toward positive or negative behaviors is directly tied to the interrelationships between cognitive appraisals and emotional responses. Positive behaviors in rehabilitation contexts include treatment compliance (Duda, Smart, & Tappe, 1989), use of psychological skills (Ievleva & Orlick, 1991), and use of social networks (Duda et al., 1989). Additionally, the effort and intensity components of motivation with which athletes pursue their rehabilitation can have far-reaching effects on recovery, practice return, and postinjury wellness as they enable physical and psychosocial recovery.

The interrelationships among emotional, cognitive, and behavioral responses are involved in two fundamental psychological characteristics of athletic injuries: anxiety and motivation. While anxiety is both an antecedent and a consequence of injuries, motivation is primarily a consequence that can affect rehabilitation adherence, the effectiveness of psychological interventions, and ultimately practice return. The following is an overview of these concepts.

DEVELOPMENTAL CONSIDERATIONS

As specified by Wiese-Bjornstal et al. (1998), age is a personal factor that impacts injury response and rehabilitation. With the increasing demands for ATCs in middle and high school settings, it is becoming more important to adopt a developmental perspective. Generalizing intervention strategies across age is becoming inappropriate because of emerging research on developmental differences in injury response (Brewer, 2003). For example, adolescents tend to have stronger athletic identities that are more closely tied to their self-worth (Brewer et al., 2003). Although adolescents may feel a greater loss when recovering from especially long-term injuries, athletic identity seems to have positive effects on adherence compliance. Compared to adults, younger patients recovering from ACL surgery were adherent more when they were highly invested in the athlete role. In contrast, adolescents also tend to report more postoperative pain, state anxiety, distress, and irrational thoughts 24 hours after surgery (Udry, Shelbourne, & Gray, 2003). Based on this research, athletic trainers should be prepared to influence adolescents with pain management, cognitive restructuring, and stress management techniques, which are discussed later in this chapter.

Developmental sport psychology research specifically on injured athletes is sparse, with most of it focusing on athletes in late adolescence and early adulthood. As highlighted by Wiese-Bjornstal (2004) in an exhaustive review of literature, the interaction of cognitive, emotional, and behavioral responses vary with age and status of development. For example, perceptions of stress increase as a function of age and increasing practice expectations, which subsequently can lead to injury and attrition. "Young athletes are also socialized with increasing age into accepting the sport normative expectations of playing with pain and injury, which in turn, increases injury vulnerability and disrupts psychological management of injury once it occurs" (p. 525). Considering childhood and adolescent age groups in postinjury cognitions, emotions, and behaviors is an important step in helping athletic trainers adopt a developmental perspective.

Two common categories of postinjury cognitions among children and adolescents are 1) preparation to receive medical treatment and 2) increasing compliance with medical advice (Wiese-Bjornstal, 2004). Several factors affect children's ability to cope with their impending treatments (Brannon & Feist, 2004). Children will not have a comprehensive understanding of their injury, medical tests, diagnosis, or associated treatments. Prior unpleasant medical experiences may also be generalized into the current context, which may amplify negative emotions and expectations. Moreover, parents can amplify their children's distress by constantly providing reassurance. It is not surprising that children who experienced higher anxiety and stress levels also experienced more pain (Palermo & Drotar, 1996).

To overcome these treatment compliance barriers, using appropriate diagrams can facilitate understanding of the injury and treatment. Giving children an opportunity to express their fears or describe previous experiences and reassuring that each injury is different while providing empathy can reduce negative thoughts and associated feelings. Because parents are often close by during rehabilitation, they can also be the focus of preparation strategies. For example, keeping them informed about the procedures, recommending attentional distractions they can use with their children, and enabling them to provide their children with choices over rehabilitation procedures (e.g., which exercise to start with) can be helpful.

A sense of invincibility and level of cognitive ability distinguishes adolescents from adults and helps to explain their frequent unwillingness to comply with medical directives and push harder when injuries cause them to fall behind in their progress. Adolescents may be unable to foresee the negative consequences of noncompliance, assuming their condition will simply diminish on its own. The athletic trainer should be prepared to highlight that every injury is different, requiring specific treatments regardless if aches, pains, and other extraneous symptoms are similar to previous injuries experienced by the athlete.

There are emotional consequences of children having a limited understanding about their injury and rehabilitation procedures and these responses tend to vary across the recovery period. For example, negative thinking, agitation, anxiety, depression, confusion, anger, and fatigue are more common responses during the beginning phases of rehabilitation and tend to decline over the course of rehabilitation (Wiese-Bjornstal, 2004). Johnson and Carroll (2000) found that adolescent athletes who were highly involved in their sport as compared to older, less involved participants reported confusion about full recovery status during the middle and latter part of their rehabilitation. When it comes to chronic injuries, Aaron, Zaglul, and Emery (1999) noted intrusive and avoidance thoughts among elite athletes that mimicked those of persons with post-traumatic stress disorder.

From a behavioral standpoint, injury is the leading cause of attrition among youth sport participants, especially among adolescents in school-sponsored sports (DuRant, Pendergrast, Donner, Seymore, & Gaillard, 1991). Risk-taking behaviors, playing through pain, enduring intense practices during critical growth periods, and use of steroids contribute to injury rates. Athletic trainers should keep in mind that these factors can also parallel behaviors during rehabilitation.

ANXIETY

Anxiety is a common antecedent of injuries because anxious athletes can be easily distracted by self-doubt and negative perceptions of physiological responses. However, injured athletes also react to rehabilitation contexts with anxiety. Anxiety is one of the most common psychological responses to injuries (Larson et al., 1996). Injured athletes may experience anxiety when being evaluated or diagnosed by medical professionals, when preparing for surgery, and when preparing for practice or competition return. They may worry about pain, reaching their preinjury performance capabilities, reinjury, or their status on the team (Krane & Greenleaf, 1999). As can be seen, injured athletes vary in their anxiety experiences across situations. An understanding of this variation can be achieved by attending to conceptual distinctions and theoretical frameworks. The following overview of anxiety constructs and frameworks is designed to heighten the athletic trainer's awareness of the multidimensional nature of anxiety. Intervention recommendations are made to help guide intervention. Specific interventions are specifically described in a latter section of this chapter.

Anxiety is often used interchangeably with stress and arousal. Arousal, essential in harnessing the body's energy to enable physical activity, is generalized neural activation operating on a continuum from comatose to extreme excitement. It is not associated with positive or negative connotations. Stress refers to the interpretation of environmental demands, and anxiety is the cognitive reaction to the perceived inability to meet those demands (Krane & Greenleaf, 1999). For example, a pitcher returning to play from a shoulder injury questions his ability to pitch through the upcoming game because he is not sure of his shoulder strength. This pitcher is experiencing stress because he perceives an imbalance between the coaches' performance expectations and his ability to pitch. In the beginning of the game, arousal is experienced by the pitcher as his heart races when walking out to the mound. When he notices this physiological reaction and the associated tense muscles, queasy stomach, and shortness of breath, he has trouble concentrating and is experiencing anxiety.

Personality characteristics influence anxiety direction and intensity levels. Trait anxiety refers to a personality characteristic that predisposes individuals to experience feelings of anxiousness across a variety of situations. A trait anxious person may feel anxious in situations that do not involve high-stakes, such as being called upon by a coach in a practice situation, when explaining injury-related pain to a therapist, or while executing a volleyball serve to a coach. In contrast, anxiety experienced in specific situations when the stakes are high or unfamiliar is referred to as state anxiety. For example, athletes may experience state anxiety prior to surgery or returning to competition but are otherwise not overly anxious. While some athletes perceive anxiety as a necessary precursor to performance, trait anxious individuals have a tendency to experience higher state anxiety regardless of the situation and thus may be at greater risk for experiencing injury and needing subsequent rehabilitation.

While anxiety research specifically on injured athletes is sparse, conceptual models generally used in the athletic domain that is grounded in multidimensional anxiety theory (Martens, Burton, Vealey, Bump, & Smith, 1990) can be extended to rehabilitation contexts. Multidimensional anxiety theory considers anxiety as a composite of cognitive and somatic components. Cognitive anxiety involves negative thoughts, concerns about abilities, disrupted attention, and concentration disruptions whereas somatic anxiety includes negative perceptions of physiological reactivity to a high-stakes situation. These reactions may include shortness of breath, increased heart rate, excessive sweating, or butterflies in the stomach (Martens et al., 1990). Because of its salience to high-stakes situations, self-confidence is also considered in anxiety models. Anxiety varies in intensity and symptoms across situations and individuals. Negative thoughts seem to be highest directly after an injury, dissipate over the rehabilitation period, and emerge just prior to practice return (Quackenbush & Crossman, 1994). Initially, three relationships were specified with performance: a negative relationship between cognitive anxiety and performance, an inverted-U relationship between somatic anxiety and performance, and a positive relationship between self-confidence and performance (Martens et al., 1990). The inverted-U relationship is particularly appealing to rehabilitation contexts. Consider an over-aroused, anxious client who may push herself beyond safe levels of exertion, risking further injury during a rehabilitation exercise. However, equivocal findings among studies testing these relationships in competitive settings led to further extensions of multidimensional anxiety depicted in catastrophe and reversal theories.

In contrast, catastrophe theory specifies the relationship between anxiety and performance will differ depending on the interaction between cognitive and somatic anxiety (Hardy, 1990). When cognitive anxiety is low, somatic anxiety and performance will reflect the inverted-U relationship to a certain point, beyond which the athlete will experience a catastrophic decline in performance that is unrecoverable during that specific situation. In contrast, when cognitive anxiety is high, higher levels of somatic anxiety lead to more disruptive attention than when cognitive anxiety is low. As distractions increase, there is little attention left for the task at hand, resulting in a catastrophe (e.g., loss of coordination). By explaining the interacting effects of cognitive and somatic anxiety, catastrophe theory highlights the importance of tapping an injured athlete's anxiety experience.

Multidimensional anxiety theory proposes that high levels of anxiety always lead to performance deterioration. However, like catastrophe theory, reversal theory postulates that high levels of both cognitive and somatic anxieties will lead to poor performance whereas low cognitive and high somatic anxiety will enhance performance. According to Kerr (1990), athletes interpret their own motivation, which fluctuates with increasing levels of arousal. This interpretation is referred to as meta-motivational states that can have either unpleasant or pleasant tones. Boredom and anxiety are considered unpleasant tones whereas relaxation and excitement are pleasant tones. Guiding athletes toward pleasant tones or having positive interpretations of arousal levels, whether low or high, is ideal. Under conditions of low anxiety, athletes can potentially feel relaxed whereas high arousal is associated with excitement. Reversal theory also proposes that meta-motivational states can be changed rapidly, suggesting interventions can achieve this end.

The zone of optimal function is also applicable to rehabilitation contexts. According to Hanin's (1986) individual zone of optimal functioning (IZOF), elite athletes perform best when precompetitive anxiety is in an individually determined optimal zone. The utility of this model for injury rehabilitation contexts involving arousal measurement can be applied to rehabilitation settings. The model is based on intra-individual analysis rather than group comparisons. That is, each athlete's rehabilitation performance can be compared to his or her own IZOF. Repeating assessments of anxiety levels can aid in modifying psychological strategies and, more importantly, demonstrate progress in psychological adjustment. Two measurement methods can be used to monitor arousal levels. The first involves repeatedly assessing anxiety and the associated performance. The second involves asking the athlete to recall arousal levels associated with peak performance. In competitive contexts, measurement error associated with recall and bias is more common in the latter technique (Gould & Tuffy, 1996). Another limitation of IZOF research is the lack of multidimensional anxiety assessment; studies did not separate cognitive and somatic anxiety. Because the effectiveness of anxiety strategies are dimension specific, care should be given to anxiety measurement.

Contemporary views of anxiety indicate that anxiety is a product of personality and situations interacting equally. Thus, assessing athletes' typical reactions to nonthreatening situations can inform athletic trainers about how an athlete may respond in upcoming rehabilitation contexts. Helping athletes accept arousal as a natural consequence of a high-stakes situation is subject to keeping their perceptions positive, or at a pleasant hedonic tone level. Negative thought-stopping, goal-setting, imagery, and relaxation are possible techniques for modifying hedonic tones. Athletes have differing abilities to manage cognitive and somatic anxieties. Relaxation techniques may be a viable resource for some athletes for managing somatic anxiety, while others may use thought-stopping to reduce cognitive anxiety, which may only moderately influence somatic anxiety. When deciding the course of psychological rehabilitation, athletic trainers should investigate anxiety symptoms thoroughly.

MOTIVATION

As described in the grief response and in the dynamic model of injury response model (Wiese-Bjornstal et al., 1998), athletes encounter several dimensions of loss following an injury. Motivation is paramount for enabling athletes to comply with effective rehabilitation and is often compromised when athletes lose control of their daily training routines in the acculturation process. Harnessing motivation to overcome an injury can be challenging not only for the athlete but also for social agents who have a vested interest in the recovering athlete, including athletic trainers. Describing the basic principles of mental preparation, relaxation, and visual techniques, general personality traits, associated trait anxiety, locus of control, and athlete social environment interactions (NATA, 2006) is an expected athletic training educational competency requirement. In order to effectively use motivational techniques, athletic trainers must first develop their understanding of various motivational concepts and theories.

Motivation is defined as the direction (e.g., approach or avoidance) and intensity (e.g., low, moderate, and high) of behavior. The role of motivation in sport injuries is two-fold. Individual differences in motivational orientations influence cognitive appraisals and emotions involved in injury response and the behaviors necessary for effective rehabilitation. For example, systematic cognitive processes directed by an individual's motivational disposition are involved in behavioral choice tendencies. More specifically, a high-achieving athlete may play through pain and take risk of further injury, or an extrinsically motivated athlete may quit rehabilitation because perceptions of personal progress are less expected.

Knowing an athlete's motivational characteristics or dispositions can help guide decisions about how to implement intervention. However, situational circumstances are also important in fostering motivation with interventions. Behaviors of the team, the coach, and the athletic trainer can influence whether or not motivation is enhanced. The following discussion on select models of motivation present ways individuals can be expected to vary in their motivational characteristics and lays the groundwork for subsequent discussion of interventions related to motivation.

Achievement and Competence Motivation

One of the ways athletes vary in dispositions is the way they define success and pursue competence in achievement contexts. Knowing these differences and presenting the rehabilitation settings as an achievement context can enhance rehabilitation adherence and intensity of effort. A high need to achieve, or achievement motivation, is common among successful athletes who derive a great deal of satisfaction from their successes. A primary tenet of achievement motivation is that success is in the eye of the beholder; success and failure depend on an individual's interpretation of their effort put forth in achievement (Roberts, 1992). Working with a high achiever who exerts extra effort and defines success as a result of effort and skill can be very different than working with a low achiever who tends to perceive low effort and lack of talent as a personality characteristic. High achievers 1) take responsibility for the outcomes of their own actions, 2) have less intense physiological symptoms of stress, 3) prefer to know about their success or failure immediately after performance, 4) give extra effort in achievement settings, 5) experience more pleasure in success, 6) prefer situations with some element of risk, and 7) are conscious of their responsibility for their progress. If a particular level of progress is viewed as a result of the person's effort and skill, then its outcome is interpreted as success. However, if poor effort is associated with the level of progress, then a sense of failure will occur.

Injured athletes may fall into a pattern of perceptions consistent with low achievement motivation. Behaviors such as low rehabilitation intensity and attrition can be explained by the perception that any effort put forth is outweighed by a low probability of success. Lack of effort is often used as a scapegoat for slow progress. Some athletes may have a high need to achieve but as a result of frequent past failures have a low motive to achieve (Duda, 1993). It is plausible that injured athletes having just experienced some degree of failure through their injury may transfer the ensuing avoidance motive, or fear of failure, into the rehabilitation setting. Setting goals in a systematic manner is a recommended strategy that can help both low and high achievers.

Competence motivation, the internal need to deal with the environment, may help buffer injured athletes from negative motivational states such as fear of failure, avoidance, and low levels of intensity. According to Harter (1981), demonstrating mastery is highly motivating and success at mastery subsequently develops confidence. Compared to athletes who have low perceptions of competence and control, those who are high in these characteristics are known to exert more effort, persisting longer at tasks and experiencing more positive feelings. Fostering competence and self-control can be achieved systematically by presenting tasks to master in measurable terms with deadlines and providing feedback about progress.

From several studies of athlete personalities, researchers have devised a psychological profile of high and low achievement individuals in competitive contexts that can be applied to rehabilitation settings. The profile encompasses goal orientation, attributional tendencies, preferred goals, task choice, and performance outcomes in evaluative situations.

Goal Orientation

Goal orientation, a disposition central to both need achievement and competence motivation, refers to the degree to which an athlete is motivated by setting and meeting goals. The type of goals set by athletes heavily relies on perceived ability, and both are tied to subsequent self-evaluations of performance. Athletes with high goal orientations will select and persist at a task with high effort until the goal is achieved, set realistic and achievable goals, and feel certainty about meeting those goals. There are two types of goal orientations that describe the thought processes involved in the need to feel competent: task and ego involvement. Task involvement refers to perceptions of competence that are influenced by improving one's current ability over time or self-competition. For example, 1 week after an ACL surgery, a soccer player who has consistently engaged in the recommended amount of quad sets is now ready to advance to 10 straight-leg raises and extends the repetitions by 5 because she feels her leg is strong enough. In contrast, ego involvement refers to demonstrating competence by out-performing others or performing similarly with less effort. Ego-involved individuals may feel less successful with their rehabilitation progress because they cannot always control how others will perform. For example, a second soccer player in the same training room similarly recovering from ACL surgery but with weaker quad strength tries to out-perform her teammate in the number of straight leg raises, which delays her rehabilitation progress.

An athlete may follow one type of involvement over another depending on the situation. When it comes to adherence, those who emphasize more mastery or task-involved goals (Duda et al., 1989) and are self-motivated (Duda et al., 1989) show higher adherence tendencies. In contrast, ego orientation and low self-esteem have been linked to missing more treatment appointments (Lampton & Lambert, 1993).

According to Duda (1993), situations involving perceptions of low ability combined with assessing competence based on outcome result in low competence motivation. The keys to enhancing motivation in light of differing goal orientations include the following:

- Reinforcing an athlete's current ability regardless of outcome
- Emphasizing effort and improvement
- Setting performance goals (i.e., improving the range of motion and strength of the athlete's knee so he can walk without crutches) rather than outcome goals (i.e., the rehabilitation protocol dictates the athlete should be running at 4 weeks postsurgery)
- Helping athletes formulate accurate perceptions of their ability
- Helping athletes think positive thoughts about their future performance
- Avoiding excuses for poor progress
- Providing systematic instruction on how to improve a particular exercise

Causal Attributions

The theoretical basis underlying the content of injury attributions is borrowed from Weiner's (1985) causal attribution models for performance. Causal attributions involve speculation over probable causes of success and failure and these explanations affect future motivation and performance. Much like after an athletic performance, athletes may collect their thoughts and engage in reflection after an injury, formulating probable causes for their injury or developing causal attributions. Injured athletes may also engage in similar reflections concerning the cause of their injury, progress of their rehabilitation, and practice return.

Locus of causality, stability, and the addition of controllability are seminal components of causal attributions. Locus of causality refers to whether the cause is within or external to the athlete such as personal effort (internal) or the effort of the opponent (external). This dimension can be considered a disposition where those who have a tendency to explain outcomes from an external cause have the following characteristics: feel that events are beyond their control, are not affected by external feedback or outcomes that are otherwise explained by luck or chance, set less challenging goals, have relatively short persistence, and are less upset by failure. External locus of causality is more common among younger age groups, females, and those who are less academically successful. In contrast, those with an internal locus of causality perceive both positive and negative events as consequences of their own actions, are easily upset from criticism in skill situations, prefer situations where they can exert skill rather than chance situations, set high performance goals, and persist longer at task. Based on these characteristics, it is important to take note of these characteristics and strive to change external causes to internal ones.

Causes can be either stable or unstable. Stability refers to change of the cause of performance over time. For example, ability and task difficulty are relatively stable when compared to luck and effort, which are unstable. Controllability is the third dimension and refers to the extent the athlete takes on responsibility for outcome and is reinforced by the result of the outcome. For example, rehabilitation attrition can result when an athlete perceives little or no progress, which is accompanied by negative emotions and personal responsibility for the lack of progress with little hope of change in the future.

Because the content of causal attributions influences future motivation and performance effectiveness, athletic trainers can play a powerful role in influencing how athletes formulate their injury-related attributions. While it may be inappropriate to expect athletes to take responsibility for their performance outcomes in rehabilitation settings, athletic trainers can strive to shift external locus of control to that which is more internal. This can be achieved by providing more specific ("nice job holding that stretch for 20 seconds") rather than general feedback ("good"), setting attainable goals, and pointing out the progress achieved once the goal is met. Focusing on improvement rather than outcome and on instructional input rather than critical feedback can also help clients learn to define success within their means. Finally, messages sent to the client must be credible in order for the messages to serve as incentive: feelings of security and mastery over exercises. Moving an athlete from an external to internal locus of causality can take extensive and long-term commitment.

Psychomotor Interventions

As in any sport context, there is an art (application) and science (theoretically based content) that enhances athletes rehabilitating an injury. Using psychological interventions with athletes are competency expectations. An athletic trainer who is informed about the theoretical underpinnings of why athletes may need specific interventions as described in previous sections of this chapter and is empathetic with effective communication skills has the potential to impact not only the rehabilitation process but also subsequent training and learning endeavors. Injured athletes should be encouraged to use some of the same mental skills while injured as they do in training (Ford & Gordon, 1998). Although most athletes will have some psychological skills from their sport involvement, few will be knowledgeable about the breadth of each skill and know how to use them systematically given the myriad of issues involved in response to injuries.

Psychological skills are abilities that improve with practice and can enhance the rehabilitation process by affecting compliance and carry over to practice and competitive contexts. For many athletes, developing psychological skills stems from social support that begins with the athletic trainer and can extend to other social agents. The following presentations of psychological skills are consistent with the NATA's competency-based expectations and those identified as important in the injury rehabilitation literature.

GOAL-SETTING

Among athletes in general, goal-setting has been shown to influence performance across age and ability levels by enhancing confidence and motivation and reducing anxiety (Gould, 2001). In a study of injured athletes, goal-setting was perceived as the most valuable psychological adjunct to physical therapy when compared to imagery and counseling, especially among female participants (Brewer, Jeffers, Petitpas, & Van Raalte, 1994). Although athletes and their coaches are well-known for setting their own goals, often goals are inappropriate incomplete or lack systematic properties such as providing goal-related feedback. Goals are usually long-term, such as winning the championship, and if short-term goals are set, they are usually vague or unrealistic with little to no planning for modification. Educating clients about various goal types is a good starting point for implementing a systematic goal-setting program that could potentially transcend the rehabilitation setting and be applied in other training and life domains.

A goal is defined as achieving a specified level of proficiency on a task by a specified time. Setting a time limit and following up to evaluate goal attainment are common oversights in goal-setting environments. Although specifying recovery time should be avoided because it can give athletes false hopes of progress and jeopardize the credibility of health professionals, incorporating specific physical criteria (e.g., improved strength, full range of motion, hop without pain) with goal-setting can help direct recovery. Four types of goals have been specified in the goal-setting literature:

1. Subjective goals: Goals lacking an objective measuring system (e.g., trying one's best, having fun)

2. General objective/outcome goals: Setting a performance standard focusing on the results of a contest (e.g., getting back to preinjury wellness, making the team, winning the championship, beating someone)

3. Specific objective/performance goals: Self-referent goals indicating improvement relative to one's past performance (e.g., lifting an additional 10% in 2 weeks, increasing stableometer balancing time by 15 seconds, pitching 10 throws without feeling pain)

4. Process goals: Specifying the procedures the performer will use during performance (e.g., focus on keeping your elbow glued to your side during 10 external rotations, keep your knee extended on each of your 12 straight-leg raises).

Overwhelming evidence indicates that goal-setting improves performance (Kylo & Landers, 1995), influences athletes to work hard, and reduces off-task behaviors (Wanlin, Hrycaiko, Martin, & Mahon, 1997). It is also clear that goal types vary in their effectiveness for enhancing performance (Kylo & Landers, 1995; Locke & Latham, 1990). Athletes are extremely accustomed to setting outcome goals because of the social norms surrounding athletics in North American culture. Accordingly, it may be difficult to refocus an athlete on the individual steps necessary for successful rehabilitation. Outcome goals are least effective for a variety of reasons. They distract athletes from task-relevant strategies and can cause worry, especially during competitive situations. Because outcomes are contingent on a concert of individual efforts, individuals have limited control over outcome situations. Outcome goals are also limited in flexibility and they lack specificity (Kylo & Landers, 1995). Despite these weaknesses, outcome goals help athletes set priorities and can be particularly motivating during rehabilitation periods when away from competition.

In contrast, process (i.e., biomechanical efficiency instructions) and performance goals (i.e., self-referent comparisons) are most effective for directing efforts toward task-relevant strategies because they can enhance rehabilitation confidence, efficiency, and effectiveness. These types of goals can be thought of as building blocks for achieving outcome goals and are similar to short-term and long-term goals, respectively. By emphasizing a combination of process, performance, and outcome goals, health care professionals can provide greater opportunities for meeting the successful needs of rehabilitation. Clients who meet their goals in one area (e.g., physical rehabilitation-specific goals) can be directed to strive toward completing goals in other areas, such as mentally practicing sport skills or strategies. Most coaches will agree that injured athletes should be kept immersed in regular training regimes. Directing athletes' efforts toward practicing physical skills (albeit mentally) can be highly motivating, enhance memory of strategies, and maintain some neuromuscular pathway activity involved in physically performing the skill.

The following guidelines specify goal-setting characteristics that can be applied when working with clients:

- Provide athletes with realistic definitions of their rehabilitation expectations.
- Set challenging goals in a variety of specific areas (e.g., physical rehabilitation, mental practice of rehabilitation exercises and sport skills or strategies, effort).
- Emphasize effort as a necessary condition for recovery at the outset of the program.
- Set specific goals in measurable terms and provide deadlines, avoid "do your best" goals (e.g., stretch further by another 2 inches, do an additional five repetitions).
- Set short- and long-term goals using a staircase model with short-term goals on each step leading to a single long-term goal at the top, emphasize that achieving the long-term goal requires taking one step at a time.
- Set process, performance, and outcome goals.
- Set goals for physical rehabilitation as well as mental practice of rehabilitation exercises, physical skills, and strategies.
- Set positive rather than negative goals.
- Identify target dates for attaining goals other than those related to physical recovery outcomes.
- In notebooks, record goals once they have been identified, attained, or need modification.
- Provide feedback regarding goals ensuring the various types of goals and performance areas (e.g., physical rehabilitation, mental practice of physical rehabilitation, emotional skills, sport skills and strategies).
- Provide social support for goals by praising effort and progress regularly.

These principles can provide clients with valuable information concerning their progress and help them keep a realistic perspective. Involving social agents such as coaches, peers, and parents can also be used as a systematic goal-setting strategy consistent with the importance of social support in rehabilitation contexts.

IMAGERY

Describing motivational techniques (e.g., imagery) used during injury rehabilitation and reconditioning is an expectation of athletic trainers (NATA, 2006). Despite this clinical proficiency competency requirement, evidence suggests that athletic trainers are apprehensive using imagery in the rehabilitation process. This apprehension is linked to lack of knowledge about how imagery can aid physical recovery and uncertainty regarding its correct use (Wiese et al., 1991). Imagery, mental practice, and visualization are often used interchangeably, but are conceptually distinct. Imagery is a component of mental practice. It involves evoking characteristics of an object that has properties related to performance, or a performance that has taken place in the past or is anticipated to take place in the future using select senses. Visual, kinesthetic, and/or auditory senses are used most often. Accordingly, visualization refers only to the use of visual imagery, which has limited application in athletic and exercise contexts. Using imagery during rehabilitation requires thoughtful consideration of individual characteristics, what to image, and timing this image content relative to the stage of the rehabilitation process. With the goal of optimizing imagery program effectiveness, these considerations are addressed next.

Imagery is a skill that improves with practice so it is important to keep in mind that athletes will vary in their ability to image. Most individuals, especially athletes, have used imagery to some extent but as with all psychological skills are unaware of the full gamut of its properties and applications. For effective imagery use, athletes should be informed about several imagery characteristics, including use of various senses (especially visual and kinesthetic), content serving cognitive and motivational functions, the internal and external imagery perspectives, and various imagery properties.

Imagery Characteristics

Prior to recommending imagery to clients, it is important to assess the extent to which imagery is used and imagery ability. This can be done through short interviews concerning the content of images (skills, strategies, goals, motivation to achieve, arousal control) and to ensure at least the visual and kinesthetic senses are being used. For more systematic assessment of content, practitioners can use questionnaires such as the Sport Imagery Questionnaire (Hall, Mack, Paivio, & Hausenblas, 1998). To determine if athletes have the ability to image, the Movement Imagery Questionnaire-Revised (Martin & Hall, 1995) is a brief questionnaire useful for assessing visual and kinesthetic imagery abilities. These questionnaires can be obtained in full either in the original reference or by contacting the authors. Research using these instruments provides scores for groups with specific characteristics (e.g., ability level, sport type) that can be used to make individual client comparisons. Alternatively, determining where a client stands on the possible range of scores and comparing scores across the various subscales is also useful for directing interventions.

Athletes can use imagery from two different perspectives, or viewpoints: externally imaging themselves performing a skill as if they are watching a video tape of their performance, or internally seeing their performance as if they were looking through their own eyes, capturing peripheral movements in space. According to White and Hardy (1998), external imagery is beneficial for rehearsing strategies and skills. It enables the athlete to replay his or her role in the action and anticipate the role of teammates and opponents. Internal imagery can enhance the feeling and precision of movements involved in rehabilitation exercises; it allows the client to be aware of the positioning, stretch, force, and/or timing involved in movement patterns. While the internal perspective may enhance rehabilitation exercise movements, both perspectives should be encouraged for imaging sport-related skills and strategies in the absence of physical performance.

There is more to imagery than just perspective. Denis (1985) contends that for imagery to have beneficial effects, the content of the image must accurately reflect the intended outcome. Incorporating key properties of imagery during imaging sessions can help improve imagery ability. These properties include vividness, clarity, and exactness of reference, which should be considered in both rehabilitation and sport-related rehearsal contexts. The following rehabilitation-specific illustrations can be used to enhance image quality:

+ *Vividness.* Better imagers increase their potential to move effectively. Focusing on the vividness of an image can be achieved through emphasizing color and positioning relative to other body parts or things in space (e.g., athletes sees themselves participating in a real game situation with defenders, coaches, referees, cheerleaders, and crowd).

+ *Controllability.* Learning how to manipulate images so they correspond to objectives enables recovery from mistakes (e.g., even if the athlete drops the ball, he or she can always control the image and imagine him- or herself catching it using the correct technique 100% of the time).

+ *Exactness of reference.* Imaging the speed, timing, and force involved in moving body parts that can serve to protect athletes from overdoing their physical performance (e.g., athlete can imagine what it means to run 50%, 75%, or 100% to help incorporate appropriate muscle forces and protect the injured body part).

What to Image?

Although the fields of psychology and education have long studied imagery with an emphasis on the visual sense, sport imagery research and application are by and large guided by Martin, Moritz, and Hall's (1999) applied model of mental imagery. This model proposes that imagery can be beneficial in sport performance, exercise, and rehabilitation settings. Depending on the content of an image and individual imagery ability, several desired outcomes can be achieved. These outcomes include learning and performing skills and strategies, modifying cognitions, and controlling arousal and confidence.

Rehabilitation is just one area encompassed by this model and includes a variety of uses that have been supported by research. Rehabilitation imagery has been shown to be effective in preparing injured athletes for practice return (Evans, Hare, & Mullen, 2006), managing pain (Sthalekar, 1993), reducing re-injury anxiety (Cupal & Brewer, 2001), and enhancing the rehabilitation process by focusing on the injured body part (Jones & Stuth, 1997). When directing athletes concerning what to image, it is important to keep in mind that there are four types of rehabilitation imagery. Each targets a specific purpose and involves a specific process. There is little outcome variability; each type of imagery increases confidence, reduces stress, and distracts attention away from pain (Walsh, 2005).

1. *Healing imagery* (e.g., imaging tissue repair) involves envisioning the internal processes and anatomical healing that takes place during rehabilitation. This process is proposed to speed up the healing process. Ievleva & Orlick (1999) point out that imaging one's body as powerful, resourceful, and successful is an important feature of healing imagery.

2. *Pain management imagery* involves imaging pleasant images such as pleasant scenes that can distract the client (e.g., preparation for an injection). It can also involve images of reducing pain intensity or dramatized coping scenarios involving handling the pain, which can provide motivation for recovery.

3. *Process of rehabilitation imagery* refers to imagery of rehabilitation activities that can help a client anticipate these activities and cope with them.

4. *Performance imagery* involves images of practicing while injured and those related to confidence in the injured area on return. When athletes image themselves performing sport skills with the injured body part functioning perfectly, they can maintain their practice routine and their sport skills.

Although researchers indicate imagery should never be used as a substitute for physical practice, when athletes are unable to practice physically due to an injury, imagery is a valuable skill to keep in mind. Because imagery has both cognitive and motivational functions, the utility of imagery in rehabilitation contexts includes learning how to do exercises efficiently, rehearsing sport skills and strategies while injured, setting rehabilitation and practice-related goals, psyching up to attend rehabilitation sessions, and managing pain.

Timing of Imagery

Various types of imagery can be systematically applied at various points in the rehabilitation process. Taylor & Taylor (1998) recommend using relaxation and pain management techniques soon after the injury and throughout the rehabilitation process. Imaging the healing process and being confident in the rehabilitation process are also recommended during the rehabilitation. After completing the physical rehabilitation, imaging being confident in the injured area can be helpful in conjunction with images geared at circumventing re-injury stress. When attempting to cope with pain, focusing attention away from the injured body part (i.e., dissociative techniques) can be helpful. Imagery can also guard against exasperating an injury in the active state of rehabilitation as monitoring changes of pain intensity can help athletes read their bodies (Walsh, 2005).

Because mentally practicing skills, attitudes, and goals can be done anywhere and any time, imagery is certainly one of the most practical intervention techniques. Research on noninjured athletes reveals that imagery is used before, during, and after practice; between breaks; when preparing to practice; during competition; and returning from practice and competition (Munroe, Giacobbi, Hall, & Weinberg, 2000). Imagery has the potential to improve the performance and wellness of both injured and non-injured athletes. With the goal of improving injury rehabilitation effectiveness, medical professionals are advised to make their own judgments about how to delineate individual imagery capabilities, incorporate imagery abilities, and recommend appropriate image content and timing.

SOCIAL SUPPORT

Derived from health-based literature, social support is defined as the interactions between at least two individuals where the intentions of the exchange are perceived as beneficial to the recipient. The intentions of the provider could include emotional, esteem, tangible assistance, and/or informational, alone or in combination. *Emotional support* helps injured individuals feel cared for by others under situations of stress or insecurity. *Esteem support* is provided with the intent of bolstering a sense of competence or self-esteem through the provision of competence-based feedback. Tangible support involves concrete assistance, such as financial or physical assistance. Finally, informational support involves a social agent whose advice or guidance is geared at finding a solution to a problem (Brustad & Babkes, 2004). Social agents who may form a supportive network for an injured athlete include teammates, friends, family (Udry, Gould, Bridges, & Tuffy, 1997), significant others, religious leaders, peers, siblings, coaches and medical personnel, including athletic trainers. Aligned with core values in athletic training, as identified in the *2006 Educational Competencies* (NATA, 2006), athletic trainers are expected to demonstrate knowledge, attitudes, behaviors, and skills necessary to achieve optimal health outcomes for patients. This includes motivating clients through encouragement, reinforcement of rehabilitation exercises, and facilitating similar interactions between other social agents and the client.

Social support is integral to the injury rehabilitation process (Udry, 1996; Weiss-Bjornstal et al., 1998). Athletic trainers are expected to facilitate social support by using motivational techniques with athletes and others involved in physical activity. Satisfaction with social networks has been shown to improve postinjury mood (Green & Weinberg, 1998), increase rehabilitation adherence (Duda et al., 1989; Udry, 1996), and decrease the incidence of postinjury depression (Brewer, Linder, & Phelps, 1995). It is important to note that social support is not always perceived as positive by injured athletes (Quinn & Fallon, 1999) possibly because of the pressure surrounding suggested tasks and the level of emotional involvement emerging from interactions. Accordingly, it is important to consider the mechanisms underlying positive social support.

Injured athletes may benefit from social support in a variety of ways. In addition to having important implications for injury prevention, social support can be viewed as a coping resource throughout injury response and recovery processes. Social agents may reduce perceptions of stress associated with an injury and foster the likelihood that individuals will engage in appropriate problem-solving behaviors associated with rehabilitation, practice return, and re-injury. Information, encouragement, and feedback about progress can serve to enhance self-perceptions and enable the self-confidence and motivation necessary to approach rehabilitation-related behaviors.

In general, social support research has traditionally focused on sources of social support rather than the type of support (Choghara, O'Brien Cousins, & Wankel, 1998). From an applied standpoint, practitioners should attend to the needs of the client by focusing on facilitating those needs within the social network. This includes specific personal roles and fostering viable relationships with other social agents. Aligned with the important social agent roles, informational support in the form of patient education is an athletic trainer's primary role but one that is often overlooked (Wiese-Bjornstal, 2004). In the case of child clients, educating parents is also advocated. Information about the nature of the injury as well as injury prevention should be provided in a way clients can understand. Examples of tangible support include various rehabilitation modalities, but can also include preventative taping, icing, or stretching assistance.

STRESS MANAGEMENT

The idea that stress is a precursor of injuries and is associated with a myriad of emotions during the injury response is well established. Accordingly, having athletic trainers use their knowledge and skills to implement stress reduction techniques for athletes should be incorporated as injury prevention strategies as well as postinjury interventions. Stress management can help prevent injuries by giving the client ways of coping with life's uncertainties, helping the client cope and adjust to his or her injuries, and improving general wellness. Proactive development of stress management skills can provide athletes with an arsenal of skills to use in stressful situations, especially when faced with injury rehabilitation issues such as pain management or anxiety about rehabilitation and practice return.

As noted in earlier descriptions of stress and the injury response, muscular tension that is rooted in anxiety and worry and alerts the muscular system of stress occupies nerve pathways necessary for impulses involved in coordinated movement. Intense bracing of several muscles is a major factor in athletic injuries because it is distracting and can impair attentional focus, decision making, concentration, and movement coordination.

Recognizing and releasing tension before it is magnified to have debilitating effects is a fundamental aspect of stress management. Educating athletes about the potential sources of stress that are highlighted in the stress response models is essential. Regular assessment of stressors for those that are within and beyond one's control can help safeguard energy resources. Minimizing perceptions of stressors that are beyond one's control enables the athlete to place more energy into coping with those that are within one's control. Coping involves thoughts and behaviors used to manage stressful demands and regulate emotions. It is important to note that coping effectiveness is contingent on social and cognitive development and thus may vary across individuals. Athletes who are less mature will have difficulty differentiating between sources of support and recognizing links between current behavior and long-range outcomes because they are motivated by self-centered needs (Lazarus, 1999).

Several strategies including those discussed thus far have implications for stress reduction. For example, goal-setting helps an athlete control their worries because it structures time, enabling systematic completion of tasks and charting of progress. Using self-referent goals helps build confidence, which buffers stress and anxiety. Similarly, imagery can be used as a distraction strategy and is particularly helpful in building confidence if image content pertains to task mastery and goal achievement (Moritz, Hall, Martin, & Vadocz, 1996). However, relaxation strategies are the most common stress management technique because they can target stress components that are cognitive, somatic (physiological), or both. Allowing the CNS to rest subsequently allows regeneration of physical, mental, and emotional states.

Once the nature of the stressor is ascertained, practitioners can tailor relaxation techniques to match the specific symptoms. Behavioral medicine (Lehrer, Carr, Sarganaraj, & Woolfolk, 1993) and sport psychology research (Maynard, Hemmings, & Warwick-Evans, 1995; Maynard, Warwick-Evans, & Smith, 1995) support the notion of matching showing greater reduction in muscular indicators of stress following muscular interventions and greater reduction in cognitive stress following those that were cognitive. The premise of relaxation is learning a self-referent feeling of zero, or no activation. Relaxation strategies are categorized into two categories: mind to body, or cognitive-based strategies; and body to mind, or somatic-based strategies. These are presented next.

Cognitive-Based Strategies

What athletes say to themselves can influence future thought processes and behavior. Worry, accompanied by negative and irrational thoughts, is intricately involved in the progressive reactions of injured athletes that can lead to anxiety and decreased motivation. Thought stoppage, reframing, desensitization, and disassociation are cognitive restructuring techniques that can help circumvent, or at least reduce, worry and doubt— common anxiety-based cognitions. The use of cognitive techniques can reduce the impact of stress and shorten rehabilitation time (Ievleva & Orlick, 1991).

Thought-Stoppage and Reframing

Negative inner dialogue, or self-talk focusing on weaknesses, is common among injured athletes and can influence subsequent thought processes and behavior and lead to anxiety and/or loss of motivation. Helping athletes reframe thoughts such as "I can't do this" or "This is a waste of time" into productive, positive thoughts or goals that are within the athlete's control can influence rehabilitation compliance and athlete wellness. Thought stopping is geared at eliminating negative thoughts that are linked to the spiraling effects of anxiety by stopping the negative thought and replacing it with a positive one using positive self-talk.

There are three steps to stopping negative thoughts: 1) identify and acknowledge the negative thought; 2) upon noticing the negative thought, encourage the athlete to interrupt that thought by saying or thinking "Stop!"; and 3) replace the negative thought with

Table 6-2

Common Negative Thoughts and Appropriate Replacement Thoughts

Negative Thought	Replacement Thought	Context
"I'll never get back to my playing ability."	"Little by little I can achieve this."	Watching practice
"I can't handle this pain."	"Hang in there, be tough."	While icing knee
"I'm too tired."	"Just a few more minutes."	During leg extension exercises
"I'm too weak."	"I am stronger than last week."	During leg extension exercises
"I'm not going to rehab today/anymore."	"Rehab will make me stronger."	Just before getting out of bed
"My teammates will forget about me while I'm injured."	"My knee is healing and I will play as well as before, and maybe even better."	While traveling to practice

Adapted from Krane, V., & Greenleaf, C. (1999). Counseling for the management of stress and anxiety. In R. Ray & D. M. Wiese-Bjornstal (Eds.), *Counseling in sports medicine* (pp. 257-274). Champaign, IL: Human Kinetics.

a productive positive thought. Common negative thoughts and their replacements are presented in Table 6-2.

Krane and Greenleaf (1999) recommend tracking the context of where specific negative thoughts occur and encouraging athletes to log these contexts, the associated thoughts, and assigned positive replacement thoughts within a logbook. Reviewing these entries can help athletes realize common situations and help practitioners anticipate their occurrence—enabling social support. Athletic trainers can remind or cue athletes to replace negative thoughts at relevant times.

Desensitization

Desensitization is a common treatment for anxieties and phobias in clinical psychology settings. It is particularly useful in rehabilitation contexts with athletes who encounter a pronounced fear of re-injury while doing a sport-skill that caused a prior severe injury (e.g., a defensive back returning to a play after suffering a brachial plexis injury). Desensitization helps individuals expose themselves to the feared situation by systematically recalling attributes of the sport situation through imagery and then using relaxation techniques to reduce anxiety. Athletes can be taught to self-administer this technique that involves three steps: 1) relaxation, 2) constructing an anxiety hierarchy, and 3) pairing relaxation with the situations described in their hierarchy.

Achieving a relaxed state of mind is the goal of the first step and any variation of progressive relaxation can be used. Construction of an anxiety hierarchy involves a temporally organized set of attributes of the sport situation (e.g., 1) driving to practice, 2) getting equipment on, 3) warming up, 4) hearing the play called by the coach, 5) approaching the line, 6) the snap of the ball, 7) approaching the defensive player, and 8) making contact). The attributes should be organized to represent a well-spaced sequence of anxiety with sufficient detail, enabling not just a visual image but a full experience of each attribute involving all of the senses. Each attribute is then written on an index card and a score of 0 to 100 is assigned to each card where 100 = highest anxiety level and 0 = no anxiety. This is followed by ranking the order of the cards by anxiety level.

The goal of the pairing procedure is to reduce the anxiety each attribute evokes. A maximum of three attributes should be considered in one session, and attributes should be used in consecutive order of the hierarchy (e.g., session 1, attributes 1 through 3; session 2, attributes 4 through 6, etc.). Each session should last no longer than 30 minutes, practiced twice a week to two times a day depending on ambition. In subsequent sessions, the first card will be the last card read during the previous session. Next, the athlete imagines him- or herself in that situation for 10 to 30 seconds, longer for those who can tolerate more anxiety. The image is then stopped, anxiety evaluated on the scale of 0 to 100, followed by re-establishing relaxation for 30 seconds. The situation is then re-read again for a tolerable time followed by the anxiety evaluation. If anxiety is still present, the attribute is re-read again until no anxiety is felt. Once this has been achieved, the athlete moves on to the next item in the hierarchy. Each session of three attributes ends in several minutes of relaxation. Desensitization is most effective when skill deficits are not the cause of the anxiety (Richmond, 2005).

Dissociation

Dissociation is based on distraction and increasing the client's pain threshold. It is a common pain management strategy used to prepare clients to deal with impending pain and may be less effective in helping clients deal with the sudden impact of pain (Fisher, 1999). Dissociation begins with a focus on breathing where the goal is to sustain slow, deep breaths. Once breathing is under control, other distractions such as listening to music, watching videos, or using imagery can also serve to direct attention away from pain sensations and associated thoughts.

Meditation

The goal of meditation is to achieve a deep state of relaxation by disciplining the mind against intruding thoughts. As thoughts enter consciousness, they are gently blocked to enable attention to refocus on achieving the relaxed state. There are four components to meditation: a quiet environment, a comfortable position, a passive attitude, and a mental device, or mantra. A mantra is a quieting, meaningless, one- or two-syllable sound repeated rhythmically to deter feelings associated with stimulation and arousal; allowing a passive, "let it flow" attitude. Various body areas should be relaxed. Meditation can be done with eyes closed or open, gazing at a specific location or object. It is common for disrupting thoughts to surface during meditation but refocusing on the mantra can gently turn them away.

Relaxation Response

The relaxation response is a meditative technique developed by Benson (1984) with an emphasis on relaxing muscle groups and specifying the word "one." According to Williams & Harris (2001), achievement-oriented athletes may find the word "one" stimulating because it can be associated with arousal that accompanies winning or being the best. They suggest using alternate words such as "calm."

Autogenic Training

Autogenic training is another relaxation technique based on efferent nerve control that involves achieving a state of warmth and heaviness through self-hypnosis. A passive approach is also important in this technique. There are 5 stages in training: learning to experience heaviness and warmth, regulating the heart rate through autosuggestion, awareness of breathing rate, self-regulation of the visceral organs, and kinesthetically imagining the effect of a cool cloth placed on the forehead. Visualization can accompany autogenic training to achieve a relaxed state associated with a desired outcome, such as regaining preinjury performance or recalling a perfect performance. Achieving the full effects of autogenetic training requires long-term commitment where each phase is practiced for 10 to 40 minutes per day over six 1-week periods. While this time frame may preclude typical injury recovery time frames, the technique can be used in non-injury settings (Schultz & Luthe, 1959).

Somatic-Based Strategies
(Adapted from Williams & Harris, 2001)

Breathing Exercises

Regulating breathing is an effective relaxation strategy that is applicable in situations immediately following an injury and during other rehabilitation stages. Stress disrupts breathing patterns in one of two ways: it causes athletes to hold their breath or breathe from the upper part of their chest slowly. These irregular behaviors exasperate tension and can lead to deteriorating concentration and performance. Deep, diaphragmatic breathing helps regulate breathing patterns and facilitates the amount of oxygen carried to muscles and the removal of waste products. Diaphragmatic breathing can be confirmed by having the athlete place one hand on the abdomen and the other on the chest. If the hand on the abdomen moves out with the inhalation and in with the exhalation, while the hand on the chest is relatively still, the athlete is breathing from the diaphragm.

Taking slow, deep, complete breaths triggers the relaxation response; learning how to achieve this efficient breathing pattern can be done through a variety of exercises proposed by Mason (1980). These exercises include: rhythmic breathing, concentration breathing, 1:2 ratio, and 5:1 count.

Rhythmic Breathing

This exercise involves learning how to maintain breathing to a specific count. A four-count hold is a good place to start. Have the athlete breathe in for four counts and out for another four counts. The rhythm of breathing can be altered by changing the count.

Concentration Breathing

Concentration breathing is a good exercise for athletes who have problems with distracting thoughts. Concentrating on breathing rhythm helps athletes focus their attention and prohibits the mind from wandering to thoughts unrelated to the breathing rhythm. The rhythm pattern acts as an anchor to return to if outside thoughts intrude. With each exhalation, athletes should be directed to feel an increasing level of relaxation as they maintain their focus on the rhythm of their breathing.

1:2 Ratio

Compared to the rhythmic breathing exercise, a 1:2 count involves inhaling for half of the exhale count. For example, inhaling for a count of 4 and exhaling for a count of 8. With practice, the count can be increased to 5:10 and 6:12.

5-to-1 Count

This exercise incorporates imagery of numbers as athletes count backwards, breathing rhythmically to a specified count. Have athletes image the number 5 and inhale for a count of five followed by a complete exhale. Next, move to imaging the number 4, inhaling for a count of four and exhaling completely. Continue down to the number 1. After completing the exhalation of each count, have the athlete declare, "I am more relaxed now than I was at number four." This exercise is particularly effective for preparing for surgery or a demanding rehabilitation session.

Progressive Relaxation

Progressive relaxation (Jacobson, 1930) is based on the premise that it is impossible to be nervous or tense if muscles are completely relaxed. This technique involves systematic, purposeful tension followed by release or relaxation of predetermined muscle groups. One of the goals of progressive relaxation is to experience differential feelings of having tense and then relaxed muscles and to decrease the amount of time it takes to feel completely relaxed in all muscle groups.

Like most psychological skills, relaxation is a skill that improves with practice. Adapted from Jacobson's method, six phases of relaxation training that vary in relaxation context, time it takes to relax, duration of phase, and number of muscle groups can be followed to improve an athlete's ability to relax. Because athletes can range on a continuum of relaxation ability, it may be more appropriate to choose one of the phases as a starting point in rehabilitation contexts. However, when the goal of relaxation training is to improve relaxation ability, to achieve best results individuals must master each preceding phase. Progressing too quickly through the program can compromise knowing the feeling of relaxation and being able to instantaneously relax (Table 6-3).

Conclusion

The proliferation of school-sponsored and organized sport will continue to affect the number of athletes across a broad range of development seeking treatment for athletic injuries. Implementing developmentally appropriate psychological interventions is becoming an increasingly important expectation in the allied health professions. When making intervention decisions, attending to personal and situational factors involved in the progressive reaction periods involving cognitive, emotional, and behavioral aspects of injury response can increase the marketability of athletic trainers, but more importantly increase rehabilitation compliance and overall wellness of injured athletes.

Chapter Exercise

Devise a developmentally appropriate course of psychological intervention for each athlete in the following examples, addressing the scenario characteristics as related to progressive injury reactions and personal and situational factors.

   a. Two soccer players are recovering from similar ankle sprains, one is a male collegiate player and the other is a 12-year-old female player. Both athletes are preparing for league championships. Identify sources of anxiety throughout the phases of rehabilitation that would affect each player and how each player may differ in motivation orientation.

Table 6-3
Six Phases of Progressive Relaxation

A. Phase I (takes 20 to 25 minutes, need a dark quiet room)
1. Lying on the floor, focus on breathing rhythm. Concentrate while taking several long, deep breaths.
2. Tense and relax individual muscle groups
   a. Begin by tensing the right fist.
   b. Hold the tension for 5 seconds, concentrating on how the muscle feels.
   c. Slowly and completely release the tension.
   d. Note the difference between the feelings of tension and relaxation.
   e. While releasing muscular tension, repeat a cue word such as "calm," "peace," "release," or "relax."
   f. Repeat steps a though e two or three times.
   g. Repeat the above steps with the left fist.
   h. Repeat each of the above steps with all remaining muscle groups, always focusing on the cue word while continuing slow, deep breathing. For example:
      i. Left biceps – relax – repeat; right biceps – relax – repeat
      ii. Shrug shoulders – relax – repeat
      iii. Tense neck muscles by touching chin to chest – relax – repeat
      iv. Tense facial muscles including clenching of teeth and closing eyes – relax – repeat
      v. Tense stomach muscles – relax – repeat
      vi. Arch lower back – relax – repeat
      vii. Tense buttocks – relax – repeat
      viii. Tense left thigh – relax – repeat; right thigh – relax – repeat
      ix. Tense left calve - relax – repeat; right thigh – relax – repeat
      x. Curl toes – relax – repeat
      xi. Tense all muscle groups noted above – relax – repeat

B. Phase 2 (takes 10 to 15 minutes, done on the floor in a lighted room)
1. Repeat Phase 1, but tense left and right muscle groups simultaneously where relevant.
2. Focus on the cue word and continue slow, deep breathing.
3. Repeat two or three times per muscle group.
C. Phase 3 (takes 5 to 10 minutes, done while sitting in a lighted room)
1. Repeat Phase 2, but only tense each muscle group once.
2. Focus on cue word and continue deep breathing.
D. Phase 4 (takes 1 to 2 minutes, done while sitting in lighted room)
1. Relax each muscle group without any contraction, using the same muscle sequence as in Phase 1.
2. Focus on the cue word and continue deep breathing.
3. Scan the body for any areas of tension and relax this area.
E. Phase 5 (takes 1 to 5 seconds, done during rehabilitation/practice)
1. Take one slow, deep breath.
2. Recall the cue word and the feeling associated with relaxation and let it quickly flow through the body.
F. Phase 6 (done instantly during rehabilitation/practice)
1. During stressful situations (e.g., preparing for surgery, holding a stretch in an injured leg)
2. Anytime a client feels tense
   a. Take one deep breath.
   b. Think of the cue word.
   c. Relax.

b. In the midst of football season, a 16-year-old quarterback sustained a painful ACL injury during his first time executing a new play during practice. He is a multi-sport athlete. His parents are pressuring his rehabilitation in hopes of being well enough for baseball season. He is very focused on the images of the injury and feels anxious about the likelihood of full recovery.

References

Aaron, J., Zaglul, H., & Emery, R. E. (1999). Post-traumatic stress in children following acute physical injury. *Journal of Pediatric Psychology, 24,* 335-343.

Benson, H. H. (1984). *Beyond the relaxation response.* New York, NY: Times.

Brannon, L., & Feist, J. (2004). *Health psychology: An introduction to behavior and health* (5th ed.). Belmont, CA: Wadsworth.

Brewer, B. W. (1994). A review and critique of models of psychological adjustment to athletic injury. *Journal of Applied Sport Psychology, 6,* 87-100.

Brewer, B. (2003). Developmental differences in psychological aspects of sport injury rehabilitation. *Journal of Athletic Training, 38,* 152-153.

Brewer, B. W., Anderson, M. B., & Van Raalte, J. L. (1999). Psychological aspects of sport injury rehabilitation: Toward a biopsychosocial approach. In D. I. Motsofsy & L. D. Zaichkowsky (Eds.), *Medical aspects of sport and exercise.* Morgantown, WV: Fitness Information Technology.

Brewer, B. W., Cornelius, A. E., Van Raalte, J. L., Petitpas, A. J., Pohlman, M. H., Krushell, R. J., et al. (2003). Age-related differences in predictors of adherence to rehabilitation after anterior cruciate ligament reconstruction. *Journal of Athletic Training, 38,* 158-162.

Brewer, B. W., Jeffers, K. E., Petitpas, A. J., & Van Raalte, J. L. (1994). Perceptions of psychological interventions in the context of sport injury rehabilitation. *Sport Psychologist, 8,* 176-188.

Brewer, B. W., Linder, D. E., & Phelps, C. M. (1995). Situational correlates of emotional adjustment to athletic injury. *Clinical Journal of Sports Medicine, 5,* 241-254.

Brustad, R. J., & Babkes, M. L. (2004). Social influence on the psychological dimensions of adult physical activity involvement. In M.R. Weiss (Ed.), *Developmental sport and exercise psychology: A lifespan perspective* (pp. 313-332). Morgantown, WV: Fitness Information Technology.

Chogahara, M., O'Brien, Cousins, S. & Wankel, L.M. (1998). Social influences in physical activity in older adults: A review. Journal of Aging and Physical Activity, 6, 1-17.

Cupal, D. D, & Brewer, B. W. (2001). Effects of relaxation and guided imagery on knee strength, re-injury anxiety and pain following anterior cruciate ligament reconstruction. *Rehabilitation Psychology, 46,* 28-43.

Denis, M. (1985). Visual imagery and the use of mental practice in the development of motor skills. *Canadian Journal of Applied Sport Sciences, 10,* 4S-16S.

Duda, J. L. (1993). Goals: A social cognitive approach to the study of motivation in sport. In R. N. Singer, M. Murphy, & L. K. Tennant (Eds.), *Handbook of research in sport psychology* (pp. 421-436). New York, NY: McMillan.

Duda, J. L., Smart, A. E., & Tappe, M. K. (1989). Predictors of adherence in the rehabilitation of athletic injuries: An application of personal investment theory. *Journal of Sport and Exercise Psychology, 11,* 367-381.

DuRant, R. H., Pendergrast, R. A., Donner, J., Seymore, C., & Gaillard, G. (1991). Adolescents' attrition from school-sponsored sports. *American Journal of Diseases in Children, 145,* 1119-1123.

Evans, L., & Hardy, L. (1995). Sport injury and grief responses: A review. *Journal of Sport and Exercise Psychology, 17,* 227-245.

Evans, L., Hare, R., & Mullen, R. (2006.) Imagery use during rehabilitation from injury. *Journal of Imagery Research Sport Physical Activities, 1,* 1-19.

Fisher, A. C. (1999). Counseling for improved rehabilitation adherence. In R. Ray & D. M. Wiese-Bjornstal (Eds.), *Counseling in sports medicine* (pp. 257-274). Champaign, IL: Human Kinetics.

Ford, I. W., & Gordon, S. (1998). Guidelines for using sport psychology in rehabilitation. *Athletic Therapy Today, 2,* 41-44.

Gould, D. (2001). Goal setting for peak performance. In J. Williams, (Ed.). *Applied Sport Psychology: Personal Growth to Peak Performance* (4th ed., pp. 190-205). Mountainview, CA: Mayfield.

Gould, D., & Tuffy, S. (1996). Zones of optimal functioning research: A review and critique. *Anxiety, Stress and Coping, 9*, 53-68.

Green, S. L., & Weinberg, R. S. (1998). The relationship between athletic identity, coping skills, social support and the psychological impact of injury. *Journal of Applied Sport Psychology, 10*(Suppl.), S127.

Hall, C. R., Mack, D., Paivio, A., & Hausenblas, H. (1998). Imagery use by athletes: Development of the Sport Imagery Questionnaire. *International Journal of Sport Psychology, 29*, 73-89.

Hanin, Y. (1986). State trait anxiety research on sports in the USSR. In C. D. Spielberger & R. Diaz (Eds.), *Cross-cultural anxiety* (vol. 3, pp. 45-64). Washington, D.C.: Hamisphere.

Hardy, L. (1990). A catastrophe model of anxiety and performance. In J. G. Jones & L. Hardy (Eds.), *Stress and performance in sport* (pp. 81-106). Chichester, England: Wiley.

Harter, S. (1981). The development of competence motivation in the mastery of cognitive and physical skills: Is there still a place for you? In G. C. Robers & D M. Landers (Eds.), *Psychology of motor behavior and sport—1980* (pp. 3-29). Champaign, IL: Human Kinetics.

Hedgpeth, E. G., & Gieck, J. (2004). Psychological considerations for rehabilitation of the injured athlete. In W. E. Prentice (Ed.), *Rehabilitation techniques for sports medicine and athletic training* (4th ed.). New York, NY: McGraw-Hill.

Heil, J. (1993). Sport psychology, the athlete at risk and the sports medicine team. In J. Heil (Ed.), *Psychology of sport injury* (pp. 1-13). Champaign: Human Kinetics.

Ievleva, L., & Orlick, T. (1991). Mental links to enhanced healing: An exploratory study. *Sport Psychologist, 5*, 25-40.

Ievleva, L., & Orlick, T. (1999). Mental paths to enhanced recovery from a sports injury. In D. Pargman (Ed.), *Psychological basis of sport injuries* (2nd ed.). Morgantown, WV: Fitness Information Technology.

Jacobson, E. (1930). *Progressive relaxation.* Chicago, IL: University of Chicago Press.

Johnson, L., & Carroll, D. (2000). Coping, social support, and injury changes over time and the effects of pain and exercise involvement. *Journal of Sport and Rehabilitation, 9*, 291.

Jones, L., & Stuth, G. (1997). The uses of mental imagery in athletics: An overview. *Applied and Preventative Psychology, 6*, 101-115.

Kerr, J. H. (1990). Stress in sport: Reversal theory. In J.G. Jones & L. Hardy (Eds.), *Stress and performance in sport* (pp. 107-131). Chichester, England: Wiley.

Krane, V., & Greenleaf, C. (1999). Counseling for the management of stress and anxiety. In R. Ray & D. M. Wiese-Bjornstal (Eds.), *Counseling in sports medicine* (pp. 257-274). Champaign, IL: Human Kinetics.

Kubler-Ross, E. (1969). *On death and dying.* New York, NY: Macmillan.

Kylo, L. B., & Landers, D. (1995). Goal-setting in sport and exercise: A research synthesis to resolve the controversy. *Journal of Sport and Exercise Psychology, 17*, 117-137.

Lampton, C., & Lambert, M. (1993). The effects of psychological factors in sports medicine rehabilitation adherence. *Journal of Sports Medicine and Physical Fitness, 33*, 292-299.

Larson, G. A., Starkey, C., & Zaichkowsky, L. D. (1996). Psychological aspects of athletic training injuries as perceived by athletic trainers. *Sport Psychologist, 10*, 37-47.

Lazarus, R. S. (1999). *Stress and emotion: A new synthesis.* New York, NY: Springer.

Lehrer, P. M., Carr, R., Sarganaraj, D., & Woolfolk, R.L. (1993). Differential effects of stress management therapies in behavioral medicine. In P. M. Lehrer & R. L. Woolfolk (Eds.), *Principles and practice of stress management* (2nd ed., pp. 571-605). New York, NY: The Guilford Press.

Locke, E. A., & Latham, G. P. (1990). *A theory of goal-setting and task performance.* Englewood Cliffs, NJ: Prentice-Hall.

Malina, R. M., Bouchard, C., & Bar-Or, O. (2004). *Growth, maturation, and physical activity* (2nd ed.). Champaign, IL: Human Kinetics.

Martens, R., Burton, D., Vealey, R., Bump, L., & Smith, R. (1990). Development and validation of Competitive State Anxiety Inventory—2. In R. Martens, R. Vealy, & D. Burton (Eds.), *Competitive anxiety in sport* (pp. 117-190). Champaign, IL: Human Kinetics.

Martin, K., & Hall, C. (1995). Using mental imagery to enhance intrinsic motivation. *Journal of Sport and Exercise Psychology, 17*, 54-69.

Martin, K. A., Moritz, S. E., & Hall, C. R. (1999). Imagery use in sport: A literature review and applied model. *Sport Psychologist, 13*, 245-268.

Mason, L. J. (1980). *Guide to stress reduction.* Cluver City, CA: Peace Press.

Maynard, I. W., Hemmings, B., & Warwick-Evans, L. (1995). The effects of a somatic intervention strategy on competitive state anxiety and performance in semi-professional soccer players. *Sport Psychologist, 9,* 51-64.

Maynard, I. W., Warwick-Evans, L., & Smith, M. J. (1995). The effects of a cognitive intervention strategy on competitive state anxiety and performance in semi-professional soccer players. *Journal of Sport and Exercise Psychology, 17,* 428-446.

McDonald, S.A., & Hardy, C.J. (1990). Affective response patterns of the injured athlete: An exploratory analysis. The Sport Psychologist, 4, 261-274

Moritz, S. E., Hall, C. R., Martin, K. A., & Vadocz, E. (1996). What are confident athletes imaging? An examination of image content. *Sport Psychologist, 10,* 171-179.

Munroe, K., Giacobbi, P. R., Hall, C. R., & Weinberg, R. (2000). The four W's of imagery use: Where, when, why and what. *Sport Psychologist, 14,* 119-137.

National Athletic Trainers' Association. (2006). *Athletic Training Educational Competencies.* Dallas, TX: NATA.

Palermo, T. M., & Drotar, D. (1996). Predictions of children's postoperative pain: The role of pre-surgical expectations and anticipatory emotions. *Journal of Pediatric Psychology, 21,* 683-698.

Prentice, W. E. (2006). *Arnheim's principles of athletic training: A competency-based approach.* Boston, MA: McGraw-Hill.

Quackenbush, N., & Crossman, J. (1994). Injured athletes: A study of emotional responses. *Journal of Sport Behavior, 17,* 178-187.

Quinn, A. M., & Fallon, B. J. (1999). The changes in psychological characteristics and reactions of elite athletes from injury onset until full recovery. *Journal of Applied Sport Psychology, 11,* 210-229.

Richmond, R. L. (2005). *A guide to psychology and its practice.* Retrieved on October 25, 2005, from http://www.guidetopsychology.com/sysden.htm

Roberts, G. (1992). *Motivation in sport and exercise: Conceptual constraints and convergence.* Champaign, IL: Human Kinetics.

Roh, J. L. C., & Perna, F. M. (2000). Psychological counseling: A universal competency in athletic training. *Journal of Athletic Training, 35,* 458-465.

Schultz, J. H., & Luthe W. (1959). Autogenic training: A psycho-physiological approach in psychotherapy. New York, NY: Grune and Statton.

Sthalekar, H. A. (1993). Hypnosis for relief of chronic phantom pain in a paralyzed limb: A case study. *Australian Journal of Clinical Hypnotherapy and Hypnosis, 14,* 75-80.

Taylor, J., & Taylor, S. (1998). Pain education and management in the rehabilitation from sport injury. *Sport Psychologist, 12,* 68-88.

Udry, E. M. (1996). Social support: Exploring its role in the context of athletic injuries. *Journal of Sport Rehabilitation, 5,* 151-163.

Udry, E. M., Gould, D., Bridges, D., & Tuffy, S. (1997). People helping people? Examining the social ties of athletes coping with burnout and injury stress. *Journal of Sport and Exercise Psychology, 19,* 368-395.

Udry, E., Shelbourne, K. D., & Gray, T. (2003). Psychological readiness for anterior cruciate ligament surgery: Describing and comparing adolescent and adult experiences. *Journal of Athletic Training, 38,* 167-171.

Walsh, M. (2005). Injury rehabilitation and imagery. In T. Morris, M. Spittle, & A. P. Watt (Eds.), *Imagery in sport.* Champaign, IL: Human Kinetics.

Wanlin, C.M., Hrycaiko, D.W., Martin, G.L. & Mahon, M. (1997). The effects of a goal-setting package on the performance of speed skaters. Journal of Applied Sport Psychology, 9, 212-228.

Weiner, B. (1985). An attribution theory of achievement motivation and emotion. *Psychological Review, 92,* 548-573.

White, A., & Hardy, L. (1998). An in-depth analysis of the uses of imagery by high-level slalom canoeists and artistic gymnasts. *Sport Psychologist, 12,* 387-403.

Weiss, M. R. (2003). Psychological aspects of sport-injury rehabilitation: A developmental perspective. *Journal of Athletic Training, 38,* 2, 172-175.

Wiese-Bjornstal, D. M. (2004). From skinned knees and peewees to menisci and masters: Developmental sport injury psychology (pp. 525-568). In M.R. Weiss (Ed.), *Developmental sport and exercise psychology: A lifespan perspective.* Morgantown, WV: Fitness Information Technology.

Wiese-Bjornstal, D. M., Smith, A. M., Schaffer, S. M., & Morrey, M. A. (1998). An integrated model of response to sport injury: Psychological and sociological dimensions. *Journal of Applied Sport Psychology, 10,* 46-69.

Wiese, D. M., Weiss, M. R., & Yukelson, D. P. (1991). Sport psychology in the training room: A survey of athletic trainers. *Sport Psychologist, 5,* 25-40.

Williams, J.M. (2001). Psychology of injury risk prevention. In R.N. Singer, H.A. Hausenblas & C.M. Jannelle (eds.) Handbook of Sport Psychology, Second Edition. New York, NY: Wiley and Sons.

Williams, J. M., & Anderson, M. B. (1998). Psychosocial antecedents of sport injury: Review and critique of the stress injury model. *Journal of Applied Sport Psychology, 10,* 5-25.

Williams, J., & Harris, D. (2001). Relaxation and energizing techniques for regulation of arousal. In J. Williams (Ed.), *Applied sport psychology: Personal growth to peak performance* (4th ed., pp. 229-246). Mountain View, CA: Mayfield.

Williams, J. M., Rotella, R. J., & Scherzer, C. B. (2001). Injury risk and rehabilitation: Psychological considerations. In J. M. Williams (Ed.), *Applied sport psychology: Personal growth to peak performance* (4th ed., pp. 456-479). Mountain View, CA: Mayfield.

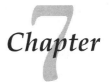

Chapter

MENTAL HEALTH ISSUES FOR ATHLETIC TRAINERS

H. Ray Wooten, PhD

Chapter Objectives

- ❖ Examination of the positive benefits of athletic involvement.
- ❖ Examination of mental health risks.
- ❖ Understanding the assessment of mental health difficulties.
- ❖ Clarification of specific mental health disorders.

NATA Educational Competencies

Psychosocial Intervention and Referral Domain

1. Describe the basic principles of general personality traits, associated trait anxiety, locus of control, and patient and social environmental interactions.

2. Describe the basic signs and symptoms of mental disorders (psychoses), emotional disorders (neuroses, depression), or personal/social conflict (family problems, academic or emotional stress, personal assault or abuse, sexual assault, sexual harassment); the contemporary personal, school, and community health service agencies, such as community-based psychological and social support services that treat these conditions; and the appropriate referral procedures for accessing these health service agencies.

Medical Conditions and Disabilities Domain

1. Describe and know when to refer common psychological medical disorders from drug toxicity, physical and emotional stress, and acquired disorders (e.g., substance abuse, eating disorders/disordered eating, depression, bipolar disorder, seasonal affective disorder, anxiety disorders, somatoform disorders, personality disorders, abusive disorders, and addiction).

Mental health problems are common in the United States at the rate of 1 in 5 adults having a diagnosable mental disorder in a given year as reported by the National Institute of Mental Health. The National Alliance for Mental Illness reported that the percentage of college students diagnosed with depression increased from 10.3% in fall 2000 to 14.9% in spring 2004. Reasons why students are struggling to such a degree are complex; however, the challenges student athletes face are well documented in the literature (Hinkle, 1994; Lanning, 1982; Remer, Tongate, & Watson, 1978; Wittmer, Bostic, Phillips, & Waters, 1981; Wooten & Miller, 2001). Regardless of how positive athletic competition may be for athletes, the challenges of balancing sport and academics can often be overwhelming and detrimental.

Valentine and Taub (1999) noted that student athletes have been the most recognized, yet unofficial, special population on college campuses. Faculty, students, and the general public have been inundated with selective reports for both male and female student athletes of the "dumb jock" image that is all too prevalent across college campuses, resulting in the devaluation of the student regardless of his or her athletic or academic ability. Ferrante, Etzel, and Lantz (1996) suggest that the general stereotype of college student athletes is privileged, lazy, out of control, and motivated solely to participate in athletics. The idea of "special population," privileged, and the like has been grossly misperceived and created a variety of deleterious stereotypes that have retarded efforts to adequately create awareness and programs that can effectively meet the needs of these individuals. The result has been to grossly under-serve the student athletes' mental health in favor of athletic enhancement, mental toughness training, and teamwork.

Benefits of Athletic Involvement

Historically, human beings have generally considered displays of physical prowess to be markers of the truly great, the best of the best. Virtually every culture in the world lifts up individuals who can run faster, jump higher, fight harder, carry more weight, etc. than others. Examples include Greek Olympiads, medieval knights, samurai, Native American hunters, and, of course, modern professional athletes. Members of these groups are or were given special honors and privileges. Typically, popularity and prestige increase a person's self-esteem. The same is true for athletes today of every level, from junior high school students to college intramural participants, and from recreational marathon runners to top draft picks for professional teams. Being able to excel in anything builds self-worth and being able to perform physical feats is especially valued by society, so it is a great boon to a person's overall happiness and mental well-being.

Self-Esteem and Athletic Involvement

Numerous empirical studies have been done comparing self-esteem and other markers of mental health for athletes and nonathletes (Edwards, Edwards, & Basson, 2004; Dykens, Rosner, & Butterbaugh, 1998; Hudd et al., 2000; Pedersen & Seidman, 2004; Wilkins & Boland, 1991). Overall, these studies conclude that sport participation is good for a person's self-esteem. More importantly, a recent empirical study of 571 college students was conducted to examine global psychiatric symptoms in athletes as compared to nonathletes. They concluded that athletes showed "less severe global psychiatric symptoms" than nonathletes, and that this held true regardless of whether the athletic involvement was competitive or recreational (Donohue et al., 2004).

These studies, however, do not clearly determine whether athletic involvement causes an increase in mental health or if those with greater mental health choose athletics. There are several potential explanations for these outcomes. One explanation is simply that athletic involvement requires mental stability, and those with mental or emotional instability participate in athletics at a much lower rate. While possible, that explanation adds little to clinical experience of providing mental health care to athletes, particularly those who are experiencing mental health disturbances. A more precise explanation of the specific aspects of athletic involvement that are beneficial is needed. Some of the aspects of athletics that do promote mental well-being are increased exercise, social support, and insulation from certain stressors. These possibilities will be explored later in the text. Furthermore, there currently are athletes needing mental health treatment, and guiding framework for clinical work with these athletes is lacking.

The Mental Health Model (Raglin, 2001) is a reasonable starting place for possible explanations. The Mental Health Model states that there is a negative correlation between mental disorders and athletic performance, meaning that when one is high the other is low. This correlation allows for the observed fact that some athletes do indeed have mental disorders and need treatment to continue their athletic endeavors because their performance suffers in relationship to that mental disturbance. Likewise, athletes with more mental stability are better able to have successful athletic performance. This is particularly important for elite athletes and potentially great athletes who do develop psychopathological symptoms. Though the Mental Health Model of sport performance may seem somewhat obvious, mental health care for athletes is frequently overlooked. When clinical care is needed, best practice in treating athletes requires that the mental health professional be knowledgeable about aspects of athletic involvement that promote mental well-being, such as exercise, social support, and anything that reduces an athlete's stress.

BENEFITS OF EXERCISE

Exercise does promote mental health (Edwards et al., 2004; Dykens et al., 1998; Hanin, 2000; Van Raalte & Brewer, 2002). Even small amounts of aerobic exercise can elevate a person's overall mood. For years, mental health professionals have recommended increased exercise, such as taking a walk for 15 to 20 minutes per day, to depressed clients because it has been repeatedly proven helpful. Using muscles requires a person to breathe more deeply to have enough oxygen in a person's body. Increased oxygen, then, also moves into the person's brain, which promotes emotional calming and stability. Furthermore, exercise releases the same neurotransmitters that are released naturally when people are having fun and feeling happy. These neurotransmitters help to stabilize a person's mood and, therefore, promote mental health in general. Clinically, in working with athletes, this principle is particularly important because mental health treatment should absolutely include discussions about appropriate exercise regimens. Care should be taken not to overdo the exercise, as some mental disorders common to athletes involve excessive exercise, but continuing some exercise is vital to successful mental health care for athletes. If athletes reduce their exercise too much, their bodies will actually be receiving less of these positive benefits from oxygen and neurotransmitters than normal.

SOCIAL SUPPORT

Another common mental health recommendation is to increase clients' access and usage of their own network of social support. Increased social support provides an inoculation from the ill effects of negative experiences in life, including those relevant to athletes with psychopathology (Murphy, 1995). Athletes may not be comfortable sharing their mental health concerns with some of their usual social support network. Clinical work with athletes must involve training athletes to access their social network in a way that still preserves the confidentiality of their mental health care. Athletes can call upon their teammates and coaches for support, with or without revealing specifics of any clinical symptoms. They can workout with a friend, participate in fun activities, celebrate victories, and commiserate losses with others. In addition, mental health professionals who do work with athletes need to be active in educating the athletic community in general about the intrinsic link between mental well-being and successful athletic performance. Increased education will add credibility to mental health care for athletes and decrease the stigma of mental disorders within this community.

ATHLETIC PRESTIGE

The extreme stigma against psychopathology is due in part to both the narrow focus on physical well-being and the prestige associated with being a successful athlete. This prestige also can be used to promote mental well-being. With prestige comes a protection from certain stressors that are experienced by peers who do not hold that same powerful position; it buffers some stress. For example, student athletes may have tutoring arranged for them to ensure that they are passing their classes so that they can continue to compete. Peak athletes are often considered leaders and as such may be given "idiosyncrasy credit" (Wren, 1995, p. 91) to explain what would otherwise be perceived as unusual behavior. One clinical description of a psychiatrist's work with athletes stated, "It may be difficult to differentiate the person from the athletic 'persona'. Although not common, emotional maturity may be delayed because of an athlete's 'iconization,' placing the athlete 'on a pedestal,' and having others insulate them from the stresses and problems of daily life" (Glick & Horsfall, 2001). Professional football player Ricky Williams describes using the prestige of his position, even in college, to mediate his social anxiety. He describes having his unusual behavior explained away by people who wanted to preserve his reputation, "If I didn't want to honor an obligation,... I knew someone would cover me... A lot of people made it easy for me to hide" (Wertheim, 2003). Clearly prestige, whether from athletic involvement or some other source, can be used as part of mental health care to protect clients from excessive stress until they are more capable of dealing with it. However, as in the case of Ricky Williams, avoiding stress cannot continue indefinitely; the athlete must also be treating the real problem causing the stress, particularly if that problem is psychopathology.

Mental Health Risks of Athletic Involvement

Despite all of the benefits of participating in athletics and the public perception that the athletes are the best of the best, professionals working with student athletes would be highly remiss in their obligation to those athletes if they did not also fully recognize and address the potential risks to athletes' mental health. Most of the risks to student athletes are intrinsically linked to the benefits, especially the benefit of prestige. As prestige increases, pressure mounts, not only to maintain one's performance but to improve it. Student athletes, as others, can handle various amounts of pressure, depending upon the individual. Therefore, inevitably, some student athletes are going to succumb to the stressors and manifest mental health anomalies in response to that pressure. In addition, prestige also brings opportunities for participating in drug and alcohol abuse, either as a method to cope with pressure or in celebration of successes. Also, no athlete is going to succeed all the time, and failures can be truly devastating. Athletic involvement cannot make people immune to mental disorders that they are inclined to develop; they still ultimately have clinically significant symptoms of psychopathology.

Challenges Unique for Student Athletes

Etzel, Ferrante, and Pinkney (1996) suggest that student athletes have a qualitatively different educational experience than nonathletes that include adjustment to competing demands, response to negative stereotypes, and need for unique support services. Etzel et al. (1996) go on to suggest that competitiveness, physical regimen, and extreme emotional demands associated with college athletics make athletes more vulnerable to developmental crises and psychological distress problems than nonathletes. Other researchers have also found negative effects of athletic participation. Sedlacek and Adams-Gaston (1992) suggest that the athletic environment is exploitive, developmentally damaging, socially alienating, and generally nonsupportive. Likewise, Hinkle (1994) suggests that student athletes have an increased level of anxiety due to the threat of evaluation from others, lack of self-confidence, and unreasonable expectations from coaches and fans.

The athletic environment is one of competing demands for the student athletes. Lack of balance in negotiating athletic and academic demands is replete in the literature (Lanning, 1982; Remer et al., 1978; Wittmer et al., 1981; Wooten, 1994). Juggling the physical, mental, and emotional demands of sport, as well as the demands from the classroom, may leave some student athletes developmentally and psychologically vulnerable. Petitpas (1978) described identity foreclosure as a significant developmental vulnerability of many student athletes. Given the seduction of sport celebrity and prestige along with the pressures from parents and community, many student athletes fail to participate in developmentally appropriate activities, resulting in a premature decision of "who they are" and what they want to do in life. This premature decision or "foreclosure" is based on a lack of developmental exploratory activities and information and inadequate insight to make an informed choice. Consequently, student athletes may suffer from low self-efficacy, external locus of control, and difficulty in dealing with complicated tasks or situations. The tumult of coping with athletic expectation, possible injury, and the realization that inevitably participation in sports will end can be harrowing. Many student athletes they face existential dilemmas of making meaning of their lives and anticipating the future for the first time. For those athletes that have foreclosed on identity or have not adequately prepared for life after sport, the stress is overwhelming.

The athletic milieu may in fact inadvertently foster difficulty in adapting to a variety of social challenges by the demands from practice, training, meetings, and competition. Student athletes are required to sacrifice substantial amounts of time that they could otherwise use to be engaged in extra-curricular and social activities. Parham (1993) noted that student athletes are often estranged from their peers and campus community. Nonathletes may not be very sympathetic toward the requirements of the athletic culture like time commitments, maintaining body weight, and responsibility to one's teammates. Fellow athletes may be so occupied with handling their own pressures that they may not be available for needed support, or athletes struggling with mental health concerns may feel vulnerable if they exposed these difficulties to fellow athletes.

Other noted areas of increased vulnerability include managing athletic success and failure, coping with physical injury, and being "cut" or terminated from sport. This trio is largely due to an inordinate amount of stress to perform athletically and academically and results in increased mental health vulnerability. Coping with athletic success translates into increased expectations and pressure to perform consistently at higher levels. Likewise, performing below expectation or "potential" may lead the athlete to overtrain and have an increased susceptibility to injury or mental health disorders. The injury can be another major stressor in that the athlete cannot practice to perfect the skill, subsequently missing competition and having the opportunity to "prove one's self." Overtraining syndrome is perhaps one of the best examples of how athletic involvement can exacerbate depression (Hanin, 2000; Murphy, 1995). In fact, the symptoms of overtraining syndrome are so similar to the diagnostic criteria for a major depressive episode that the most prominent distinction between them is simply being actively involved in physical training of some form and noticing a decrease in physical performance. Furthermore, many of the same neurotransmitters are indicated in both overtraining syndrome and major depression (Armstrong & VanHeest, 2002). Among swimmers who are overtraining, psychological hardiness has been shown to mediate mood disturbances, including depression and anxiety (Goss, 1994). Depression can appear independently or as an aspect of many other mental disorders, often appearing comorbidly with anxiety (Schofield, Dickson, Mummery, & Street, 2002), and substance abuse (Longman, 2003).

Coinciding with student athlete vulnerability and distress is their reluctance to disclose problems and utilize counseling services. Recent research (Brewer, Van Raalte, Petitpas, Bachman, & Weinhold, 1998; Maniar, Curry, Sommers-Flanagan, & Walsh, 2001) have shown that student athletes are averse to employ mental health counseling as well as sport psychology services. Instead, student athletes are more inclined to call upon coaches, teammates, family, or friends (Selby, Weinstein, & Bird, 1990). This reluctance to access mental health professionals mirrors a shame of mental health disorders in the general public. This is magnified by the fact that athletes are in the spotlight and open to critique from many sources. Furthermore, athletes are in peak physical condition, and often society expects that their physical health should correspond to health in all aspects of their lives. It, therefore, should come as no surprise that athletes avoid professional mental health support.

Consequently, student athletes can be considered "at risk" or "high risk" for increased physical, mental, emotional, learning, and developmental anomalies. This is largely due to conditions that demand excessively high levels of effort, both academically and athletically, without supportive mechanisms that would facilitate effective coping. The "at risk" or "high risk" connotation is likewise appropriate given the statistical likelihood of student athletes experiencing a mental health disorder or dysfunction. Given the nuances of the athletic milieu as described earlier, student athletes are vulnerable to inordinate amounts of environmental and life stress events that directly affect their personal homeostasis. This effect is often described as the diathesis stress model. The diathesis stress model is an advantageous heuristic proposing that individuals have a diathesis or predisposition of risk factors that arise given the amount of acute or chronic stress experienced and lack accompanying coping abilities. In this case, the student athlete may be vulnerable to a variety of mental health anomalies (e.g., depression, anxiety, and substance abuse). For example, Green, Uryasz, Petr, and Bray (2001) found that almost 81% of student athletes had used alcohol in the year 2000. The researchers also found that college student athletes had significantly higher rates of heavy drinking than nonathletes. The results confirmed an earlier study that college student athletes drink more alcohol than other students (Leichliter, Meilman, Preseley, & Cashin, 1998). Likewise, Johnson, Powers, and Dick (1999) conducted a NCAA survey and found that the appearance-related and performance-related drives to thinness are devastating illusions that are counterproductive and dangerous to male and female athletes. In the study, Johnson et al. discovered that 58% of female athletes were at risk for an eating disorder and that 9% warranted medical attention. Among male athletes, 38% were at risk for an eating disorder and 1% warranted medical attention. These are only a few statistics that illuminate the need for more awareness of mental health problems and frontline aggressive efforts to identify, assess, and refer student athletes to appropriate care.

Assessment of Mental Health Difficulties

The athletic trainer is often the first to recognize mental health anomalies of student athletes. Athletic trainers have a day-to-day experience with the athlete and can create a mental health baseline for the athlete. It is important that the athletic trainer create an atmosphere conducive for a relationship to enable the baseline to be created. The baseline can be created from signs that the athletic trainer experiences and from the athlete's disclosure of symptoms. Signs are observed by an outside party such as the athletic trainer, while symptoms are reported by the person experiencing them. Signs may include mood (e.g., happy, sad), emotion (e.g., flat affect, animated), and physiology (e.g., head down and slumped shoulders, restlessness). Symptoms may be disclosed in form of comments or complaints about sleeping patterns, eating patterns, and general or specific somatic complaints. All information from signs and symptoms can be used to create a profile when further assessing the athlete. Accurate diagnosis requires an open mind to observe all signs and ask about all symptoms, so as to not prematurely foreclose on a specific diagnosis before all other possibilities are ruled out. Choosing a diagnosis before enough information is gathered will impair observation to the exclusion of other possibilities. This can lead to wrong conclusions and ineffective discussion with the counseling professional. Always keep several possibilities open when assessing and consult with peers and other professionals.

Assessment must be done within a safe, healthy, nonjudgmental context. This listening relationship is created with gentle but direct questions to gain clarity of the athlete's experience. A template to help conceptualize and understand the athlete's mental health functioning is the Mental Status Exam (MSE). The MSE is an outline of specific mental health criteria that takes only minutes to administer. The MSE is a combination of signs and symptoms that can guide attention to relevant details and interviewing questions. Listed are a variety of signs and symptoms to assess. This is not an exhaustive list of the MSE but some guidelines to help in creating an assessment template. Secondly, observations from this list may help alert those in the athlete's support system to recognize that the athlete may need further attention from a mental health professional. Some important signs include the following:

- *Appearance*: This is how the athlete looks presently.

- *Basic grooming and hygiene*: How is the athlete dressed, is it appropriate attire for the weather, how would you describe the athletes hygiene?

- *Motor coordination*: What is the athletes' posture, mannerisms; are the athlete's motor movements awkward, staggering, rigid, shuffling?

- *Eye contact*: Does the athlete make eye contact or avoids or hesitates to make eye contact?

- *Speech and expressive language*: Is the athlete's speech normal rate, pressured, slow, loud, or quiet? How does the athlete express him- or herself? (answers could include no problems expressing self, tangential, difficulty finding words, mumbling).

- *Interpersonal characteristics*: Open and friendly, cooperative, defensive, oppositional, resistant, submissive.

- *Behavioral and mood characteristics*: Alert, lethargic, anxious, depressive, distant, indifferent, angry, frightened. How does he or she feel most days (e.g., happy, sad, elevated, depressed)?

- *Orientation and alertness*: Is the athlete aware of where he or she is and the time; does he or she appear alert, sleepy, dull, or uninterested?

Several simple questions can further the assessment and allow the athletic trainer or other person doing the assessment to show concern for the athlete. These questions can include the following:

- How are you sleeping?

- Do you have trouble falling asleep, staying asleep, or waking up in the middle of the night?

- How is your eating and appetite?

- How do you feel most days?

- How has your mood been?

- What has been on your mind?

- Are there things that worry you?

Questions that are well-timed, caring, and succinct can illicit ample information to assess the athlete's level of stress and duress. The goal is to create a profile to conceptualize the athlete's level of current functioning and possible further behavioral assessment and subsequent diagnosis by other helping professionals. Some common diagnostic classifications that are important to be aware of are mood disorders, anxiety disorders, substance abuse, and eating disorders. These classifications are very common in the general population and with student athletes. The discussion below is to outline salient information that can be crucial when those close to an athlete suspect that the athlete may be suffering from a disorder.

Mood Disorders

Mood disorders are a category of diagnoses in the DSM-IV-TR that are characterized by gross deviations in mood or overall attitude and feeling. There are some fundamental building blocks, namely major depressive episode and mania, that individually or in combination make up this category. These building blocks appear quite different and yet can be correlated. Accurate diagnosis requires attention to the possibility of both.

Depressive Disorders

A major depressive episode is not merely being "down in the dumps" or having a "blue day" but a syndrome of mood, cognitive, and physical complaints that are more severe and require medical and psychological attention. The DSM-IV-TR criterion for depression is a 2-week period of notably depressed mood accompanied by cognitive and physical difficulties. However, sometimes depression impacts a person's mood by causing him or her to feel irritable or frustrated rather than sad. Also, depression can be marked by a sense of restlessness. Either way, clearly the person's mood is more negative than usual. Thoughts of death, suicide, or harming one's self are recurrent among depressed individuals. If a person seems to be saying goodbye to his or her loved ones, giving away treasured belongings, or other types of activities that signify the idea that his or her life is over, refer the person immediately to a mental health professional, as they may be actively suicidal. The cognitive symptoms of depression can include symptoms of hopelessness or helplessness; they also may notice clouded thinking or an inability to focus. Some also describe feelings of guilt or worthlessness. Often, individuals suffering from depression display a loss of interest or pleasure in activities of the day. Physical systems can be affected also, especially sleeping, eating, and energy levels. These physical symptoms can change either by increasing or decreasing. With appropriate assessment of symptoms (experienced and reported by the athlete) and signs (observed by someone else), it is possible to make a determination if the student athlete is experiencing a major depressive episode.

DSM-IV-TR CRITERIA FOR MAJOR DEPRESSIVE DISORDER

The criteria require that five (or more) of the following symptoms have been present during the same 2-week period and represent a change from previous functioning, and at least one of the symptoms is either (1) depressed mood or (2) loss of interest in things previously found enjoyable.

- Depressed mood most of the day
- Anhedonia (markedly diminished interest or pleasure in activities of the day)
- Weight loss (when not dieting) or weight gain
- Insomnia or hypersomnia almost every day
- Psychomotor retardation or agitation
- Fatigue or loss of interest
- Feelings of worthlessness, helplessness, or hopelessness

- Diminished ability to concentrate or make decisions
- Recurrent thoughts of death, suicidal ideation, suicide attempt

A clinical note of importance is to assess for symptoms that are directly due to a general medical condition (e.g., hypothyroidism), to the direct effects of a substance (e.g., drug of abuse, a medication), or the effects of bereavement of a loved one. In any of these cases, a different diagnosis and treatment would be in order. Depression does not have a single, independent cause, nor does it progress in the same way for all people. Depression may be precipitated by significant events. It also can be associated with illness or injuries that adversely affect a person's lifestyle, such as a disabling injury that hinders a person's mobility. However, often there is no understandable "cause" for a person's depression, because depression ultimately is the result of a chemical imbalance in the brain. It is also associated with a person's genetic history. Stress, loss, hormone changes, and even seasons of the year can trigger depression. Depression varies in intensity and duration from person to person. It also can exist alone or in combination with many other mental health disorders.

A second building block for the mood disorders is mania. Mania is often characterized as an abnormally elevated, expansive, or irritable mood. People that have experienced a manic episode describe it as exaggerated joy, too much energy, and euphoria. They become extraordinarily restless, active, requiring little to no sleep, develop grandiose plans, and if not hospitalized and treated can have deleterious effects. DSM-IV-TR also defines a less severe state of mania called hypomania. People experiencing hypomania report feeling good and the ability for high productivity in school or work. This state is far less problematic and does not usually cause marked impairment but does contribute to several mood disorders (e.g., bipolar II). Hypomania could possibly lead to a full blown manic episode or can precede a major depression.

DSM-IV-TR Criteria for Manic Episode

The criteria require that three or more of the following are observed over a period lasting at least 1 week characterized by abnormally and persistently elevated, expansive, or irritable mood:

- Inflated self-esteem or grandiosity
- Decreased need for sleep
- Flight of ideas (i.e., racing thoughts)
- Distractibility
- Excessive involvement in pleasurable activities that have high potential for painful consequences (e.g., buying sprees, sexual promiscuity, car racing, etc.)
- Psychomotor agitation
- Pressured speech

A clinical note of importance is to assess for direct effects of a substance (e.g., medication, drug abuse) or general medical condition (e.g., hyperthyroidism). Either of these effects would warrant a different diagnosis and treatment.

Bipolar Disorders

Bipolar disorders are phenomena when manic or hypomanic episodes alternate with major depressive episodes. This creates an experience of highs and lows, shifts in mood, energy, and the ability to function that creates severe mental distress. Distress usually takes the form of poor school and job performance, relationship difficulties, legal problems, and suicide. Bipolar disorders can be treated successfully with medication, combined with long-term prevention strategies, and counseling. Bipolar I is the most severe because of the manic episodes and subsequent major depressive episodes followed by bipolar II disorder, which is characterized by hypomania episodes that alternate with depression.

RELATIONSHIP ISSUES

Depression is often associated with relationship problems. People suffering with depression are often withdrawn from their family and friends. They may be so focused on their own concerns that they seem selfish. Frequently, people lose interest in activities they once enjoyed, including sexual intimacy. Sometimes, friends and family blame the person with depression for not being able to handle their emotional lives more effectively because they do not understand that depression is beyond the person's control. Another common relationship problem is the lack of motivation to participate in life. Families may be discouraged because their loved one cannot even seek out treatment, much less complete his or her household responsibilities. Depression, then, can leave family members trying to take up the slack for the depressed person. This adds to the family's stress, which compounds the mood disturbances and tends to spread around the negative mood. Commonly, if one person in the house is depressed, another may become so within a short period of time.

Any time symptoms of depression are observed in a person for more than 2 weeks, the person should be referred to a mental health professional. Untreated depression can cause serious problems in a person's life, relationships, and work. Ultimately, it can be fatal because severe depression places a person at a high risk for suicide. On the bright side though, depression is highly treatable with a combination of medication, therapy, and simple lifestyle changes.

MEDICATION FOR DEPRESSION

Depression is typically quite responsive to medication. Some types of antidepressants include tricyclics, monoamine oxidase inhibitors, selective serotonin uptake inhibitors, and the newer atypical antidepressants. Most of these take about 6 weeks to reach full potency within a person's body, although often the person begins to feel some relief within 2 to 3 weeks. If the person experiences adverse side effects, the physician will then simply try a different type of antidepressant because people do have unique responses to the different types and doses of medications. Some common, but usually mild, side effects are dry mouth, weight gain, changes in sleep patterns, or headaches. Antidepressants are typically not habit-forming and do not change people's personalities. They should, however, be taken as prescribed and should not be stopped without consulting the physician because the depression could come back worse than before if stopped prematurely.

COUNSELING TO TREAT DEPRESSION

In addition to medication, counseling is also helpful in treating depression. Often depression comes about after a prolonged period of stress in a person's life. More adaptive responses to stress and stress management typically relieve some of the symptoms of depression. Therapy can help a person work on problem-solving strategies and can change a person's beliefs or expectations about life. Counseling is useful when people are at transition points in their life, such as starting or leaving school, getting married, having children, divorcing, as children age, or even at retirement. These transitions are difficult for all people, and if there are other factors present, these are times that a person is more prone to depression. Counseling allows people to directly face these emotional difficulties and make the necessary shifts to proceed with their lives. Therapy, particularly family therapy, facilitates resolving some of the relationship issues that often are associated with depression.

People suffering with depression can also do several things themselves to treat their depression in addition to or until the medication and therapy take effect. Moderate exercise is a wonderful way to combat depression because exercise produces endorphins and neurotransmitters, which help to rebalance the chemicals in the brain. Exercise outdoors is particularly beneficial because fresh air and sunshine also encourage the body to regulate its chemical production. People suffering with depression also need to make the most of their personal support networks, such as family, friends, teammates, and mentors. Positive support helps replace the feelings of worthlessness and hopelessness often associated with depression. It is important when coping with depression to try to maintain regular eating and sleeping habits as much as possible, even when the person does not feel as hungry or tired as usual. This means people must make themselves stick to their usual routines despite wanting to deviate from those patterns. Drinking lots of water is particularly important, due to the side effect of dry mouth, to enable optimum processing of medications. Perhaps most importantly, alcohol and drugs should be avoided because of their complex, adverse interaction with the neurotransmitters connected with depression. All of these are general habits of good health that are of vital importance when coping with depression.

Referral

Depression in athletes must be recognized, referred to a mental health professional, and treated, or it will ultimately affect their athletic performance. In fact, observed decline in their athletic abilities may be the point when the athletes or their coaches recognize that there is indeed a problem. Depression is not a disorder that people can simply ignore or think their way out of, or hope it will go away. Overcoming depression is not the same as preparing the appropriate mindset for athletic competition. Untreated depression rarely improves; it usually gets worse. Athletes may lose their motivation to practice or even to try their hardest during performances. Losses or failure to achieve certain athletic goals may be unnecessarily devastating to athletes who have depression. Weight fluctuations or loss of energy may prevent them from achieving their full capabilities athletically. Finally, depression in athletes is a big problem because it so frequently occurs with other disorders like anxiety, eating disorders, and substance abuse.

The most important thing to remember about depression is that if it is suspected, the person should immediately be referred to a mental health professional for treatment. Depression can cause tremendous disruptions in a person's life and can be fatal if left untreated. Depression clearly shows physical components and may appear without any observable reason. When treated, depression usually begins to subside within 2 or 3 weeks and may be fully alleviated within 2 months. People who have mood disturbances and changes in their sleeping and eating patterns should immediately be referred to a counselor or psychiatrist to be screened for depression. If anyone ever reports having thoughts of suicide or death, someone needs to escort that person to the emergency room because he or she could be actively suicidal. Depression needs to be treated in everyone, including athletes.

Anxiety Disorders

Anxiety is often characterized as a negative mood of apprehension accompanied with physiological characteristics. Everyone experiences some level of anxiety, and it is not until that level of anxiety exceeds what might be expected for the situation that anxiety becomes a problem. When studying for a test or athletic competition, an "optimal" level of anxiety is helpful to achieve the highest possible performance. However, too much anxiety can become problematic. Over-anxious people may begin to panic at the thought that they may not perform well and catastrophize the results of such a failure. Irrationality becomes rampant and physiological alarm kicks in, creating an emotional situation that can lead to panic.

Anxiety is a part of any competitive endeavor, which certainly includes athletics. In fact, some anxiety is necessary for peak performance in competition. Physically, anxiety raises a person's energy level by getting adrenaline flowing through the person's body. Adrenaline sharpens one's senses, increases heart rate and breathing, and allows for bursts of strength and speed. Anxiety is what gives competitors this edge to their performance. Lack of anxiety typically means one of two things. First, anxiety represents a desire to perform one's best; it means the outcome of the competition matters to the person competing. To put it simply, if there is no anxiety regarding a performance, the person does not care whether he or she succeeds or fails. The second way a person could exhibit no anxiety about a performance is if he or she is completely confident that he or she will succeed no matter what. This attitude tends to lead to mistakes and errors that are not typical of the person's capabilities. So, athletes and other competitors need anxiety. However, too much anxiety is even more detrimental to peak performance.

PERFORMANCE ANXIETY

An overabundance of anxiety during competition is most commonly known as performance anxiety. When people experience performance anxiety, their bodies are in overdrive. There is so much adrenaline flowing that people become focused on their bodies or worrying about the outcome rather than giving attention to their performance in the moment. When experiencing performance anxiety, people do not achieve their peak performance levels. Sometimes, they get so anxious that they cannot even begin the competition. Other times, they may start the competition but, again, make mistakes on well-rehearsed tasks. Often, the ability to manage one's anxiety marks the difference between elite competitors and those that are merely pretty good. Another important trait of performance anxiety is that it builds as the competition nears, and then subsides, often even disappearing completely, after the event is over.

Although performance anxiety is detrimental to athletes and other competitors and may prevent them from achieving success and moving to the next level of competition, it usually does not affect their lives outside of the competitive arena. When anxiety crosses that boundary and begins to affect a person's life in multiple settings, anxiety has then become a true mental health concern. Anxiety is fear when there is no actual threat of harm to one's self. This fear can be about specific things, as in phobias, or it can be more global, as in generalized anxiety disorder. The most important distinction between good anxiety, performance anxiety, and clinical anxiety is the degree to which this fear interferes with normal daily functioning.

SIGNS AND SYMPTOMS OF ANXIETY

The symptoms of clinical anxiety are very similar to symptoms people typically associate with fear. Physical symptoms include increased heart rate or the feeling that one's heart is pounding, shortened breaths, trembling or shaking, sweating, cold hands or feet, dizziness, choking, muscle tightness, numbness, and headaches. People experiencing anxiety typically find their minds flooded with thoughts of disaster, losing control, going crazy, and even death. Typically, after the anxiety has passed, the person can recognize their fears as extreme for the situation. Nevertheless, the next time it occurs, they cannot stop those same fears from running rampant. Anxiety is essentially the body running on overdrive for no apparent reason. It resembles the opposite of depression, where the body does not have enough energy or motivation to act. Since some of the same parts of the brain are affected, many people have both anxiety and depression. For people with both, their bodies swing from one to the other.

PANIC ATTACKS

Intense anxiety is called a panic attack. People having panic attacks cannot control their panic; their bodies are in overdrive just as if they were actually in immediate mortal danger when none exists. During the panic attack, the person can recognize that logically there is no real danger, but this only adds to the thoughts of going crazy and losing control. After the panic attack is over, the person is left with a feeling of dread of having another one. This may cause the person to try to begin avoiding situations in which he or she might have a panic attack. Since the attacks themselves cannot be controlled when they are occurring, people try to avoid triggering the attacks. This begins a cycle of increased avoidance, increased general anxiety, and increased panic attacks until it escalates so much that the person can no longer function in daily life. People with untreated panic attacks often begin avoiding necessary situations like work or the grocery store. This is known as agoraphobia, which specifically means avoiding situations in which if a panic attack occurred, the person would have not be able to get out of the situation easily. In other words, there would be no ready escape route available for the person to retreat until the panic passed. Severe agoraphobia can even mean that people are afraid to leave their homes.

DSM-IV-TR describes a panic attack as a discrete period of intense fear or discomfort, in which four or more of the following symptoms develop abruptly and reach a peak in 10 minutes:

- Palpitations, racing heart
- Sweating
- Trembling, shaking
- Shortness of breath
- Chest pain or discomfort
- Choking
- Nausea or abdominal distress
- Fear of losing control or going crazy
- Fear of dying
- Numbness or tingling sensation
- Chills or hot flashes
- Feeling dizzy, faint

- Derealization (feelings of unreality) or depersonalization (being detached from one's self)

Three basic types of panic attacks are described in the DSM-IV-TR: unexpected (uncued), situationally predisposed, and situationally bound (cued). Most people experience their initial panic attack as an unexpected or uncued panic attack. In many cases, the person then experiences what is called anticipatory anxiety in preparing for another attack but is unsure of what might trigger the panic attack. Situationally bound attacks are cued to a specific situation. For example, people who are afraid of heights may have a panic attack if presented with such an experience but not anywhere else. A situationally predisposed panic attack is where people anticipate that another attack may occur in a similar situation to a previous panic episode. For example, people may have a fear of heights yet some situations that involve high places may not illicit a panic episode.

Panic attacks are not the only form of clinical anxiety. Generalized anxiety can also cause great difficulty in maintaining one's daily routines. Whereas panic attacks come on very suddenly, are extremely intense, and then dissipate, generalized anxiety exists all the time at a lower level than the panic attacks. Generalized anxiety can be thought of as worrying all the time about everything. People with this disorder cannot escape the sense that something is wrong. As one might expect, this can lead to health problems such as ulcers, heart problems, and immune dysfunction.

GENERAL ANXIETY DISORDER

Another anxiety condition that deserves attention is generalized anxiety disorder (GAD). People that suffer from GAD are sometimes referred to as "worry-warts." This is not worrying about a few things that sporadically might result in a little worry, but an indiscriminate worry process that includes everything. The worry appears as if it has a life of its own, resulting in worrying about everything, becoming unproductive, and miserable. DSM-IV-TR describes the criteria for a GAD diagnosis by the following:

- Excessive anxiety and worry (apprehensive expectation) occurring more days than not for 6 months, about a number of events and activities (e.g., school, work)
- The person finds it difficult to control the worry
- The anxiety and worry can be associated with 3 or more of the following:
  * Restlessness
  * Being easily fatigued
  * Difficulty concentrating
  * Irritability
  * Muscle tension
  * Sleep disturbance

Phobia

Another type of clinical anxiety is phobia. Phobias are intense fear triggered by a certain thing, like heights, tight spaces, or spiders. The most difficult phobias are those in which the triggers are found frequently in life, such as water, dirt, germs, or even other people. The fear of people is known as social phobia. It can begin as performance anxiety, but then the embarrassment aspect becomes more powerful. Untreated, the person could then begin to apply the fear of being embarrassed to situations other than the specific performance. Social phobia can include fear of simple interactions with other people such as checking out of a store or having someone speak to them in an elevator. As with panic attacks, people with phobic disorders work very hard to avoid anything that will trigger their phobias. People may go to great lengths to avoid the feared object, which if the trigger is common, could create major disruptions in their lives. Again, at its most severe and particularly with social phobia, the avoidance behaviors can become agoraphobia.

STRESS DISORDER

Stress disorders are another type of anxiety disorder. The stress is in response to an extreme stress or trauma, such as a car accident, sexual abuse, living in a war zone, or other dangerous event. Acute stress disorder occurs immediately following the trauma. If it does not resolve, it can become post-traumatic stress disorder, which can last for the rest of the person's life. Stress disorders are characterized by fear-like symptoms, especially about anything resembling their trauma. People with stress disorders may be extremely jumpy or overly careful. They may have difficulty falling asleep, concentrating, or handling frustrations. It also includes frequent thoughts of the trauma that interfere with daily activities or with sleep as nightmares. Most noticeably, stress disorders can include flashbacks to the traumatic event. During a flashback, people are re-experiencing the trauma in their minds and will react accordingly. For example, a person who survived the trauma of a fire may have a flashback at the scent of even a small amount of smoke, like from a candle. When the person flashes back, he or she may cough, cover his or her mouth, and cry out in pain. To that person, he or she is actually back in the fire. Stress disorders do not get better without treatment, and anyone close to a trauma survivor should watch him or her closely for any signs of a stress disorder.

OBSESSIVE-COMPULSIVE DISORDER

A final type of anxiety disorder is obsessive-compulsive disorder. Obsessions are persistent anxious thoughts, and compulsions are repeated actions in response to obsessions. Obsessive thoughts are considered inappropriate and cannot be stopped no matter how hard the person tries. Some common obsessions include thoughts of being contaminated, doubts about security or accuracy, an excessive need for order, or even aggressive or sexual thoughts. Compulsions attempt to relieve the anxiety of the obsessive thought, and they do temporarily. However, then the obsessions return, and the compulsion must be repeated to relieve the anxiety. These disruptive thoughts and actions take a significant amount of time, at least an hour or more per day, away from the person's normal life. Some compulsions are hidden from even the person's closest friends, and the person considers them a burdensome part of his or her daily routine. The source of obsessions is ultimately anxiety, and this disorder must be treated like any other anxiety disorder for it to improve.

TREATMENT

Treating anxiety disorders usually involves medication and therapy, especially cognitive behavioral therapy. As with depression, there are varieties of medications used to treat anxiety disorders, and a physician must moderate the dosage according to the individual's reactions to it. The medication stabilizes the chemicals in the person's brain, and side effects are usually well tolerated by most people. However, people with anxiety disorders have also learned maladaptive behavior over time, and they must take the time to learn more appropriate behaviors in addition to taking the medication. Cognitive behavioral therapy is used to directly address both the feelings of fear and the avoidant behaviors. The therapist works with the client to decrease the frequency of the problematic behavior and to replace it with more adaptive responses. People undergoing therapy for anxiety behaviors are gradually exposed to the object of their fear, and as they gain success in handling it, the intensity of the exposure is increased. For example, a person with social phobia would be asked first to imagine having a successful, nonthreatening social encounter. Then he or she might be asked to practice the encounter with a doll in the therapy session and then to practice with the therapist. Next, the person could be asked to rehearse with a friend or family member out in public. Finally, the person would try a small, simple encounter with a stranger. Slowly, this would teach the person a healthier response. Each step of this process would include training the person in relaxation methods to help control the physiological responses to the anxiety. To address the fears during deep relaxation, hypnosis may be used in conjunction with the other forms of therapy. Anxiety disorders are highly responsive to treatment, and often people experience complete relief of their symptoms.

Anxiety impacts athletes in several important ways. The most obvious way is that many athletes suffer from performance anxiety. This prevents them from achieving their potential athletically and is something that therapy can help them overcome. However, clinical anxiety causes problems outside of the sports arena and definitely requires therapy. Some medications used to treat anxiety are not allowed in sports, which places even more emphasis on the therapeutic options. If an athlete has achieved success, the development of an anxiety disorder can be devastating. Successful athletes are expected to manage their anxiety in their sports, and often this is carried over into their lives outside of their sports. Succumbing to anxiety is shameful to many competitors, and it can be very difficult to separate the inevitable anxiety that is part of competing from clinical anxiety. Clinical anxiety, though, will get worse unless it is treated, even for elite athletes.

Adjustment Disorder

As mentioned previously, people can exhibit signs and symptoms of mood disorders in response to difficult life experiences, such as loss, moving, employment difficulties, or another major stressor. In those cases, adjustment disorder is the primary focus. The DSM-IV-TR lists the following criteria for adjustment disorder:

- The development of emotional or behavioral symptoms in response to an identifiable stressor(s) occurring within 3 months of the onset of the stressor(s).

- These symptoms of behaviors are clinically significant as evidenced by either of the following: 1) marked distress that is in excess of what would be expected from exposure to the stressor and 2) significant impairment in social or occupational/academic functioning.

- The stress-related disturbance does not meet the criteria for another specific Axis I disorder and is not merely an exacerbation of a pre-existing Axis I or Axis II disorder.

- The symptoms do not represent bereavement.

- Once the stressor (or its consequences) has terminated, the symptoms do not persist for more than an additional 6 months.

Adjustment disorder can occur with either depressed mood, anxiety, mixed anxiety and depressed mood, disturbance of conduct, or mixed disturbance of emotions and conduct. In simple terms, people meet the criteria for adjustment disorder if they feel they need additional assistance in managing the stress of life or if those around them describe significant distress. Adjustment disorder can occur in response to many different stressful stimuli, such as relationship difficulties, academic problems, illness, financial struggles, or simply unexpected change. Athletes may display adjustment disorder after an injury, losing an important competition, being "cut" from their team, or the realization that they will not be able to continue to achieve higher levels of success in their sport. Any stressor can trigger adjustment disorder.

Conclusion

Athletes face a myriad of difficulties and stressors that are unique to this population. These men and women often appear invincible as athletes, yet as humans are extremely vulnerable. The aforementioned literature is explicit that due to the demands and stressors these individuals face they are indeed in need of services to help them cope. A misperception exists between their athletic persona and public image that has resulted in miscommunication, lack of understanding, and apathy when it comes to helping the athlete. This chapter has illuminated aspects of athlete development and stressors that can result in mental health anomalies. A variety of mental health issues impact athletes at all levels of competition and often go unrecognized and untreated until the athlete is in crisis. The athletic trainer can play a pivotal role in the preliminary assessment and referral of these mental health issues. The athletic trainer is in a wonderful position to be a first line responder in assessing athletes and potentially preventing the issue from exacerbating. Athletic trainers can learn to appreciate and recognize the mental health needs of athletes by developing a new awareness of their role and knowledge about the mental health of athletes.

Chapter Exercises

1. Divide the class into small groups of five persons each. Ask each group to brainstorm a list of the mental health benefits of participation in athletics or in a physical fitness program. Give each group 10 minutes to do this. Next, ask each group to prioritize the top three items from their list. Allow another 5 minutes for this. Lastly, have the groups compare and discuss their lists in the total class.

2. Ask a counselor from your institution's counseling center to come and speak to the class regarding mental health issues faced by students on campus. Prior to this individual's visit, have each student prepare one question regarding a mental health issue and send it to the counselor so she or he can focus on some specifics for the class members.

3. Divide the class into groups of five and have each group report on one of the following :
    a. Depressive disorders
    b. Anxiety disorders
    c. Adjustment disorders.

    In this report they should include sources from the following:
    a. A psychology textbook
    b. A psychology journal article
    c. A web-based source such as Web MD

4. Ask a professional from a local mental health center to come to class and speak about the treatment services available to individuals in the community and discuss the intake procedures for an individual that may be referred to that agency.

5. Present the film Fear Strikes Out, depicting the impact mental illness had on the baseball player Jimmy Piersall. It is suggested that the film be previewed and discussion questions be developed for the students prior to showing the film.

6. Have students conduct a web search regarding the quarterback Terry Bradshaw and his battle with depression. Students could then read his biography and prepare a report on his experiences.

7. Have students contact various mental health agencies in your community and develop a resource guide for referring individuals for mental health assistance. Secure the following information from these contacts:

    a. Population served
    b. Fees for services
    c. Insurance coverage policies
    d. Referral procedures
    e. Hours of operation
    f. Contact personnel

References

Armstrong, L. E., & VanHeest, J. L. (2002). The unknown mechanism of the overtraining syndrome: Clues from depression and psychoneuroimmunology. *Sports Medicine, 32*(3), 185-209.

Brewer, B. W., Van Raalte, J. L., Petitpas, A. J., Bachman, A. D., & Weinhold, R. A. (1998). Newspaper portrayals of sport psychology in the United States, 1985-1993. *Sports Psychologist, 12,* 89-94.

Diagnostic and statistical manual of mental disorders (4th ed., text revision). (2000). Washington, DC: American Psychiatric Association.

Donohue, B., Covassin, T., Lancer, K., Dickens, Y., Miller, A., Hash, A., et al. (2004). Examination of psychiatric symptoms in student athletes. *Journal of General Psychology, 131*(1), 29-36.

Dykens, E. M., Rosner, B. A., & Butterbaugh, G. (1998). Exercise and sports in children and adolescents with developmental disabilities: Positive physical and psychosocial effects. *Child & Adolescent Psychiatric Clinics of North America, 7*(4), 757-771.

Edwards, D. J., Edwards, S. D., & Basson, C. J. (2004). Psychological well-being and physical self-esteem in sport and exercise. *International Journal of Mental Health Promotion, 6*(1), 25-32.

Etzel, E. F., Ferrante, A. P., & Pinkney, J. W. (1996). *Counseling college student athletes: Issues and interventions* (2nd ed.). Morgantown, WV: Fitness Information Technology.

Ferrante, A. P., Etzel, E. F., & Lantz, C. (1996). Counseling college student athletes: The problem, the need. In E. F. Etzel, A. P. Ferrante, & J. W. Pinkney (Eds.), *Counseling college student athletes: Issues and interventions.* Morgantown, WV: Fitness Information Technology.

Glick, I. D., & Horsfall, J. L. (2001). Psychiatric conditions in sports. *Physician and Sportsmedicine, 29*(8), 44-52.

Goss, J. D. (1994). Hardiness and mood disturbances in swimmers while overtraining. *Journal of Sport and Exercise Psychology, 16*(2), 135-149.

Green, G. A., Uryasz, F. D., Petr, T. A., & Bray, C. D. (2001). NCAA study of substance use and abuse habits of college athletes. *Clinical Journal of Sports Medicine, 11,* 51-56.

Hanin, Y. L. (2000). *Emotions in sport.* Champaign, IL: Human Kinetics.

Hinkle, S. J. (1994). *Sports counseling: Helping student athletes.* ERIC Document Reproduction Service, No. ED 379 532.

Hudd, S. S., Dumlao, J., Erdmann-Sager, D., Murray, D., Phan, E., Soukas, N., et a.. (2000). Stress at college: Effects on health habits, health status, and self-esteem. *College Student Journal, 34*(2), 217-228.

Johnson, D., Powers, C., & Dick, C. (1999). Athletes and eating disorders: The national collegiate athletic study. *International Journal of Eating Disorder, 26*, 179-188.

Lanning, W. (1982). The privileged few: Special counseling needs of athletes. *Journal of Sport Psychology, 4*, 19-23.

Leichliter, J. S., Meilman, C. A., Presley, C., & Cashin, J. R. (1998). Alcohol use and related consequences among students with varying levels of involvement in college athletics. *Journal of American College Health, 46*, 257-262.

Longman, J. (2003, November 26). An athlete's dangerous experiment. *New York Times*, p. D1.

Maniar, S. D., Curry, L. A., Sommers-Flanagan, J., & Walsh, J. A. (2001). Student-athlete preferences in seeking help when confronted with sport performance problems. *Sport Psychologist, 15*, 205-223.

Murphy, S. M. (1995). *Sport psychology interventions*. Champaign, IL: Human Kinetics.

National Alliance for Mental Illness (2004). Mental illness profiles among college students. Retrieved July 24, 2007, from http://www.nami.org

Parham, W. (1993). The intercollegiate athlete: A 1990's profile. *The Counseling Psychologist, 21*, 411-429.

Pedersen, S., & Seidman, E. (2004). Team sports achievement and self-esteem development among urban adolescent girls. *Psychology of Women Quarterly, 28*(4), 412-422.

Petitpas, A. (1978). Identity foreclosure: A unique challenge. *Personnel and Guidance Journal, 56*, 55-56.

Raglin, J. S. (2001). Psychological factors in sport performance: The Mental Health Model revisited. *Sports Medicine, 31*(12), 875-890.

Remer, R., Tongate, F. A., & Watson, J. (1978). Athletes: Counseling the over-privileged minority. *Personnel and Guidance Journal, 56*, 626-629.

Schofield, G., Dickson, G., Mummery, K., & Street, H. (2002). Dysphoria, linking, and pre-competitive anxiety in triathletes. *Athletic Insight: Online Journal of Sport Psychology, 4*(2), 78-92.

Sedlacek, W. E., & Adams-Gaston, J. (1992). Predicting the academic success of student-athletes using SAT and noncognitive variables. *Journal of Counseling and Development, 70*, 724-727.

Selby, R., Weinstein, H. M., & Bird, T. S. (1990). The health of the university athlete: Attitudes, behaviors, and stressors. *Journal of American College Health, 39*, 11-18.

Valentine, J. J., & Taub, D. J. (1999). Responding to the developmental needs of student athletes. *Journal of College Counseling, 2*, 164-179.

Van Raalte, J. L., & Brewer, B. W. (2002). *Exploring sport and exercise psychology* (2nd ed.). Washington, DC: American Psychological Association.

Wertheim, L. J. (2003). Prisoners of depression. *Sports Illustrated, 99*(9), 70-76.

Wilkins, J. A., & Boland, F. J. (1991). A comparison of male and female university athletes and nonathletes on eating disorder indices: Are athletes protected? *Journal of Sport Behavior, 14*(2), 129-144.

Wittmer, J., Bostic, D., Phillips, T. D., & Waters, W. (1981). The personal, academic, and career problems of college student athletes: Some possible answers. *Personal and Guidance Journal, 60*, 52-55.

Wooten, H. R., & Miller, G. (2001). Sports counseling preparation at CACREP institution. *Academic Athletic Journal, 15*, 6-10.

Wooten, H. R. (1994). Cutting losses for transitioning student-athletes: An integrative transition model. *Journal of Employment Counseling, 31*, 2-9.

Wren, J. T. (1995). *The leader's companion: Insights on leadership through the ages*. New York, NY: The Free Press.

Chapter

CATASTROPHIC INJURIES AND THE ROLE OF THE ATHLETIC TRAINER

Timothy D. Malone, MD
Bryan D. Fox, PhD
Ashley Mulvey, MS, ATC

Chapter Objectives

- ❖ Define catastrophic injuries.
- ❖ Identify normal and pathological responses to catastrophic events.
- ❖ Discuss clinical strategies to aid athletic trainers in making the appropriate mental health interventions and referrals.
- ❖ Discuss the essential components of the therapeutic relationship and expanded role of the athletic trainer as the front line mental health counselor.
- ❖ Present case vignettes to illustrate the application of the interventions found in the chapter.

NATA Educational Competencies

Psychosocial Intervention and Referral Domain

1. Describe the acceptance and grieving processes that follow a catastrophic event and the need for a psychological intervention and referral plan for all parties affected by the event.

Medical Conditions and Disabilities Domain

1. Explain the possible causes of sudden death syndrome.

At its inception, the role of the athletic trainer was to come to the aid of an injured athlete and apply immediate treatment and subsequent rehabilitation in order to speed the athlete's return to participation. This role has greatly expanded over the years. The athletic trainer now manages critical incidents extending from a wide variety of injuries. These include injuries both on and off the field due to, for example, auto accidents, environmental tragedy, and personal illness. In addition, managing the aftermath and early psychological adjustment to career-ending injuries as well as emotional adjustments to the death of a player are other examples of situations increasingly being managed at least in part by the athletic trainers.

In the past, the need for psychological interventions in athletics was often overlooked. May and Sieb (1987) suggest the following reasons for this oversight:

- Emotional responses are seen as obvious and normal and therefore are taken for granted.

- Training and treatment in sports medicine are mechanistic and technical and ignore the psychosocial aspects.

- Athletes are often reluctant to admit their psychosocial distress.

In many cases, athletic trainers are thought of as the first responder with respect to the athletes under their care. It is therefore important for the athletic trainer to wear multiple hats and be able to address both the psychological as well as the physical needs of their athletes. This is particularly important regarding catastrophic injury or illness. The serious impact such events have on the athlete's coping ability both on and off the field highlights the need for education in this area.

Catastrophic injury or illness may have a devastating impact on both the athletes and all those associated with him or her. Whether the catastrophe occurs as a result of competition, physical illness, or an emotional traumatic event, the athlete may display significant physiological and psychological symptoms that impede recovery for all those involved. In response to the evolution of these developments, health care administrators in secondary schools, collegiate, and professional settings must now establish specific protocols to address catastrophic events and avoid any complications. The NATA has incorporated educational objectives for responding to catastrophic events as part of required didactic and clinical experiences of undergraduate students. Sports medicine professionals are now looking to be more proactive and less reactionary to catastrophic events that may paralyze an athletic team, sports medicine program, university, or entire athletic department.

It is intuitively clear that no one is immune from catastrophic events. Recent data suggest that traumatic events on the whole are increasing throughout our culture (Norris, 1992). The prevalence of catastrophic injury in athletic populations is certainly no less than the general public. However, considering the increased potential of serious injury in contact sports such as football, soccer, rugby, and ice hockey, the risk may actually exceed that of the general public. When confronting a catastrophic event, it is alarming to learn the breadth and depth of educational preparation that many athletic trainers and other allied health professionals receive on this topic. The prevailing misconception of athletes as "super human," and thus immune from such troubling events, compounds the problem. Athletic departments are often unprepared to implement a comprehensive plan to address issues relevant to a catastrophic event. When constructing a plan, it is important for athletic trainers to realize that individuals will respond to catastrophic events based on their unique personalities. How an athlete will respond to a catastrophic injury will be no different than someone from the general population. Individuals may have reactions ranging from no response to moderate to a very significant response to a trauma (Breslau, Davis, Andreski, & Peterson, 1991). It is the job of the athletic trainer to recognize these patterns and counsel the athletes accordingly. The development of post-traumatic stress disorder (PTSD) is linked to factors such as a high stress lifestyle, a previous trauma, a poor support system, and a poor premorbid functioning correlating with a significantly poor prognosis for recovery (Kessler, Sonnega, Bromet, Hughes, & Nelson, 1995). Examples of poor premorbid functioning include a history of poor coping skills, negative personality traits, and prior mental health illness as described by the DSM-IV Diagnostic Manual (American Psychiatric Association [APA], 2000). These include borderline, antisocial, and dependant traits (APA, 2000). In addition, prior diagnoses of major depression, anxiety disorders, substance abuse disorders, and PTSD are precursors of a potentially poor prognosis regardless of the significance of the trauma (APA, 2000).

Response to Trauma

The psychological response to injury has historically been described on a stage model thought to portray the evolution of normal coping. There are a number of these models. The most famous of which was presented by Kubler-Ross in 1969 in an attempt to describe the psychological response to death and dying. It is actually quite easy to see the connection of catastrophic injuries to the grieving process. The stages described by Kubler-Ross (1969), Ogilvie (1987), and Pedersen (1986) utilize a variation on the theme of shock, denial, anger, bargaining, depression, and acceptance. It is suggested that post-traumatic stress disorder patients may move in and out of these various stages from moment to moment or day by day, rather then following a sequential progression. Brewer (1994) suggested that cognitive appraisal models used to describe general responses to stress may be more appropriate as a model for athletes. Weiss and Troxell (1986) indicated that an injury should be conceptualized as a stressor and that the relevant psychological processes are those related to increase coping. Asken (1999) highlights four general reactive responses by athletes to catastrophic injuries:

1. Stage of reaction to catastrophic events with a special emphasis on critical nature of the injury or illness immediately after injury or after diagnosis
2. Depression as a result of injury
3. The potential for post-traumatic stress symptoms when trauma is involved
4. The social impact on the athlete, family, teammates, and others

GRIEVING PROCESS

One of the most challenging issues facing the allied sports medicine professional is telling an athlete they will never play again. Career-ending injuries can precipitate grief reactions in athletes. Pederson's (1986) three-phase model of grieving has been utilized by athletic trainers and other allied health professionals to work with individuals experiencing grief. According to Pederson (1986), the first phase of the grieving process is characterized by the athlete experiencing shock, resulting in disbelief and doubt about his or her diagnosis. For example, an athlete who has been disqualified as a result of a spinal stenosis may be unwilling to accept the team physician's diagnosis. The idea of no longer being able to play in one's sport can be a traumatic event for an athlete. During this time, the patient experiences an emotional separation between himself and the significant dream that has been lost. In addition, the individual experiences disbelief about the injury and begins doubting and mistrusting the diagnosis of the injury (Asken, 1999; Heil, 1993; Pedersen, 1986). This phase parallels the sense of denial, as mentioned earlier in the chapter. The athlete does not believe or imagine that what he is told is true. Physical symptoms such as crying, seeming dazed or lost, nausea, and a sense of having no control or grasp of reality can be experienced (Pedersen, 1986). This lack of control and sense of crisis overwhelms the individual and taxes one's coping strategies (Asken, 1999).

In the second phase, preoccupation with the injury becomes a major sense of focus for the patient (Pedersen, 1986). During this time, it is common for the athlete to constantly replay the injury in one's mind. The athlete often will talk in detail about the event, the play, and the exact position he was in, reflecting on numerous specifics regarding the injury event. "Daymares" and nightmares are common. Physical signs such as insomnia, anorexia, excessive crying, and utter fatigue are common during this phase (Pedersen, 1986).

The focus of the third phase involves a personal reorientation (Pedersen, 1986). The athlete attempts to return to a normal life without the sport. The individual attempts to re-engage in social activities while making an effort to return to the person he or she was prior to the injury (Pedersen, 1986).

DENIAL

Asken (1999) notes that denial is "the repudiation of minimization of the implications for the situation" (p. 296). It represents the mind's way of delaying hurt (Heil, 1993). The athletic trainer needs to realize athletes who say "it doesn't hurt" or "it's not that bad" may be coping through the process of denial. Denial can be characterized as both positive and negative. How each athlete perceives his or her own unique situation will determine whether his or her denial is inhibiting or growth promoting (Heil, 1993). Denial is positive when it allows the athlete to manage a potentially overwhelming situation. Positive denial allows the athlete to function and move on with daily activities, thus inhibiting the idea and memories of the catastrophic event. Denial can also have a negative impact when it impedes the athlete's ability to rehabilitate the physical and psychological factors of a major injury (Heil, 1993).

As a part of the denial process, the patient may enter a crisis stage in which the feelings of loneliness, loss, being out of control, and possibly being unable to breathe (coupled with the sense of a loss of reality) surface (Asken, 1999; Kubler-Ross, 1969; Pederson, 1986). It is essential that the athletic trainer let the athlete know assistance is available during a time of crisis. Here is a place to incorporate the helping skills noted in Chapter 2. It is not uncommon for the athlete to experience despair, anguish, and hopelessness during this time. The athletic trainer can be a positive support person for the athlete and may need to seek consultation regarding the referral of the athlete to a mental health professional as discussed in Chapter 3.

Common Diagnoses

There are three main DSM-IV-TR psychiatric conditions that may be seen in the days and weeks following the initial trauma (APA, 2000).

ADJUSTMENT DISORDER

Adjustment disorder is the most common diagnosis associated with traumatic injury. This is a disorder that is associated with clinically significant emotional and behavioral symptoms that develop in response to a specified stressor. The symptoms appear within 3 months of the stressor's onset and are clinically significant as evidenced by either marked distress in excess of what is expected or significant impairment of social, occupational, or academic functioning. Primary disturbance of mood, anxiety, and personal conduct or any mixtures of the three may also be present. In fact, mixed symptoms are most common with most adults. Manifestations may include primary anxiety depression as well as assaulting behavior, reckless driving with excessive drinking, or disregarding academic or legal responsibilities. As the name implies, the disorder tends to be time limited. Symptoms usually resolve within 6 months, although they may last longer if the stressor becomes more chronic.

MAJOR DEPRESSIVE DISORDER

Major depressive disorder (MDD) is the second condition that can occur during the postinjury phase of genetically susceptible individuals. Unlike adjustment disorder, MDD requires not only a psychosocial stressor but also a biological genetic vulnerability that is the pathophysicology of the disorder. MDD is one of the most common psychiatric disorders with lifetime prevalence as high as 25% (Kessler et al., 2003; Paradise & Kirby, 2005). In fact, the World Health Organization currently rates MDD as fourth on the global disease burden index and is projected by the year 2020 to rise to the number two position (World Health Organization, 2001). Multiple biological factors appear to be the basis for this disorder, including derangements of norepinephrine, serotonin dopamine, neuroendocrine regulation, thyroxin, and growth hormone, just to name a few (Rush, Crismon, & Toprac, 1998). The DSM-IV-TR (APA, 2000) describes MDD as a significant loss of psychosocial functioning with associated depressed mood or lost interest or pleasure. In addition several pathognomonic symptoms must be present, some of which include hopelessness, helplessness, insomnia, loss of appetite/energy, inability to concentrate, and recurrent thoughts of suicide or death. The athletic trainer may notice changes in the athlete consistent with the above symptoms as well as personality changes, weight fluctuations, and increased avoidant behaviors.

Suicide

Regarding suicide, the athletic trainer must consider the findings that note in 2001, 30,622 people committed suicide in the United States. This figure is the equivalent to more than 83 suicides a day or one every 20 minutes. Self-directed violence resulted in 116,639 medical emergency department visits (National Center for Injury Prevention and Control, 2004). This is complicated by the fact that many suicidal people do not voluntarily divulge their self-harm intent. They are, however, more likely to discuss these issues with someone with whom they feel comfortable. Be aware that athletes, due to the amount of time spent with athletic trainers, may discuss such issues with the athletic trainer. It is certainly understandable that the athletic trainer may hesitate asking the athlete about suicidal thoughts. Multiple concerns come to mind, including embarrassment to the athlete as well as feeling uncomfortable to discuss the topic. Also, many athletic trainers are unsure what to do in light of an athlete's discussion about suicide. Some hold the misconceived notion that asking the question may initiate feelings of self-harm, resulting in an avoidance pattern that may place the athlete in a potentially lethal situation. This is an area where appropriate protocol should be discussed and a policy developed for all with access to the injured athletes. The importance of this is quite obvious; any reports of self-harm or suicidal ideation should be appropriately documented and referred to a qualified mental health professional immediately. Again, in Chapter 3 one can find information about the referral process. A mnemonic (Sad Persons), noted by Patterson, Dohn, and Bird (1983), can be used to assess suicide risk, highlighting the following factors for the athletic trainer to consider:

- Sex (male)
- Age (adolescent early adult or elderly)
- Depression
- Previous suicide attempts
- Ethanol abuse (substance abuse)
- Rational thinking lost (psychosis)
- Social support lacking
- Organized plan to commit suicide
- No spouse (divorced, widowed, single)
- Sickness (physical illness)

Athletic trainers should be aware of factors that may also lead to individuals harming themselves. Keep in mind these are factors to consider and not causes of suicide attempts. In 1999 the Department of Health and Human Services (DHHS) noted the following factors to watch:

- Previous suicide attempt(s)
- History of mental disorders, particularly depression
- History of alcohol and substance abuse
- Family history of suicide
- Family history of child mistreatment
- Feelings of hopelessness
- Impulsive or aggressive tendencies
- Barriers to accessing mental health treatment
- Loss (relational, social, work, or financial)
- Physical illness
- Easy access to lethal methods
- Unwillingness to seek help because of the stigma attached to mental health and substance abuse disorders or suicidal thoughts
- Cultural and religious beliefs
- Local epidemics of suicide
- Isolation, a feeling of being cut off from other people

POST-TRAUMATIC STRESS DISORDERS

PTSD tends to develop in the aftermath of an extreme traumatic stressor. The individual reacts to this experience with fear and helplessness and tends to persistently re-experience the event. It is also associated with significant attempts to avoid all reminders of the event. The lifetime prevalence of PTSD is estimated to be 1% to 3% of the general population (Norris, 1992; Resnick, Kilpatrick, Dansky, Saunders, & Best, 1993). The hallmark of this disorder involves persistent nightmares or daytime experiences of the trauma. Avoidant behavior and increased arousal are also defining symptoms. PTSD tends to follow more severe or extreme cases of both physical and emotional trauma. For the athletic trainer, attention should be placed on recognizing the athlete that suddenly appears to avoid his or her teammates or the practice field on which he or she was injured. In addition, reports of increased nightmares or subtle signs of anxiety including sweating, tachycardia, or elevations in blood pressure during routine treatment may be observed. It is important to recognize this condition because it also suggests the need for an appropriate, prompt referral to a qualified mental health professional as noted in Chapter 3.

Counseling as an Intervention

The similarities of catastrophic sports injuries and traumatic events in our daily lives have already been drawn. In keeping with this tenant, the basic principles of good intervention with athletes and the general public alike involves the use of counseling. Counseling is defined as a helping process in which one person facilitates exploration, understanding, and actions about the problems presented in order to help an individual to make decisions or cope with challenges. Taylor and Taylor (1997) have shown that good psychological intervention leads to better rehabilitation adherence and improved recovery. The athletic trainer practicing within the educational and ethical guidelines of the profession knows that his or her role does not include providing extensive counseling services to patients. Short-term care regarding psychological issues may be applied by the athletic trainer, primary care physician, physical therapists, and coaches. Since these individuals have access to the injured player, they can provide some counseling-related interventions on a daily basis. Such interventions may include the following (Vanguard University & Zeigler, 2006):

- Providing social support
- Providing information about choices
- Helping the patient establish goals
- Encouraging decision making based on identified alternative choices
- Screening for more serious psychoemotional problems
- Making referral to mental health professionals when appropriate

Based on the information in Chapter 2, counseling implies that the counselor attempts to listen and provide appropriate information and feedback in order to set goals in action toward the future. The therapeutic relationship is useful in working with athletes and patients and includes six basic tenants that appear to facilitate an effective relationship (Pedersen, 1986):

1. Be aware
2. Be there
3. Be sensitive

4. Be human
5. Be ready
6. Be patient

When being aware, the athletic trainer recognizes that emotional reactions to the experienced trauma are a part of the course of the recovery program. Being there involves setting aside the time needed to assist the athlete with problem solving. Being sensitive relates to being able to be patient with the athlete's expression of his or her feelings with a sense of empathy. Being human is to take an objective approach to the concerns expressed by the athlete, despite moments of selfishness or triviality. Being ready relates to being willing to be called back for future sessions, while being patient sets the tone that many repeated sessions may be required while the individual adapts to his or her new condition.

While athletic trainers may play an integral role in assisting athletes, there are specific considerations they must make:

- Delving into areas in which one does not have expertise
- Lack of personal energy or time
- Conflict of interest
- Having professional knowledge that could potentially break confidentiality

Athletic trainers are not prepared to engage in extensive counseling with their patients, even though they may be able to use basic counseling skills while working with their patients. It is important for athletic trainers to utilize additional health care professionals and make a quick and effective referral of issues outside of their scope of practice. In addition to the information in Chapter 3 regarding referral, the athletic trainer can use the following information suggested by May and Sieb (1987) as indications for referral:

- When presenting problem requires intervention beyond the skill of the sports medicine professional
- When aspects of the athlete's personality require support or intervention beyond that of general counseling
- When a clinical situation does not seem to be improving
- When a situation seems to be worsening
- When discomfort reactions or personal bias on the part of the sports medicine professional compromise objective treatment of the athlete

One special consideration needs to be made regarding family interventions. It is well known that families do react quite emotionally to catastrophic illnesses and do so in a myriad of different ways. At times, depending on the severity of the illness or comorbid dysfunctional behaviors within the family, family therapy may be indicated. This type of situation would warrant a referral to a family counseling specialist who has an appreciation of the role athletics and physical activities have in the lives of patients. With the consent of the athlete, and in the case of a minor permission of the parents or guardian, the athletic trainer can inform the family counselor about the situations faced by the patient. The goal of the athletic trainer regarding the family is to provide information that will facilitate the rehabilitation process and avoid the pitfalls of the family members becoming over-protective, becoming codependent, and consciously or unconsciously avoiding discussion of the issues impacting the patient.

Action Plan

In order to effectively address catastrophic injuries/events, it is advisable to have a well-developed plan of action. Quick response both in assessment of needs and subsequent intervention is crucial to successfully navigating a catastrophic event.

Borrowing from the counseling profession, Schwitzer (2003) proposed the use of a combination model that incorporates the use of the DSM-IV-TR (APA, 2000) to determine target mental health concerns, along with the tripartite response model of Drum and Lawler (1988) for determining appropriate interventions. This model was developed to guide therapists in addressing mental health concerns such as eating disorders and large scale traumatic incidents. The value of this model lies in its simplicity and versatility. It can easily be adapted to the athletic setting, serving as a guide for athletic trainers in assisting their athletes who have experienced a catastrophic event.

The model consists of two main components, assessment and responses. These are further subdivided as follows:

- Assessment:
  - Nonpathological responses
  - Adjustment disorders
  - Acute stress/post-traumatic stress disorder
- Responses:
  - Preventative interventions
  - Immediate interventions
  - Advanced interventions

Generally, the athletic trainer will be responsible for assisting athletes at the initial level of non-pathological responses and preventative interventions. In some cases, the athletic trainer may be equipped to assist with intermediate interventions, but only under the supervision of a trained mental health practitioner. It is imperative that the athletic department have a plan and that the athletic trainer be familiar with the goals and protocols for each level of the model prior to an event.

In the following description of the model and its application to the athletic setting, it may be helpful to think of the team and athletic department in general as a distinct community. The individual athletes that make up each team all come from various backgrounds and bring with them individual experiences and personality traits that influence the way they react to traumatic events. Therefore, it is very likely that even on a small athletic team, the athletic trainer is likely to encounter individuals who react and need assistance at each level of the model.

In order to pair an individual with the appropriate level of intervention, it is important to understand and be able to recognize each level of response. Those individuals experiencing non-pathological responses will demonstrate very little disturbances in their daily lives beyond what is normally expected. Sadness and grief are normal reactions to catastrophic incidents and generally present mild disruption to daily functioning. Typically this is short-term, and these individuals will resume their normal routines relatively quickly following an event. These individuals often demonstrate a high degree of resiliency and resistance to daily life stress. They typically have a well-developed social support system in place as well. Minimal intervention beyond efforts to normalize their reactions is necessary.

Another segment of the community (team) will experience stress reactions at such a level that disruptions in functioning are in excess of what is expected. These individuals may experience significant mood disturbances such as depression and anxiety related to the trauma. Impairments can often be seen in academic performance, athletic performance, and/or relationships. Reckless behavior such as fighting, truancy, or increased substance use is not uncommon. Symptoms most often emerge immediately following the incident and last up to 6 months afterwards.

Acute stress/PTSD occur in reaction to extreme stress. Typically, this affects those individuals who are most directly involved in the catastrophic event, including the first responders. These individuals will experience intense feelings of fear and/or helplessness following the event. Additionally, those dealing with PTSD will re-experience the trauma through flashbacks and nightmares. Most areas of life are negatively impacted by PTSD, thus severely compromising one's level of functioning. Symptom onset is typically within 1 month of the event. The course of symptoms and treatment are usually long-term.

TRIPARTITE RESPONSE MODEL

The tripartite response model proposed by Drum and Lawler (1988) provides a useful guide for taking appropriate actions in the event of a catastrophic incident. The athletic trainer can provide the initial assistance for athletes facing a trauma. The utility of the tripartite model is that it addresses each level of need with specific targets an intervention strategies.

Preventative Interventions

A unique feature of the model is that the first level of responses is preventative interventions. The primary target at this level is the community (team) as a whole. The purpose of efforts is to pre-empt the onset of problematic responses to the stress of a traumatic event. Preventative measures can equip members of the team with new skills and attitudes to effectively deal with moderate levels of stress. Specifically, these interventions are aimed at providing education to raise awareness of typical responses and available resources and promoting functional responses (behaviors). Direct efforts include lectures, presentations, and workshops to help engage the athletes in preparing for potential events. Indirect methods include having posters or brochures available in the training room, residence halls, and locker rooms. Indirect efforts can be a good way to present the message without encountering typical resistance. Athletic trainers can play a vital role in establishing preventative interventions.

The second target of the preventative interventions is those individuals who are most vulnerable to problematic responses. Informal discussions with athletes about how they handle normal daily stress can be helpful in identifying those individuals who are more susceptible to high levels of stress. Those athletes who have previously experienced some trauma (injury) or who are currently dealing with a particular mental health issue are more likely to experience moderate to high dysfunctional reactions to stress. The overall goal of this level is to utilize psychoeducational interventions to prepare athletes for their own responses to catastrophic events.

Intermediate Interventions

The intermediate level of interventions is aimed at assisting the athlete with the psychological adjustment to a traumatic event. These interventions should be implemented for those individuals who demonstrate some impairment in functioning; typically meeting DSM-IV-TR criteria for an adjustment disorder, but falling short of severe impairment of daily functioning (APA, 2000).

⊕The targets for the intermediate level of interventions are those individuals who have a deeper emotional connection to the event or those who are directly involved (e.g., the best friend of an athlete experiencing a career-ending injury). Other targets of this level are those athletes who have previously suffered a serious injury or are currently experiencing other emotional distress.

Severe reactions to trauma have been linked to maladaptive thinking prior to the event (Ehlers & Clark, 2000; Bryant & Guthrie, 2005). Dysfunctional self-appraisals (unrealistic expectations about one's ability, or distorted self-image) tend to be the strongest predictors of PTSD in individuals whose identity is tied to their image of competence, which is common for athletes, military, and emergency personnel (Solomon, 1989). As first responders to traumas in the athletic domain, athletic trainers may also fit into this category. Therefore, each athletic trainer should take steps to ensure his or her own needs are being addressed as well.

⊕The goals of this level of interventions are to promote self-assessment and increased awareness of the event and their reactions to it, as well as to develop appropriate problem-solving skills. In addition, providing psychosocial support in the wake of the trauma gives athletes an opportunity to discuss concerns and fears and helps normalize their reactions.

Typically, these interventions involve brief, short-term counseling sessions. One-time workshops could be utilized to facilitate healthy coping with the larger community. Brief interventions with trained mental health practitioners should be stressed with the athletes. These efforts help reduce some of the natural resistance to help-seeking brought on by the culture of toughness found in the athletic world. Research has shown that individuals with high levels of resistance and lower motivation to seek help respond best to brief interventions (Seligman, 1996).

Advanced Interventions

The final phase of the tripartite response model involves advanced interventions. ⊕These interventions are aimed at those individuals who are experiencing extreme life dysfunctions due to severe reactions to the stress of trauma. These individuals are typically those directly involved in the incident, eyewitnesses, and first response workers. (Keep in mind that this often includes the athletic trainer responding to a catastrophic injury.) Interventions at this level involve long-term psychotherapy with highly trained mental health practitioners and/or licensed psychologists and psychiatrists. The role of the athletic trainer in this instance will be to make appropriate referrals. Knowing what resources are available and how to access them quickly are essential to providing necessary care.

Catastrophic injuries and events are rare; however, being prepared to handle them systemically is crucial. Each athletic department should have an action plan and protocols for dealing with catastrophes. Keep in mind that all members of the community (team) are affected, not simply those directly involved. When developing an action plan for dealing with catastrophic injuries, it is important for the athletic trainer to gain input from all appropriate members of the sports medicine team. At a minimum, this plan should include options and resources for addressing athletes at an intermediate level and protocols for making referrals for those needing advanced interventions.

SPECIFIC INTERVENTION FOR A CATASTROPHIC EVENT

Debriefing

Debriefing was originally a form of crisis intervention and not a specific form of psychotherapy. As a treatment modality, however, it can be quite powerful, if not in fact necessary for promoting emotional processing in response to traumatic events. Normally in response to traumatic injury athletes will tend to ventilate and normalize their reactions on their own, and for the majority this can be successful. Individuals to whom debriefing appears to be most helpful are those that have demonstrated some abnormal response to the trauma, including acute stress, anxiety, sleep or appetite disturbance, depression, as well as pathological denial. The primary goal of debriefing is to avoid pathologic labels and promote a sense of normalization of the event. In other words, the athlete begins to understand that he or she is a normal person that has experienced an abnormal event.

Critical incident stress debriefing (CISD) was first described by Mitchell (1983). However, Dyregrov (1998) detailed the seven stages and interpreted the technique as follows:

1. *The introduction.* This is the stage that essentially requires participants to discuss their reactions to the trauma and identify methods to deal with them to prevent future problems. Participants are encouraged to engage the discussion only when they feel at ease to do so. Finally, the focus of the discussion is on the impressions and reactions of the participants.

2. *Expectations and facts.* At this stage, the focus is on the detail of what happened without incorporating impressions or emotional reactions. Individuals are encouraged to express their own experiences.

3. *Thoughts and impressions.* This stage focuses on assisting the individual in reconstructing a more realistic version of the trauma. The goal here is to construct a picture of the trauma and to put individual reactions into prospective.

4. *Emotional reactions.* At this stage, the facilitator attempts to aid in the release of emotions by demonstrating common reactions during trauma and attempting to normalize feelings such as frustration, anger, guilt, anxiety, helplessness, and fear.

5. *Normalization.* This is an extension of stage four, where further work is aimed at normalization of emotions. In addition, the facilitator attempts to describe future symptoms that may develop in an attempt to normalize them. These may include avoidance of feelings/thoughts, depressed mood, anxiety, nightmares, shame, guilt, intrusive thoughts, and hypervigilance.

6. *Future planning/coping.* This very important stage focuses on ways to help the athlete develop coping skills as future symptoms or problems arise. In addition, the seed is planted here for the possibility of additional support should they have excessive problems coping with little resolution.

7. *Disengagement.* At this stage, additional information is given to firm up the athlete's knowledge on when, where, and how to seek further assistance by a mental health professional. Extreme psychological symptoms that do not decrease after 4 to 6 weeks are positive indicators toward the need for additional counseling.

Goal Setting

As noted in Chapter 2, goal setting is a vital component for working with patients. Athletes are used to setting goals in relation to their physical performance. Similarly, this skill can be very useful when facing a catastrophic injury or event. Achievement goal theory (Nichols, 1984) describes two preferences that individuals use when approaching achievement situations. Individuals taking a task-orientation focus mainly on their own performance, effort, and improvement. Individuals with an ego-orientation focus primarily on comparing their performance against others, with little interest in mastery of a skill. Research has determined that task-oriented individuals tend to persist in the face of a challenge, whereas ego-oriented individuals tend to avoid challenges and look for excuses for poor performance.

Athletic trainers, coaches, and parents can foster a task-oriented environment when facing a catastrophic injury. This can be vital to getting an athlete to adhere to a rehabilitation program. Athletic trainers can foster this by helping athletes set realistic rehab goals, reinforce effort over results, and measure progress in self-referent terms rather than comparison with others (Duda, 1992). Generating a task-oriented approach to a catastrophic injury can greatly improve the individual's reaction to the event by facilitating personal responsibility for the rehabilitation, effective problem-solving and planning strategies, and reducing anxiety. Emphasizing the control the athlete has over the rehabilitation process can help to counter the loss of control stemming from the event/injury.

These strategies can also be very helpful for other athletes associated with the catastrophic event. Fear of injury/reinjury will be high among associated athletes. Encouraging those athletes to approach their athletic involvement in terms of task-oriented goals will help limit comparisons with the injured teammate, facilitate an internal locus of control, and reduce anxiety and fear of injury.

Imagery

Imagery is another psychological skill most athletes are familiar with and probably use regularly. Imagery can be used to increase motivation and confidence, set and achieve goals, and manage emotions (Hall, Mack, Paivio, & Hausenblas, 1998). In the face of a catastrophic injury, imagery may be most useful for assisting to regulate anxiety and for relaxation. Traumatic events frequently result in individuals replaying the trauma mentally. This is similar to a VCR being stuck in a negative replay loop. Through regular contact with the athlete, the athletic trainer can help train the athlete to stop the negative image and replace them with positive ones. This can lead to a reduction in the anxiety and fear of reinjury because the athlete can stop re-experiencing the catastrophe. The key to helping athletes change their imagery is to encourage them to reflect on successful past events and focus on being confident and emotionally in control. Understand that each individual will have a unique interpretation of a given image (Ahsen, 1984). Therefore, it is important to explore with each athlete to determine the most effective image.

Arousal Regulation

Anxiety is a common emotion experienced following a catastrophic injury/event by any athlete associated with the event. Anxiety can manifest as physical symptoms (racing heart rate, sweating, nausea, dizziness), cognitive symptoms (intense worry, concentration disruption, difficulty making decisions), emotional symptoms (irritability, paranoia, crying spells, anger outbursts), and behavioral symptoms (isolation, shifting of activities, avoidance).

There are several methods for reducing an athlete's anxiety following a traumatic event. At the most basic level, the athletic trainer can provide factual information and be a sympathetic listener. This will lessen the fear of the unknown and normalize the athlete's reactions. Should anxiety persist, there are various approaches for managing it by reducing the associated physical and cognitive symptoms. Progressive muscular relaxation (PMR) involves systematically tensing and releasing muscle groups while engaging in deep diaphragmatic breathing. This helps bring awareness of the contrast of tension and relaxation so that the athlete can train him- or herself to achieve a relaxed state. Often imagery can be used, either in conjunction with PMR or alone, to facilitate relaxation. This is particularly effective if there is a high degree of cognitive disruption or rumination, as it provides a means of refocusing the mind and allowing the athlete to "let go" of troubling thoughts. A more advanced method of relaxation involves biofeedback. This involves using physiological measures (heart rate or galvanic skin response) to provide information as to how an individual experiences anxiety. The athlete can then learn to control their autonomic nervous system response and manage the response to the anxiety (Benson & Klipper, 2000).

While it may seem daunting to deal with the psychological responses along with the physical consequences of a catastrophic injury/event, understanding the interaction between the two is critical to successfully managing the event. The psychological skills presented here are not meant to serve as quick fixes, but rather to provide techniques that can augment other interventions and can easily be integrated into the athletic trainer's repertoire. Keeping the interventions short and targeted is the key. Some athletes will possess the skills necessary to cope effectively and may only need periodic reinforcement to utilize them. In other cases, the athletic trainer may need to briefly teach such skills. Psychological skills, much like physical skills, improve dramatically with regular practice.

Conclusion

Catastrophic injuries in athletes occasionally present physical challenges but in all cases present some psychological issues that may over shadow the physical ones. In this chapter the potential problems that can occur when these psychological interventions are not instituted have been discussed. Importantly, the chapter has given information on how athletic trainers may manage the psychological aspects of the injury. The hope is that this chapter will increase the curiosity of athletic trainers to continue to educate themselves in obtaining counseling skills, such as active listening, emotional support, goal setting, self-monitoring, and relaxation training. Increased knowledge of counseling and psychology will assist the athletic trainer in making referrals to mental health professionals, as well as increasing the collegial interaction to improve the overall wellness of athletes.

Chapter Exercises

1. Antoine is a rather shy but talented defensive back on a mid-western Division 1 football team. While playing in his senior year, Antoine has assisted in turning his team into one of the best defensive threats in the conference. He has in 2 consecutive years been named all conference and had attracted the attention of several NFL scouts. Antoine is the son of a broken home. He is extremely close to

his mother and has very infrequent contact with his father. Antoine has few social outlets at school, and this year moved home with his mother who lives just blocks from the university. Antoine sustained a complicated neck injury due to incidental spearing during the second to the last game of the season. As a result of the spearing, Antoine fractured his C3 vertebrae and was left partially paralyzed.

Discussion: In this case involving Antoine, there are long- and short-term goals for interventions. The immediate issue involves assisting Antoine with his anxiety, fear, and shock. Debriefing at this point should primarily be focused on allowing him to discuss what happened when it happened and how it happened with as much emotion and feeling as he cares to display. This is important as an early intervention to keep him focused on the reality of his injury and yet to begin the grieving process. In addition, this reality-based discussion will assist in combating the onset of pathological denial. The second important short-term intervention should involve improving his social support system. Maintaining an appropriate connection with his mother and improving his relationships with his teammates and peers will be critical in helping him overcome this injury. In addition, the athletic trainer should assist in increasing Antoine's support system by encouraging the coaches, assistant coaches, and other support members including administration to become involved with Antoine's recovery. Long-term goals should involve the institution of goal-setting, as these may be quite different from his previous goals. At the appropriate time discussions about his future as it relates to athletics should be discussed. Arousal regulation and guided imagery are intermediate, and long-term goals of counseling to improve his mood regulation and assist with rehabilitation are needed. Debriefing may also be utilized with teammates that maybe traumatized by this injury. The athletic trainer should be on the look out for other individuals displaying disturbing behaviors in the aftermath of the injury.

2. Mark is an 18-year-old starting mid-fielder for a southeastern soccer team. His father is one of the assistant coaches for the team. Despite not being overly talented, Mark is quite well-loved by all of this teammates. He is an articulate outgoing young man who has plans of playing college soccer in his pursuit of a law degree in the fall. While returning home from spring break in Puerto Rico, Mark is killed when his commuter plane goes down in route to his home. The entire team is not expected to return to school for a few more days, and preparations are being made to notify the team when they return to school on Monday.

   Discussion: In this tragic case the athletic trainer must become a counselor for the deceased player's teammates and coaches. This is also a situation where the athletic trainer must take an inventory of his or her own feelings and coping skills. The use of group debriefing sessions would be highly recommended in this situation. Administration should be involved in providing the time and appropriate additional mental health specialists to assist with this counseling. The goal of the session would be to allow everyone to vent their feelings about their loss but also focus on education. Specifically participants should be educated about the natural and pathologic course of grieving and be encouraged to seek further counseling should they notice problems in their ability to cope.

3. Larry is a 29-year-old professional hockey player who sustained a high femur fracture a year ago while playing in the final playoff game. He has been slated to return to the team on multiple occasions; however, the latest second opinion from the orthopedist suggests a developing avascular necrosis. If this is the case,

his hockey career certainly will be over. He has struggled greatly with his year away from the sport. He is isolated away from the team and away from his family. There are rumors that he is drinking. He has spoken to the athletic trainer on several occasions about having trouble sleeping and having recurring nightmares. His wife has been calling the office in order to get information regarding the latest second opinion. He, however, refuses to sign the consent, stating, "I will deal with things on my own."

Discussion: In this case, Larry appears to be severely impaired to the point that a mental health referral is indicated at this time. Multiple factors are evident in this case, including the likelihood that this injury will be career ending. In addition, factors suggesting possible substance abuse, the onset of post-traumatic stress symptoms, and depression further complicate this case and make it an unlikely case for the athletic trainer to engage in counseling, as referral is the best course of action to take. In addition significant loss of psychosocial support appears to be present—evidenced by his lack of involvement with the team and apparent estrangement from his wife. Nonetheless, interventions by the athletic trainer are needed in this case but need to be largely focused on improving the social support system, perhaps by contacting his wife and fellow teammates. In addition, because of the serious concerns for suicide it would be recommended protocol that the athletic trainer at least assess Larry for safety, and if concerns exist report them immediately to an experienced mental health provider.

4. Scott is a 16-year-old member of a New Jersey area high school basketball team. Scott is an important member of the team but has had many difficulties over the past year. His parents are currently getting a divorce, and he and his siblings have suddenly been separated. It is rumored that Scott has been experimenting with marijuana. On Friday, Scott was in the athletic trainer's office discussing problems with poor sleep, poor energy, feelings of guilt, and worthlessness. In addition, he had a big altercation with his teammates and now appears to be at odds with other members of the team as well as the coach. It is now Monday morning, and the athletic trainer's office is being notified that Scott attempted to take his own life on Sunday night by an overdose. The report is that he will make a full recovery.

    Discussion: In this case the immediate attention again should be placed on Scott's teammates and coaching staff. Initial debriefing should involve each of these groups to uncover their feelings about Scott's suicide attempt.

These feelings are likely to include feelings of anxiety, fear, grief, and anger. In this situation, multiple sessions may be necessary in order to completely process each individual's issues. In particular, time should be spent on dealing with any teammate's feelings of guilt or responsibility for Scott's suicide attempt. Again, education is important to assist each member with appropriate referrals if he or she should develop more pathological symptoms. Community support groups and self-help books may also be recommended.

References

Ahsen, A. (1984). ISM: The triple code model of imagery and psychophysiology. *Journal of Mental Imagery, 8,* 15-42.

American Psychiatric Association. (2000). Diagnostic and Statistical Manual of Mental Disorders, 4th edition, Text Revised (DSM-IV-TR). Washington, D.C.: American Psychiatric Press.

Asken, M. (1999). Sports psychology and the physically disabled: Interview with Michael D. Goodling, OTR/L. *Sports Psychologist, 3,* 166-176.

Benson, H., & Klipper, M. (2000). *The relaxation response.* New York, NY: Harper Torch.

Breslau, N., Davis, G. C., Andreski, P., & Peterson, E. (1991). Traumatic events and post-traumatic stress disorder in an urban population of young adults. *Archives of General Psychiatry, 48,* 216-222.

Brewer, B. (1994). Review and critiques of models of psychological adjustment to athletic injury. *Journal of Applied Sport Psychology, 6,* 87-100.

Bryant, R. A., & Guthrie, R. M. (2005). Maladaptive appraisals as a risk factor for posttraumatic stress. *Psychological Science, 16*(10), 749-752.

Department of Health and Human Services. (1999). *The Surgeon General's call to action to prevent suicide.* Washington, DC: Department of Health and Human Services. Retrieved March 2, 2006 from http://www.surgeongeneral.gov/library/calltoaction/default.htm.

Drum, D. J., & Lawler, A. C. (1988). *Developmental interventions: Theories, principles, and practice.* Columbus, OH: Merrill Publishing.

Duda, J. L. (1992). Motivation in sport settings: A goal perspective approach. In G. C. Roberts (Ed.), *Motivation in sport and exercise* (pp. 161-176). Champaign, IL: Human Kinetics.

Dyregrov, A. (1998) Psychological debriefing—An effective method? *Traumatology, 4*(2), Article 1. Retrieved June 13, 2007, from http://www.fsu.edu/~trauma

Ehlers, A., & Clark, D. M. (2000). A cognitive model of posttraumatic stress disorder. *Behavior Research and Therapy, 38,* 319-345.

Hall, C. R., Mack, D., Paivio, A., & Hausenblas, H. A. (1998). Imagery use by athletes: Development of the Sport Imagery Questionnaire. *International Journal of Sport Psychology, 29,* 73-89.

Heil, J. (1993). *Psychology of sport injury.* Champaign, IL: Human Kinetics Publishing

Kessler R. C., Berglund, P., Demler, O., Jin, R., & Koretz, D. (2003). The epidemiology of major depressive disorder: Results from the National Comorbidity Survey Replication (NCS-R). *Journal of the American Medical Association, 289,* 3095-3105.

Kessler, R.G., Sonnega, A., Bromet E., Hughes, M., Nelson, C. B., Merikangas, K. R., et al. (1995). PTSD in the national comorbidity survey. *Archives of General Psychiatry, 52,* 1048.

Kubler-Ross E. (1969). *On death and dying.* London: MacMillan.

May, J., & Sieb, G. (1987). Athletic injuries: Psychological factors in the onset, sequence, rehabilitation, and prevention. In J. May & M. Asken (Eds.), *Sport psychology: The psychological health of the athlete* (pp. 157-185). New York, NY: PMA.

Mitchell, J. T. (1983). When disaster strikes. *Journal of Emergency Medical Services, 8,* 86-89.

National Center for Injury Prevention and Control. (2004). Suicide: Fact sheet. Retrieved March 2, 2006 from http://www.cdc.gov/ncipc/factsheet/suifacts.htm

Nichols, J. G. (1984). Achievement motivation: Conceptions of ability, subjective experience, task choice, and performance. *Psychological Review, 91,* 328-346.

Norris, F. (1992). Epidemiology of trauma: Frequency and impact of different potentially traumatic events on different demographic groups. *Journal of Consulting and Clinical Psychology, 60,* 409-418.

Ogilvie, B. (1987). Counseling for sports career termination. In J. May & M. Asken (Eds.), *Sport psychology: The psychological health of the athlete* (pp. 213-230). New York, NY: PMA.

Paradise L., & Kirby, P. (2005). The treatment and prevention of depression: Implications for counseling and counselor training. *Journal of Counseling and Development, 83,* 116-119.

Patterson, W. M., Dohn, H., & Bird, J. (1983). Evaluation of suicidal patients: The Sad Person Scale. *Psychosomatics, 24*(4), 343-349.

Pedersen, P. (1986). The grief response and injury: A special challenge for athletes and athletic trainers. *Athletic Training, 21,* 312-314.

Resnick, H., Kilpatrick, D., Dansky, B., Saunders, B., & Best, D. (1993). Prevalence of civilian trauma and post-traumatic stress disorder in a representative national sample of woman. *Journal of Consulting and Clinical Psychology, 61*(6), 984-991.

Rush, A. J., Crismon, M. L., & Toprac, M. G. (1998). Consensus guidelines in the treatment of major depressive disorder. *Journal of Clinical Psychiatry, 59*(suppl 20), 73-84.

Seligman, L. (1996). *Diagnosis and treatment planning in counseling* (2nd ed.). New York, NY: Plenum Press.

Schwitzer, A. (2003). A framework for college counseling responses to large-scale traumatic incidents. *Journal of College Student Psychotherapy, 18*(2), 49-66.

Solomon, Z. (1989). Untreated combat-related PTSD – why some Israeli veterans do not seek help. Israeli Journal of Psychiatry and Related Sciences, 26, 111-123.

Taylor, J., & Taylor, S. (1997). *Psychological approaches to sports injury rehabilitation*. Gaithersburg, MD: Aspen.

Weiss, M.R. & Troxell, R.K. (1986). Psychology of the injured athlete. Athletic Training, 21, 104-109.

World Health Organization. (2001). *World Health Report 2001: Mental health: New understanding, new hope*. Geneva, Switzerland: Author.

Vanguard University, & Zeigler, T. (2006). *Role of the sports medicine professional*. Retrieved March 2, 2006, from http://search.vanguard.edu

Bibliography

Andersen, M. B., & Williams, J. M. (1988). A model of stress and athletic injury: Prediction and prevention. *Journal of Sport and Exercise Psychology, 10*, 294-306.

Augsburger, N. (2001, February 12-13). Providers need time, help to recover from trauma. *NATA NEWS*.

Barefield, S., & Mcallister, S. (1997). Social support in the athletic training room: Athletes' expectations of staff and student athletic trainers. *Journal of Athletic Training, 32*, 333-338.

Mueller, F., & Cantu R. (2004). *22nd Annual Report Fall 1982-Spring 2004*. National Center for Catastrophic Sport Research. Retrieved February 26, 2006, from http://www.unc.edu/depts/nccsi/allsport.htm

Mueller, F. (2003). Catastrophic sports injuries; who is at risk? *Current Sports Medicine Reports, 2*(2), 57-58.

Perna, F. M., & Antoni Mschneiderman, N. (1998). Psychological intervention prevents injury/illness among athletes [abstract]. *Journal of Sport Psychology, 10*, S53.

Nutrition and Supplements: A Scientific Review for the Athletic Trainer

Thomas D. Armsey, MD
John P. Batson, MD, FAAP
James M. Mensch, PhD, ATC

Chapter Objectives

* ❖ Educate athletic trainers about anabolic steroids and several common nutritional supplements.
* ❖ Discuss the physiological impact and legal implications associated with nutritional supplements.
* ❖ Examine the potential benefits and possible adverse reactions of nutritional supplements.
* ❖ Discuss the importance of proper nutrition as an ergogenic aid.
* ❖ Discuss the athletic trainer's role when consulting with athletes and physically active individuals on the use of nutritional supplements.

NATA Educational Competencies

Psychosocial Intervention and Referral Domain

1. Identify and describe the sociological, biological, and psychological influences toward substance abuse, addictive personality traits, the commonly abused substances, the signs and symptoms associated with the abuse of these substances, and their impact on an individual's health and physical performance.

Nutritional Aspects of Injuries and Illnesses Domain

1. Describe the principles, advantages, and disadvantages of ergogenic aids and dietary supplements used in an effort to improve physical performance.
2. Explain the principles of weight control for safe weight loss and weight gain, and explain common misconceptions regarding the use of food, fluids, and nutritional supplements in weight control.

Pathology of Injuries and Illnesses Domain

1. Identify the normal acute and chronic physiological and pathological responses (e.g., inflammation, immune response, and healing process) of the human body to trauma, hypoxia, microbiological agents, genetic derangements, nutritional deficiencies, chemicals, drugs, aging, and the musculoskeletal system adaptations to disuse.

Stories regarding anabolic steroids and nutritional supplements have received unremitting media attention largely due to recent drug scandals in major league baseball, track and field, and professional football. Although this attention has enlightened some to the prevalence of drug abuse in professional sports, the problem reaches much farther into the core of American society. According to The Council for Responsible Nutrition, the retail sale of dietary supplements generated $3.3 billion in 1990 (Cowart, 1992) and revenues have increased each year. This enormous spending is due in large part to aggressive advertising aimed at high school, collegiate, and recreational athletes. These supplements claim to produce quick strength increases without years of hard training or appropriate nutrition. Because of this advertising, nutritional supplements and anabolic steroids appeal to millions of consumers seeking physical gains that seem too good to be true.

The reality is that most nutritional supplements have little or no scientific proof of efficacy and no safety regulation by the FDA. None of these supplements have been subjected to the type of scientific scrutiny that is required of over-the-counter and prescription drugs. Given the financial influence of the supplement industry, it is unlikely that the FDA will ever be able to effectively monitor this growing business.

This lack of responsible regulation allows many supplement companies the opportunity to partake in unscrupulous advertising, ignore impurities in manufacturing, and fail to report potentially dangerous adverse reactions. Therefore, athletic trainers and other sports medicine specialists must become experts regarding the risks and possible benefits of supplements in order to educate their athletes, coaches, administrators, and parents. Although it is difficult to compete with slick advertisements and the exaggerated claims of a supplement's power, we must become familiar with the scientific research if we are to make a difference in this potentially devastating epidemic. The purpose of this chapter is to educate athletic trainers about anabolic steroids and several common nutritional supplements, their mechanism of action, potential benefits and possible adverse reactions, and overall scientifically based recommendation. With this knowledge, athletic trainers can intelligently counsel their athletes who are already using or interested in trying anabolic steroids or nutritional supplements.

Anabolic Agents

ANABOLIC ANDROGENIC STEROIDS

Steroids as ergogenic aids (i.e., substances that enhance energy production, use, or recovery to provide an athlete with a competitive advantage) have been utilized by athletes primarily to enhance performance in strength- and power-oriented events. Testosterone is the "prototype" anabolic steroid and was first isolated in 1935 (Sturmi & Diorio, 1998; Blue & Lombardo, 1999). It and similar anabolic substances were used by German soldiers to increase strength and aggressiveness in World War II (Metzl, 2000).

As early as the 1950s it is believed many eastern block athletes used anabolic steroids in power lifting events (Metzl, 2000; Sturmi & Diorio, 1998). The first documented usage of anabolic steroids by athletes was in the 1972 Montreal Olympics (Sturmi & Diorio, 1998). Their popularity grew in the late 1970s and 1980s in activities such as football, powerlifting, and body building. In the 1990s, health and ethical concerns surrounding anabolic steroids contributed somewhat to a curbing of the trend of usage. Despite a decrease in popularity, it is still estimated that more than 1 million Americans either use or have used anabolic androgenic steroids (AAS). Steroid use among recreational weight lifters has been estimated at 15% and anywhere from 30% to 75% for elite or professional athletes and body builders (Sturmi & Diorio, 1998). An NCAA survey of football players found a 3% user rate for anabolic steroids (NCAA, 1997). Many studies in adolescent athletes in grades 9 through 12 have documented usage rates of 3% to 12% and one recent study of athletes in grades 5 to 7 reported almost 3% of both male and females using steroids (Faighenbaum et al., 1998; Greydanus & Patel, 2002; Sullivan & Anderson, 2000).

Physiological Impact of Steroids

Steroid hormones are derivatives of cholesterol. In males, testosterone is secreted primarily by the Leydig cells of the testes. Females secrete a small amount of testosterone from their ovaries and adrenal glands. Natural and synthetic anabolic steroids are both derived from the testosterone molecule. These products are available as injectable, oral, and transdermal preparations. Typical doses used by athletes as an ergogenic aid can be as much as 10 to 40 times that of therapeutic doses used for medicinal purposes (Greydanus & Patel, 2002; Sturmi & Diorio, 1998). Athletes often "stack" or "pyramid" doses of steroids. Stacking refers to combining different steroids at the same time to augment certain effects or target different receptors in the body. Pyramiding refers to increasing the steroid dose with time to lessen potential side effects. Athletes often cycle the drugs 4 to 12 weeks at a time during intense training and avoid times when they are subject to drug testing. Steroid hormones have both anabolic and androgenic effects on the body (Sturmi & Diorio, 1998). The desirable anabolic effects include the following:

- Increased muscle mass
- Increased body weight
- Decreased body fat
- Increased bone mass
- Stimulation of red blood cell production

At the cellular level, these changes occur as a result of increased protein synthesis (Blue & Lombardo, 1999; Sturmi & Diorio, 1998). The undesirable androgenic properties affect the development of secondary sexual characteristics and reproductive ability. Additional ergogenic properties of anabolic androgenic steroids include anticatabolic (anti-stress) properties (Sturmi & Diorio, 1998). This potentially allows athletes faster recovery after workouts or injuries and allows increased tolerance of high intensity training. Steroids also appear to induce aggression and a state of euphoria, both of which can potentially convey an athletic edge in the right situation (Sturmi & Diorio, 1998).

There are numerous side effects associated with the use of anabolic steroids (Blue & Lombardo, 1999; Greydanus & Patel, 2002; Sullivan & Anderson, 2000). These include the following:

- Premature growth plate closure
- Collagen dysplasia
- Potential tendon weakness
- Testicular atrophy
- Clitoral enlargement
- Decreased sperm function and production
- Prostate enlargement
- Liver dysfunction
- Neoplasm

Certain cardiovascular side effects have been reported and are as follows:

- High blood pressure
- Elevated total cholesterol
- Decreased HDL ("good" cholesterol)
- Glucose intolerance
- Cardiomyopathy
- Sudden cardiac death

More obvious external side effects include male pattern baldness, acne, increased facial hair, gynecomastia, deepening of the voice, emotional liability, and aggressive behaviors. Though many of the side effects are transient and resolve with cessation of use, certain side effects can be permanent. Of note, women and children appear to be more susceptible to the permanent side effects (Blue & Lombardo, 1999). Synthetic anabolic steroids are designed with the goals of maximizing the anabolic properties and minimizing any possible side effects. Injectable steroids carry the additional risk of blood-borne diseases such as hepatitis and HIV. Unhealthy lifestyle behaviors have also been documented in young athletes taking steroids, including risk-taking behaviors and additional drug usage (stimulants and diuretics) (Blue & Lombardo, 1999; Greydanus & Patel, 2002).

Potential Benefits and Clinical Effectiveness of Steroids

A generation of athletes heard from the medical community "steroids do not enhance muscle development, muscle size, or athletic performance." For those who knew athletes taking high doses of anabolic steroids, the reality was quite different and obvious—steroids did positively affect muscle size and development, as well as intensity of workouts. This discrepancy was primarily because of poor study design in early clinical trials, and the early studies failed to administer the supraphysiologic doses of steroids similar to the amount athletes were actually taking (Sturmi & Diorio, 1998). Recent studies with participants taking high doses of testosterone have shown increased fat-free mass, muscle size, and muscle strength (NCAA, 1997; Sturmi & Diorio, 1998). This effect is most pronounced with added strength training and adequate protein intake (Sturmi & Diorio, 1998). The American College of Sports Medicine has officially stated "anabolic androgenic steroids, in the presence of an adequate diet, can contribute to increases in body weight, often in the lean mass compartment" and "the gains in muscular strength achieved through high-intensity exercise and proper diet can be increased by the use of anabolic steroids in some individuals." Of note, no clinical trials have documented enhancement of aerobic capacity in athletes (Sturmi & Diorio, 1998).

Legal Implications

Anabolic steroids are banned from most major athletic organizations, including the International Olympic Committee (IOC), the NCAA, the NFL, Major League Baseball (MLB), and the National Basketball Association (NBA). In 1990, congress passed the Anabolic Steroids Control Act that classified steroids as Schedule III federally controlled substances and made it a felony to either posses or distribute (Sturmi & Diorio, 1998). Most universities at the Division I level utilize random urine testing to detect their usage. Gas chromatography/mass spectroscopy is considered the "gold standard" technique to detect anabolic steroids and is used by the IOC. Of note, often no testing is conducted on athletes during the off season and testing is rarely, if ever, done at smaller universities. High school athletes currently are not subject to drug testing despite well-documented usage for over 10 years.

STEROID PRECURSORS (PROHORMONES)

Dehydroepiandrosterone and Androstenedione

Dehydroepiandrosterone (DHEA) and androstenedione (Andro) became popular in the late 1990s as a potential "natural" and "safer" alternative to anabolic steroids. Sales of these steroid precursors skyrocketed after the endorsement of multiple professional athletes and aggressive marketing by the supplement industry. For example, sales of Andro alone increased over 500% after Mark McGwire's 1998 baseball season and his association with the supplement (Koch, 2002).

These substances are sold as dietary supplements without any regulation from the FDA. Few studies have looked at user rates with these steroid precursors, but according to those in the supplement industry, they are among the supplements most requested by young individuals (Johnson, 2001). A survey by the NCAA (1997) found that 1% of 13,914 NCAA collegiate athletes were using DHEA.

Physiological Impact of DHEA and Andro

DHEA and Andro are steroid precursors that are produced in the adrenal cortex and the testes. With respect to DHEA, levels tend to peak in young adulthood and taper down as one ages. Andro is further "downstream" in the testosterone synthetic pathway than DHEA. The theory behind both DHEA and Andro is that these prohormones are taken orally and converted in the body to testosterone. Because levels of DHEA decrease naturally as one ages, many thought this may be a "fountain of youth" prescription to ward off the negative effects of aging. The proposed ergogenic effect of DHEA and Andro are similar to anabolic steroids, including the following:

- Increased protein synthesis
- Increased lean muscle development and strength
- Faster postworkout and postinjury recovery

Potential side effects are likewise similar to anabolic androgenic steroids. In addition, athletes taking these steroid precursors may test positive for certain steroid metabolites in the urine, leading to disqualification and public humiliation.

Potential Benefits and Clinical Effectiveness of Dehydroepiandrosterone and Androstenedione

As opposed to true anabolic androgenic steroids, clinical data substantiating the effectiveness of DHEA and Andro are currently lacking. Studies have shown that with oral administration of DHEA, it is possible to increase serum levels of both DHEA and Andro (Armsey & Green, 1997; Brown et al., 1999). Despite this, it is important to point out that in younger healthy subjects no positive effect was seen on serum testosterone levels (Brown et al., 1999). Brown et al. (1999) went on to show that despite the increase in serum Andro concentrations, no significant strength gains in young healthy subjects were observed as compared to subjects strength training without DHEA. Some studies have shown increases in serum testosterone levels in postmenopausal women when given DHEA as a supplement (Brown et al., 1999; Morales et al., 1994; Mortola, 1990). No studies have documented the long-term effects of DHEA supplementation on serum DHEA, Andro, or testosterone levels.

With respect to Andro, some studies have documented a rise in serum levels after it is taken orally. A dose dependent elevation in serum testosterone has also been demonstrated (Armsey & Green, 1997; Leder, Longcope, Catlin, et al., 2000; Rubinstein & Federman, 2000). Despite this, two important points should be made. First, at higher doses Andro appears to undergo favorable conversion to biologically active estrogen and similar compounds (King et al., 1999; Leder et al., 2000; Rubinstein & Federman, 2000). Second, this rise in estrogen likely negates any potential ergogenic effect from the elevated Andro or testosterone levels as no studies have demonstrated a significant increase in strength, increase in muscle mass, or histologic changes in the muscle tissue (Earnest, 2001; King et al., 1999; Rasmussen, Volpi, Gore, et al., 2000; Wallace, Lim, Cutler, et al., 1999). The rise in estrogen and estrogen-like molecules may lead to the unwanted permanent feminizing side effects when Andro is taken in large doses.

Legal Implications

Both DHEA and Andro were banned by the FDA in 1996 and 2004, respectively. They continue to be available as "nutrition supplements." Their use is banned by most major sports governing organizations, including the IOC, NCAA, NHL, MLB, and the NFL. Drug testing inconsistencies have caused authors to voice concern that these prohormones may increase urinary concentrations of steroid-like substances and result in a positive drug screen (elevated testosterone to epitestosterone ratio) (Armsey & Green, 1997). The supplement industry has failed to make the public and elite athletes aware of this consequence.

CREATINE MONOHYDRATE

Creatine monohydrate is a naturally occurring substance that exists in free and phosphorylated forms (attached high energy phosphate). It is consumed in the diet from animal (meat and fish) and dairy products (typically 1 to 2 grams/day) (Greydanus & Patel, 2002; Rubinstein & Federman, 2000). In humans, creatine is synthesized by the liver, pancreas, and kidneys (Kraemer & Volek, 1999; Stricker, 1998). It is formed from the amino acids glycine, arginine, and methionine. In the human body, 95% of creatine is stored in the skeletal muscle, primarily in type 2 or fast twitch muscle fibers (Kraemer & Volek, 1999). Two thirds of the creatine in muscle is in the phosphorylated form (Greydanus & Patel, 2002).

The first reported use of creatine as an ergogenic aid was in British track athletes in the 1992 Barcelona Olympics (Stricker, 1998). Creatine has since grown in popularity and continues to be one of the more common performance-enhancing substances requested by athletes (Greydanus & Patel, 2002), especially in the high school and collegiate athletics. Recent studies have documented almost 6% of students in grades 6 through 12 using creatine and rates as high as 44% in high school seniors (Metzl et al., 2001). Surveys of NCAA athletes have shown 13% to 29% using or have used creatine (NCAA, 1997). Of note, sales of creatine topped $4 million in the late 1990s (Kraemer, 1999).

Physiological Impact of Creatine

During short-burst intense physical activity, adenosine triphosphate (ATP) is used as the primary energy substrate and is converted to adenosine diphosphate (ADP) and phosphorus. The body's ability to regenerate ATP is somewhat limited and thus the ability to do brief, high intensity physical activity is restricted. Creatine phosphate (Cr-P) in the skeletal muscle is thought to act as a substrate to donate a high energy phosphate molecule to ADP and more easily and quickly resynthesize ATP (Greydanus & Patel, 2002; Kraemer & Volek, 1999; Stricker, 1998). Cr-P is also thought to help buffer intracellular lactic acid production in that hydrogen ions are utilized when ATP is regenerated (Armsey & Green, 1997; Greydanus & Patel, 2002; Kraemer & Volek, 1999; Stricker, 1998). Thus creatine is thought to allow prolonged and more intense short-burst anaerobic type activity such as sprinting, strength training, short track cycling, or sprint swimming. Creatine is also marketed to assist with lean muscle development and weight gain. Fortunately, the side effect profile for creatine appears low and no direct cause and effect relationship between creatine and negative side effects has been established (Kraemer & Volek, 1999).

Anecdotal claims of muscle cramping, gastrointestinal distress, and nausea have been reported (Armsey & Green, 1997; Greydanus & Patel, 2002; Kraemer & Volek, 1999; Stricker, 1998). Some have concerns regarding creatine's increased solute load on the kidneys and potential for kidney disease or heat-related illness. There have been two reported cases of renal failure in adults associated with creatine supplementation. One case involved a patient with pre-existing kidney disease and the other involved persistent high-dose creatine ingestion for 4 weeks (Koshy et al., 1999; Pritchard et al., 1998). Because of these potential risks, it is advised to follow a diligent hydration plan and not use creatine while "in season" with one's particular sport, especially if there is potential for dehydration and heat-induced illness.

Potential Benefits and Clinical Effectiveness of Creatine

It has been documented that creatine ingestion can in fact increase intracellular creatine stores in certain individuals (Kraemer & Volek, 1999; Rubinstein & Federman, 2000). Data have shown that the mean creatine concentration in human skeletal muscle is

125 mmole/kg-dm (dry muscle), with a normal range between 90 and 160 mmole/kg-dm (Armsey & Green, 1997). This variance between subjects in baseline creatine stores likely accounts for certain individuals being "responders" (increased creatine stores with supplementation and subsequent improved performance) and "nonresponders" (subjects in which creatine ingestion results in little to no change in intramuscular creatine stores and subsequent athletic performance). Identification of potential "responders" is currently not readily available, but one study found vegetarians had statistically lower baseline creatine stores than their omnivorous colleagues (Armsey & Green, 1997). Therefore, vegetarians may benefit from creatine supplementation during periods of high intensity training. The most widely accepted method of creatine ingestion includes a cycle consisting of a loading phase (5 grams four times a day for 5 days), maintenance phase (2 grams a day for 2 to 3 months), and subsequent 1- to 2-month break. A continuous lower dose (3 grams per day) regimen has been shown to be equally effective at increasing intramuscular creatine stores (Stricker, 1998).

Many studies have documented short-term creatine supplementation can improve performance with activities that involve brief or repetitive bouts of strenuous physical activity (cycling, running, repeated jumping, swimming, kayaking or rowing, and weight training) (Brown et al., 1999; Greydanus & Patel, 2002; Kraemer & Volek, 1999; Stricker, 1998). The same studies have also documented statistically significant weight gain with creatine ingestion and strength training. The initial gains are thought to primarily be due to water influx into cells following the increase in intramuscular creatine stores. Long-term muscle and weight gains are thought to be due to increased training ability and intensity. Creatine supplementation does not appear to improve athletic performance in aerobic type activities. Creatine monohydrate may improve performance in activities such as soccer and football in which anaerobic bouts of sprinting are interspersed in an overall aerobic event. No studies have documented performance benefits or the health consequences of long-term creatine ingestion.

Legal Implications

Creatine monohydrate is not banned or tested for by any sports organizations. The NCAA has banned its distribution in university training facilities. The American College of Sports Medicine discourages the use of creatine in patients under the age of 18 years due to the concerns for possible side effects or adverse reactions and lack of data in pediatric patients (Terjung et al., 2000).

Additional Ergogenic Supplements

CHROMIUM PICOLINATE

Chromium is an essential trace mineral present in various foods, such as mushrooms, prunes, nuts, and whole grain breads and cereals (Cowart, 1992). It has been found that a normal American diet contains between 50% to 60% of the recommended daily allowance (RDA) of chromium. Chromium has an extremely low gastrointestinal absorption rate, therefore, manufacturers have bound chromium with picolinate, forming chromium picolinate (CrPic), to increase the absorption and bioavailability.

Chromium supplementation became popular after it was found that exercise increases chromium loss, raising the concern that chromium deficiency may be common among athletes. The function of chromium seems to be its action as a cofactor that potentiates the action of insulin, especially its role in carbohydrate, fat, and protein metabolism. Promoters of CrPic claim it increases glycogen synthesis, improves glucose tolerance and lipid lipoprotein profiles, and increases amino acid incorporation into muscle.

CrPic supplementation gained scientific credence in the early 1980s when two researchers demonstrated anabolic, "steroid-like" actions with doses of 200 mcg/day. Evans (1982, 1989) and Hasten, Rome, Franks, and Hegsted (1994) demonstrated decreased percent body fat and increased lean mass when CrPic supplementation and resistance exercise training were performed by collegiate athletes and students. Critical analysis of these studies reveal that imprecise measurement techniques may account for these "ergogenic" results rather than CrPic supplementation. Studies by Clancy et al. (1994) and Hallmark et al. (1996), utilizing more precise measurement techniques, failed to demonstrate any significant improvement in percent body fat, lean body mass, or strength.

The current consensus of scientific data seems to indicate that no improvement in percent body fat, lean body mass, or strength occurs with CrPic supplementation. Although most short-term studies reveal no side effects (except gastrointestinal intolerance) when CrPic was supplemented at doses of 50 to 200 mcg/day, there have been reports of serious adverse effects including anemia (Lefavi, 1992), cognitive impairment (Huszonek, 1993), and chromosomal damage (Stearns, Wise, Patierno, & Wetterhahn, 1995). Therefore, the use of CrPic supplementation as an ergogenic aid should be strongly discouraged and considered potentially dangerous.

AMINO ACIDS

Amino acids are the basic structural units of protein and one would therefore assume that the more amino acids ingested, the greater the potential for building skeletal muscle. According to the 1989 RDA, a normal human must ingest 0.8 grams/kg/day of protein in order to fulfill 100% of the protein requirements. Athletes, however, have traditionally been assumed to need significantly more protein than "normal" individuals to maintain their increased muscle mass. To this end, athletes commonly augment their diets with various forms of protein supplementation.

Theoretically, increasing the bioavailability of amino acids promotes protein synthesis and attenuates the muscle loss that occurs during both strength and endurance exercise. These theories have gained support through scientific experimentation in the area of protein metabolism. With regards to strength training, Fern, Bielinski, and Schultz (1991) and Lemon, Tarnopolsky, MacDougall, and Atkinson (1992) demonstrated increased protein synthesis with substantially increased protein ingestion during 4 weeks of resistance training. By tracking the nitrogen balance of these athletes, a new daily requirement of protein was developed for strength athletes in the range of 1.4 to 1.8 grams/kg/day.

Amino acid supplementation also plays a role in the endurance athlete. Lemon (1991) and Gontzen, Sutzecu, and Dumitrache (1974) demonstrated that endurance athletes who train at moderate intensity (55% to 65% VO2 max) and high intensity (80% VO2 max) for more than 100 minutes significantly increase protein breakdown unless their intake equals 1.2 to 1.4 grams/kg/day.

Although all of these studies demonstrate the necessity for higher protein intakes than the current RDA, there has yet to be a well-designed study showing performance enhancement with amino acid supplementation. Also, no scientific evidence has ever supported protein supplementation in doses greater than 2.0 grams/kg/day, which may lead to potential renal complications in normal healthy athletes. It may also be true that with adaptation to exercise over a 4- to 8-week period of training, amino acid requirements may decrease to a value much closer to the RDA.

L-Carnitine

L-carnitine is a quaternary amine whose physiologically active form is beta-hydroxyg-amma-trimethyl-amino butyric acid. This is found exogenously in meats and dairy products, as well as synthesized in the human liver and kidneys from two essential amino acids, lysine and methionine. Theoretically, L-carnitine is thought to be "ergogenic" in two ways. First, by increasing free fatty acid transport across mitochondrial membranes, carnitine may increase fatty acid oxidation and utilization for energy, which may spare muscle glycogen. Second, carnitine may prolong exercise by buffering pyruvate, and thus reducing muscle lactate accumulation (which is associated with fatigue).

Early studies by Gorostiaga, Maurer, and Eclache (1989); Wyss, Ganzit, and Rienzi (1990); and Natalie, Santoro, Brandi, et al. (1993) indirectly demonstrated an ergogenic effect of this compound. These studies showed a decreased respiratory exchange ratio (RER) with L-carnitine supplementation (2 to 6 grams per day) during exercise, which supports the argument that fatty acids are used for energy instead of carbohydrates. However, multiple methodologic problems are present in these studies, including the use of the RER as the sole measure of enhanced fatty acid oxidation. The RER is an indirect measure of lipid utilization that is influenced by many factors, such as pre-exercise diet, exercise intensity, load, duration, and training level (Krogh & Lindhard, 1920). These confounders were not controlled and may have influenced the results. A more controlled study by Vukovich, Costill, and Fink (1994) avoided these factors by directly measuring muscle glycogen and lactate levels through biopsy and serum analysis. This study failed to demonstrate any glycogen-sparing effect or reductions in lactate levels while supplementing with 6 grams per day of L-carnitine. Also, no study to date has confirmed performance enhancement with carnitine supplementation. Additionally, many currently available supplements actually contain D-carnitine, which is physiologically inactive in humans and may cause significant muscle weakness through competitive mechanisms with L-carnitine. Therefore, this agent should not be advocated by the scientific community as an ergogenic supplement.

L-Tryptophan

L-tryptophan, an essential amino acid, is commercially available in a variety of nutritional supplements and reported to remedy insomnia, depression, anxiety, and premenstrual tension. Athletes in the past decade have taken L-tryptophan based on its advertised "ergogenic" activity. Theoretically, L-tryptophan supplementation increases serotonin levels in the brain that produce analgesia and reduce the discomfort associated with prolonged muscular effort and, thereby, delays fatigue. This theoretical model gained scientific credence in 1988, when Segura and Ventura (1988) demonstrated a 49% increase in total exercise time to exhaustion when supplementing with 1.2 grams of L-tryptophan versus placebo. Such a profound improvement in human performance is difficult to imagine and these results have never been replicated. Two larger, well-designed studies by Seltzer, Stoch, Marcus, and Jackson (1982) and Stensrud, Ingjer, Holm, and Stromme (1992) failed to demonstrate any improvement in subjective or objective outcome measures when supplementing with 1.2 grams of L-tryptophan versus placebo. The results of these two studies are more consistent with the current exercise data found in the literature, and therefore suggest more reliable results.

Also, it should be noted that the use of L-tryptophan has declined among elite athletes, possibly suggesting that subjectively there is little effect. One more important note is that L-tryptophan ingestion was linked to the development of multiple cases of eosinophilia-myalgia syndrome and the death of 32 individuals (Teman & Hainline, 1991).

In summary, although one study has demonstrated substantial improvement in exercise performance, the use of this supplement should not be advocated due to the inability to reproduce these results and the risk that L-tryptophan supplementation may cause to the health of the consumer.

Beta-Hydroxy-Beta-Methylbutyrate

One of the most recent additions to the nutritional supplement market is beta-hydroxy-beta-methylbutyrate (HMB). HMB is known to be a metabolite of the essential branched-chain amino acid, leucine, and is produced in small amounts endogenously. HMB is also found exogenously in catfish, citrus fruits, and breast milk. In the early 1980s, researchers at Iowa State University hypothesized that HMB is the bioactive component of leucine metabolism that regulates protein metabolism (Nissen, Panton, Wilhelm, & Fuller, 1996). The exact mechanism of action is currently unknown, but promoters hypothesize that HMB regulates the enzymes responsible for protein breakdown. They propose that high levels of HMB decrease protein catabolism, thereby creating a net anabolic effect.

Scientific research in livestock (Gatnau, Zimmerman, Nissen, Wannemuehler, & Ewan, 1995; Nissen, Fuller, Sell, Perket, & Rives, 1994; Nissen, Morrical, & Fuller, 1992; Ostaszewski et al., 1996; Van Koevering et al., 1994) and humans seems to suggest that supplementation with HMB, may, in fact, increase lean muscle mass and strength (Nissen, Sharp, Ray, et al., 1996; Nissen, Panton, Wilhem, & Fuller, 1996). Nissen et al. has conducted two randomized, double-blinded, placebo-controlled studies to evaluate the ergogenic potential of HMB in exercising males (Nissen, Panton, et al, 1996; Nissen, Sharp, et al., 1996). In the first study, 41 untrained subjects participated in a 4-week structured resistance-training program. This study demonstrated statistically significant improvements in lean muscle mass and strength as well as significant decreases in muscle breakdown products (3-methylhistidine and creatine phosphokinase) while supplementing a controlled diet with 1.5 or 3.0 grams HMB per day versus controls. The second study evaluated both trained and untrained male subjects in a similarly designed weight training program. Both groups demonstrated significant increases in lean muscle mass and 1-repetition maximum bench press, as well as decreases in percent body fat with 3.0 grams HMB per day in comparison to controls.

Therefore, HMB supplementation (dosages of 1.5 to 3.0 grams per day) has been shown to augment resistance-training programs in novice and experienced male subjects with regard to muscle mass, strength, and percent body fat, presumably by decreasing muscle catabolism. Further studies regarding this supplement may continue to support the anabolic, "steroid-like" effects, as well as elucidate the role of HMB in protein metabolism. Currently, there are no reported side effects of HMB supplementation, but the safety profile of this agent is still unknown. Therefore, it is premature to recommend the use of HMB supplementation as a safe and effective ergogenic aid.

Nutrition as an Ergogenic Aid

In addition to affecting growth, maturation, and many health measures, it is well accepted that nutrition can positively affect athletic performance. Despite this, studies have demonstrated that many athletes, even at the elite level, lack basic nutrition knowledge and often times have less than ideal nutrition practices. Athletes at the high school and college level often look to coaches and athletic trainers for nutrition recommendations. It is very important that the information distributed is factual and follows recommended guidelines. Proper nutrition should be encouraged as an alternative to ergogenic aids for athletes found to be using them or who are interested in their usage. According to the American Dietetic Association (ADA), "there is insufficient evidence to suggest athletes need a diet substantially different from that recommended in the Dietary Guidelines for Americans" (Manore, Barr, & Butterfield, 2000) The main difference is that athletes typically require more baseline calories to support their athletic endeavors.

CARBOHYDRATES

Carbohydrates can be divided into simple and complex sugars. Simple carbohydrates include monosaccharides and disaccharides. Examples of monosaccharides include glucose, galactose, and fructose. Two sugar molecules linked together make up a disaccharide. Sucrose, lactose, and maltose are examples of disaccharides. Complex carbohydrates are longer "links" of sugar molecules and include starch, which is digestible, and fiber, which is indigestible. In the body, glucose exists in the free form in the blood stream and is stored as glycogen in the muscles and liver. Liver glycogen is responsible for maintaining a constant blood sugar in the body. Muscle glycogen supplies the necessary energy to exercising muscles.

Carbohydrates should serve as the major nutrient consumed by athletes, accounting for approximately 60% of total calories consumed. Healthy carbohydrates include wholesome breads, grains, and cereals, as well as fruits and vegetables. Lactose is the sugar molecule in dairy products such as milk, yogurt, and cheese. In addition to energy for working muscles, healthy carbohydrates have many other health benefits for athletes. Whole grains are great sources of fiber for a healthy digestive system. Fruits and vegetables are rich in antioxidants, which reduce the stress of strenuous workouts and assist with injury repair. Dairy products supply calcium and vitamin D to ensure healthy bones and teeth.

Carbohydrates can be categorized into those that have a high or low glycemic index. This becomes important for athletes in terms of the timing of meals and snacks in relation to work out schedules. High glycemic index carbohydrates cause a sharp rise in blood sugar quickly after being digested and include such items as sports drinks, plain baked potatoes, sugar snacks, and white breads. Moderate or low glycemic food items induce a slower and more sustained rise in blood sugar. Low glycemic food examples include high-fiber fruits, milk, yogurt, lentils, and beans. It is recommended the majority of carbohydrates consumed on a day-to-day basis be of low to moderate glycemic index foods. Their function is to maintain adequate baseline liver and muscle glycogen stores. High glycemic foods and drinks are primarily consumed during exercise to maintain blood sugar and immediately following exercise to replenish any depleted muscle glycogen. Athletes must experiment with both the timing and type of their food or drink in relation to exercise prior to important competitions so they will know if they "tolerate" the item. In the past it was commonplace to "carb load" prior to an endurance-oriented event, with the hopes of super-saturating muscle glycogen and ensuring more than adequate energy for working muscles. This strategy has fallen out of favor for most athletes, who instead maintain fairly constant carbohydrate intake on a day to day basis and simply taper down their training regimen 1 to 2 weeks prior to the competition. In this fashion, muscle glycogen stores are saturated and the reduced training schedule ensures the body is in optimal condition for the event.

PROTEIN

Dietary proteins are digested in the body to amino acids subsequently serve many bodily functions. Some of these functions include tissue repair and growth, and producing certain proteins, hormones, and enzymes, as well as molecules such as hemoglobin.

Dietary protein can also serve as an energy source during exercise when carbohydrate stores are low or diminishing. Examples of dietary proteins are meats, fish, poultry, beans, legumes, nuts, soy, and dairy.

The recommended daily allowance of protein for the average adult is 0.08 grams/kg/day. Athletic individuals (both strength- and endurance-oriented) require more dietary protein than sedentary individuals during times of training to maintain a positive nitrogen balance. This ensures the athlete is in a state of repair and building, rather than constant tissue breakdown. Athletes with potential deficiencies in protein intake include young athletes with the added effects of linear growth, athletes restricting certain foods or calories, those with eating disorders, vegetarians, and individuals initiating a fitness program.

Protein should account for approximately 15% of total calories consumed. The recommended amount of protein for athletes in both strength- and endurance-oriented events is approximately 1.5 to 2 grams/kg/day. It is recommended athletes consume a variety of proteins to ensure a rich amino acid "body pool" and avoid any possible deficiencies. Protein intake should be divided throughout the day in meals and snacks rather than consumed in one large quantity. A small amount of protein added to the postworkout carbohydrate snack may assist with glycogen store replenishment. Protein intakes above 1.5 to 2 grams/kg/day have not been shown to convey any athletic edge, including muscle gain or strength. Excessive protein intake may pose some theoretical health risks, including dehydration and heat illness, the risk of calcium loss in the urine, and the risk of kidney problems.

Fat

Dietary fats or lipids are insoluble in water and include products such as cholesterol, margarine, oils, and butter. Fat serves important functions in the body, including absorption of fat-soluble vitamins (vitamins A, D, E, and K), providing essential fatty acids the body cannot produce, and serving as a source of stored energy for low intensity physical activity or endurance-oriented activities. Fat also contributes to the production of hormones, cell membranes, neurons, and brain matter.

The recommended fat intake for the general population and athletes is approximately 25% of total daily calories. It is recommended the majority of fats consumed in the diet be relatively low in saturated fat and trans-saturated fat. Food items high in saturated fat such as red meat, sausage, bacon, butter, and whole milk should be limited to avoid the health risks such as high cholesterol and early heart disease. Foods high in trans-saturated fat include cakes, cookies, and chips. "Healthy" fats from items such as nuts (i.e. cashews, almonds, and walnuts), oils from cold water fish (i.e. salmon, tuna, and herring), and some vegetable oils should be included in the diet for the heart healthy benefits. It is important to point out that reducing fat intake to less than 15% to 20% of total calories consumed does not enhance performance. Athletes engaged in ultra-endurance events or large frame athletes may require a higher fat intake in the diet for adequate calorie consumption and adequate body fat stores.

Micronutrients

Micronutrients include vitamins and minerals. Studies have documented a user rate up to 40% at the high school level and 70% at the collegiate level for athletes taking a vitamin or mineral supplement. Some functions of micronutrients include energy production (direct and indirect), hemoglobin synthesis, bone formation, immune system enhancement, protection from oxidative stress, and building and repairing muscle. Most sports nutritionists agree that micronutrient supplementation is not necessary in most cases if an athlete's nutrition plan is well balanced.

With athletic performance in mind, the vitamins of interest include antioxidants, vitamin D, and the B-complex vitamins. As a general rule, fortified grains, fruits, and vegetables are excellent sources of vitamins. Antioxidants include vitamins A, E, C, betacarotene, and selenium. These nutrients play an important role in cell membrane protection, which may be subject to damage as oxidative stress increases with exercise. Some have also postulated that habitual exercise leads to an augmented antioxidant system, which could increase the amount of antioxidants necessary for optimal function. To date, studies are inconclusive whether or not athletes have a higher antioxidant requirement than sedentary subjects. B-complex vitamins, including thiamin (B-1), riboflavin (B-2), niacin (B-3), pantothenic acid (B-5), pyridoxine (B-6), and biotins, are involved in energy production. Folate and cobalamin (B-12) are also B-complex vitamins and are involved in production of red blood cells, protein synthesis, and tissue repair. Some studies do indicate the athlete's need for B-complex vitamins may be higher than the RDA. However, most experts agree this higher amount is usually met by an athlete's higher overall dietary intake. Deficiencies are possible in pure vegetarians (B-12 deficiency), dieters or picky eaters (all vitamins potentially deficient), those with poor vegetables and fruit intake (antioxidants and folate deficiency), those with poor milk intake, or indoor athletes (vitamin D deficiency).

Two of the most important minerals of interest to athletes include calcium and iron. Calcium is important for bone and tooth health, wound healing, muscle contraction, and other bodily functions. Sources of calcium include dairy products (milk, cheese, yogurt, and ice cream), fortified grains and orange juice, tofu, broccoli, and spinach. For most individuals over the age of 11 years, the RDA is approximately 1200 mg/day. Deficiencies are more common in amenorrheic female athletes, athletes with stress fractures, and athletes dieting or with poor eating behaviors. Iron is a necessary component of the hemoglobin molecule. Hemoglobin transports oxygen from the lungs to the working muscles of the body. Athletes have been shown to have an increased iron requirement due to losses in the urine, sweat, and gastrointestinal track associated with physical activity. Athletes also tend to have higher baseline hemoglobin concentrations, which increases their iron requirement. Sources of iron include beef, pork, lamb, and fortified grains. The RDA for males is 10 to 12 mg/day and for females 15 mg/day. Endurance athletes, females with heavy menses, and those dieting or with poor nutritional habits have a greater potential for deficiency. Vitamin D assists in the intestinal absorption of calcium, and vitamin C assists in the absorption of both calcium and iron. Calcium interferes with the absorption of iron and therefore these minerals should not be taken together as supplements.

Hydration

Adequate hydration is an essential aspect of training and conditioning. Approximately 60% of the typical adult body weight is water and almost 70% of lean body mass is water. Water serves many functions in the body, including cooling and preventing heat illness, nutrient transport and waste removal, digestion and nutrient absorption, and joint lubrication. Dehydration has been shown to affect perceived effort, cognitive abilities, morale, and desire to work. As one becomes dehydrated, body temperature rises, gastric emptying time decreases, sweat decreases, heart rate increases, and stroke volume decreases. All of these factors can obviously affect the athlete, and, in fact, as little as 1% to 2% dehydration has been shown to negatively affect sports performance. Certain factors can be risks for dehydration, including youth or old age, medical conditions, medications, supplements, poor conditioning or acclimatization, and a history of heat illness.

Having a hydration plan for athletes to follow can assist the coach or athletic trainer to ensure his or her athletes are functioning in a euhydrated state and avoid problems such as heat illness. Water should be easily accessible at all times during training and competitions. It is recommended athletes drink 12 to 20 ounces of water 2 to 3 hours prior to the athletic event. This should correct for any pre-game deficits and give time to use the restroom if necessary. Drinking 8 to 10 ounces of water immediately before the event and drinking regularly throughout will help correct losses occurring during the event. The athlete should again drink approximately 12 to 20 ounces after practice or competition. For events lasting well over 30 to 45 minutes, sports drinks may be preferable to water to replenish blood glucose and muscle glycogen. It can be helpful to periodically determine the amount of sweat lost in a typical game or practice to determine how much the athlete should try to drink during the event on subsequent days to avoid a deficit. This can be done by obtaining a body weight prior to practice and immediately after practice. Each pound of weight loss is equal to 1 pint or 16 ounces of fluid deficit. Weight deficits should be corrected prior to the next practice or competition. Body weight logs can serve as helpful reminders to young athletes about the importance of hydration.

The Role of the Athletic Trainer

The popularity of ergogenic aids at all levels of competition (secondary, collegiate, professional, recreational) has forced athletic trainers and other allied health personnel to enhance their knowledge and skills related to these performance-enhancing supplements. Without a certain level of knowledge or skill, communication to athletes, parents, coaches, and administrators becomes problematic. Athletic trainers play an integral part in the proper assessment, counseling, and appropriate referral of athletes/patients with maladaptive behaviors associated with nutritional supplements. Not all ergogenic aids pose a health risk to athletes. Athletic trainers must be able to provide insight and information to athletes seeking information on specific ergogenic aid. Specifically, athletic trainers must be aware of the potential health risks associated with improper use of nutritional supplements and other performance-enhancing aids. Brower and Rootenberg (1999) identify the following specific factors for sports medicine professionals to consider when treating athletes suspected of abusing nutritional supplements/ergogenic aids:

- *Understand the pressures associated with elite athletic performance.* Example: The cost of a specific collegiate athlete (e.g., football or basketball) not starting or playing in a specific game could cost the university and the athlete millions of dollars.

- *Consider yourself a part of a team.* Example: The athletic trainer must not work in isolation and keep in mind that the primary goal is to ensure a healthy athlete.

- *Recognize the competitive themes.* Example: The athletic trainer may be perceived as the "opponent" and athletes will become competitive during treatment and counseling.

- *Caution in providing special treatment.* Example: Athletic trainers should not get caught up in the performance (winning/losing or success/failure) associated with the athlete. The athletic environment can be a distraction from the overall goal (i.e., health of the athlete).

HELPFUL STRATEGIES

Specific treatment of an athlete suffering from an addiction or mental disorder associated with nutritional supplements is outside the scope of practice for an athletic trainer. Chapters 2 and 3 provide athletic trainers with general counseling strategies and a plan for referral for athletes suffering from a wide variety of psychosocial issues. In this section, three specific areas will be presented to assist athletic trainers in discussing ergogenic aids with their athletes. These focus on a knowledge component, a relationship component, and a team approach orientation for athletic trainers.

Knowledge of the Drug or Supplement

Educational competencies for athletic trainers clearly outline specific knowledge to be included in the educational experiences of accredited athletic training programs. These include specific competencies related to the physiological make-up of supplements, as well as the advantage or disadvantage and common misconceptions related to enhanced performance and supplements. Knowledge of a specific drug or supplement must also include an awareness of drug-testing policies and comprehensive list of banned substances by collegiate and professional organizations.

Example: If an athlete comes to you several times and asks for advice related to a specific supplement and you have no answer or incorrect information, it will damage your reputation and spread through the team very quickly. Athletic trainers need to provide appropriate referral or research the supplement.

Relationship Considerations

In Chapter 2, information was presented about developing a positive counseling relationship and the skills necessary to be effective in working with athletes. The athletic trainer can incorporate these skills and avoid creating conflict with athletes regarding supplement use. Both coaches and athletes will have strong opinions regarding the use of supplements and since most coaches are former players, they are well aware of the popularity and intake of specific supplements. The athletic trainer's role is not to pass judgment, but rather educate and refer if necessary so the appropriate facts are provided to those inquiring. The use of nutritional supplements and other ergogenic aids is a sensitive issue that requires excellent interpersonal skills.

Example: An athlete may use a supplement the athletic trainer knows for a fact has no nutritional value, physiological benefit, or positive influence on performance. It is important for the athletic trainer not to pass judgment, but rather educate the athlete and coaches.

Use a Team Approach

It is imperative that athletic trainers gain the trust and respect of their athletes/patients. If an athlete does not trust the athletic trainer, the information or treatment an athletic trainer is trying to provide will be useless. Whether dealing with nutritional supplements or a sprained ankle, the athlete/patient must understand that the health care professional has his or her best interest in mind. Athletic trainers should make it clear to athletes that it is important to them to enhance the performance of all athletes on the team. This may include finding the appropriate nutritional supplement with the help of a dietician, strength coach, and team physician.

Example: Be proactive and do some research to provide an athlete interested in nutritional supplements with a choice of appropriate and legal supplements. Be sure to include the strength and conditioning coaches, as they are closely involved with physiological enhancement of the athletes. Dieticians and physicians should also be consulted.

Psychosocial Influences

Dietary practices and the use of nutritional supplements are influenced by a variety of psychosocial issues. It is important to be aware of specific factors (sociological or psychological) that may contribute to the misuse of ergogenic aids. Athletic trainers must attempt to address the cause of the underlying behavior and not merely the misuse or abuse of an ergogenic aid. For example, an athlete who abuses steroids may have additional psychosocial issues that may have contributed to this behavior. In addition, the environment that surrounds the athlete may also be part of the cause. Storlie (1991) identified the following specific psychosocial influences that commonly affect an athlete's nutritional health:

- Social influences (e.g., family, friends, teammates, and coaches)
- Self-concept (e.g., body image, self-efficacy, locus of control)
- Competitive goals and commitment (e.g., realistic aspirations)
- Attitudes and philosophy toward life (e.g., need for power and control)

Similar to other issues involving health care of athletes, athletic trainers are typically in the best situation to provide initial care. Issues pertaining to supplements and ergogenic aids are no different. A clearer understanding of the benefits and potential adverse reactions to specific ergogenic aids is vital for athletic trainers charged with providing nutritional consultation to athletes and coaches.

Conclusion

This chapter presents information regarding several popular nutritional supplements and their use as ergogenic aids. Although some of these supplements discussed may have potential benefits, it is important to mention the NCAA guidelines that state, "there are no shortcuts to sound nutrition and the use of suspected or advertised ergogenic aids may be detrimental and will in most instances, provide no competitive advantage" (Benson, 1994).

The skepticism of nutritional supplements is due to a number of factors. As mentioned in this chapter, there is a paucity of properly performed scientific research to support a positive effect for many substances. In addition, the lack of rigorous FDA regulation may lead to impurities in the preparation of supplements. An example of this is the recently popularized substance melatonin. Abramowicz (1995) analyzed several commercial preparations of melatonin and found unidentifiable impurities in four out of six samples tested. Therefore, the pure supplements tested and reported in this review may not be equivalent to the forms available to the consumer.

Finally, the cost of nutritional supplements must be addressed. In this era of shrinking athletic department budgets, it makes little sense to invest in nutritional supplements that offer little or no benefit. This is an area in which an athletic trainer could take a leadership role in counseling members of the athletic department to make the best use of resources. Decisions regarding the use of nutritional supplements should only be made on the basis of proper scientific study and proven benefit to the patient.

Chapter Exercise

1. Fred is a red-shirt football athlete (offensive linemen) who will not play in games during the upcoming season. Coach has asked you and the weight coach to make sure that he gains at least 20 pounds (of muscle) prior to the start of the spring football practice.

   - What is the role of the athletic trainer in this scenario?
   - What other allied health professionals should be consulted?
   - What nutritional supplements would you recommend (if any)?

References

Abramowicz, M. (Ed.). (1995). Melatonin. *The Medical Letter on Drugs and Therapeutics, 37*(962), 111-112.

Armsey, T. D., & Green, G. A. (1997). Nutrition supplements: Science vs hype. *Physician and Sports Medicine, 25*(6), 77-92.

Benson, M. T. (Ed.). (1994). *NCAA sports medicine handbook 1994-95* (7th ed., p. 30). Indianapolis, IN: NCAA.

Blue, J., & Lombardo, J. (1999). Steroids and steroid-like compounds: Nutritional aspects of exercise. *Clinics in Sports Medicine, 18*(3), 667-689.

Brower, K. J., & Rootenberg, J. H. (1999). The role of the sports medicine professional in counseling athletes. In R. Ray & D. Bjornstal (Eds.), *Counseling in sports medicine* (pp. 179-204). Champaign, IL: Human Kinetics.

Brown, G. A., Vukovich, M. D., Sharp, R. L., Reifenrah, T. A., Parsons, K. A., & King, D. S. (1999). Effect of oral DHEA on serum testosterone and adaptations to resistance training in young men. *Journal of Applied Physiology, 87*(6), 2274-2283.

Clancy, S. P., Clarkson, P. M., DeCheke, M. E., Nosaka, K., Freedson, P. S., Cunningham, J. J., et al. (1994). Effects of chromium picolinate supplementation on body composition, strength, and urinary chromium loss in football players. *International Journal of Sports Nutrition, 4*, 142-153.

Cowart, V. S. (1992). Dietary supplements: Alternatives to anabolic steroids? *Physician and Sports Medicine, 20*(3), 189-198.

Earnest, C. (2001). Dietary androgen supplements. *Physician and Sports Medicine, 29*(5), 63-77.

Evans, G. W. (1982). The role of picolinic acid in metal metabolism. *Life Chem Rep, 1*, 57-67.

Evans, G. W. (1989). The effect of chromium picolinate on insulin controlled parameters in humans. *Int J Bios Med Res, 11*, 163-180.

Faighenbaum, A. D., Zaichkowsky, L. D., Gardner, D. E., & Micheli, L. J. (1998). Anabolic steroid use by male and female middle school students. *Pediatrics, 101*, E6.

Fern, E. B., Bielinski, R. N., & Schultz, Y. (1991). Effects of exaggerated amino acid and protein supply in man. *Experimentia, 47*, 168-172.

Gatnau, R., Zimmerman, D. R., Nissen, S. L., Wannemuehler, M., & Ewan, R. C. (1995). Effect of excess dietary leucine and leucine catabolites on growth and immune response in weanling pigs. *Journal of Animal Science, 73*, 159-165.

Gontzen, I., Sutzecu, P., & Dumitrache, S. (1974). The influence of muscular activity on the nitrogen balance and on the need of man for proteins. *Nutrition Reports International, 10*, 35-43.

Gorostiaga, E. M., Maurer, C. A., & Eclache, J. P. (1989). Decrease in respiratory quotient during exercise following l-carnitine supplementation. *International Journal of Sports Medicine, 10*, 169-174.

Greydanus, D. E., & Patel, D. R. (2002). Sports doping in the adolescent athlete: The hope, hype, and hyperbole. *Pediatric Clinics of North America, 49*, 829-855.

Hallmark, M. A., Reynolds, T. H., DeSouza, C. A., Dotson, C. O., Anderson, R. A., & Rogers, M. A. (1996). Effects of chromium and resistive training on muscle strength and body composition. *MSSE, 28*, 139-144.

Hasten, D. L., Rome, E. P., Franks, E. D., & Hegsted, M. (1994). Effects of chromium picolinate on beginning weight training students. *International Journal of Sport Nutrition, 4*, 142-153.

Huszonek, J. (1993). Letter to the editor: Over-the-counter chromium picolinate. *American Journal of Psychology, 150*, 1560-1561.

Johnson, W. (2001). Nutritional supplements and the young athlete: What you need to know. *Contemporary Pediatrics, 18*(7), 63-74.

King, D. S., Sharp, R. L., Vukovich, M. D., Brown, G. A., Reifenrath, T. A., Uhl, N. L., et al. (1999). Effect of oral androstenedione on serum testosterone and adaptations to resistance training in young men: A randomized control trial. *Journal of American Medical Association, 281*(21), 2020-2028.

Koch, J. (2002). Performance-enhancing substances and their use among adolescent athletes. *Pediatrics in Review, 23*(9), 310-317.

Koshy, K. M., Griswold, E., & Schneeberger, E. E. (1999). Interstitial nephritis in a patient taking creatine. *New England Journal of Medicine, 340*(10), 814-815.

Kraemer, W. (1999). *Advanced team physician course.* Orlando, FL: ACSM.

Kraemer, W. J., & Volek, J. S. (1999). Creatine supplementation: Nutritional aspects of exercise. *Clinics in Sports Medicine, 18*(3), 651-666.

Krogh, A., & Lindhard, J. (1920). The relative value of fat and carbohydrate as sources of muscular energy. *The Biochemical Journal, 14,* 290.

Lefavi, R. G. (1992). Sizing up a few supplements. *Physician and Sports Medicine, 20*(3), 190.

Leder, B. Z., Longcope, C., Catlin, D. H., Ahrens, B., Schoenfeld, D. A., & Finkelstein, J. S. (2000). Oral androstenedione administration and serum testosterone concentrations in young men. *Journal of American Medical Association, 283*(6), 779-782.

Lemon, P. W. (1991). Effect of exercise on protein requirements. *Journal of Sports Sciences, 9,* 53-70.

Lemon, P. W., Tarnopolsky, M. A., MacDougall, J. D., & Atkinson, S. A. (1992). Protein requirements, muscle mass, and strength changes during intensive training in novice bodybuilders. *Journal of Applied Physiology, 73,* 767-775.

Manore, M. M., Barr, S. I., Butterfield, G. E. (2000) Position of the American Dietetic Association, Dietitians of Canada, and the American College of Sports Medicine: Nutrition and athletic Performance. Journal of the American Dietetic Association, 100(12), 1543-1556.

Metzl, J. D., Small, E., Levine, S. R., & Gershel, J. C. (2001). Creatine use among young athletes. *Pediatrics, 108*(2), 421-425.

Metzl, J. (2000). Performance enhancing drugs in sports. *Presented at American Academy of Pedatrics* pre-conference in pediatric sports medicine; Hilton Head, SC.

Morales, A. J., Nolan, J. J., Nelson, J. C., & Yen, S. S. (1994). Effects of replacement dose of DHEA in men and women of advancing age. *Journal of Clinical Endocrinology and Metabiology, 78,* 1360-1167.

Mortola, J. (1990). The effects of oral DHEA on endocrine-metabolic parameters in postmenopausal women. *Journal of Clinical Endocrinology and Metabiology, 71,* 696-704.

Natalie, A., Santoro, D., Brandi, L. S., Faraggiana, D., Ciociaro, D., Pecori, N., et al. (1993). Effects of acute hypercarnitinemia during increased fatty substrate oxidation in man. *Metabolism, 42,* 594-600.

National Collegiate Athletic Association. (1997). *NCAA study of substance use and abuse habits of college student-athletes.* NCAA Committee on Medical Safeguards and Medical Aspects of Sports. Indianapolis, IN: NCAA.

Nissen, S. L., Fuller, J. C., Sell, J., Perket, P. R., & Rives, D. B. (1994). The effect of b-hydroxy b-methylbutyrate on growth, mortality, and carcass qualities of broiler chickens. *Poultry Science, 73,* 137-155.

Nissen, S. L., Morrical, D., & Fuller, J. C. (1992). The effects of the leucine catabolite b-hydroxy b-methylbutyrate on the growth and health of growing lambs. *Journal of Animal Science, 77*(suppl. 1), 243.

Nissen, S. L., Sharp, R., Ray, M., Rathmacher, J. A., Rice, D., Fuller, J. C., et al. (1996). The effect of the leucine metabolite beta-hydroxy beta-methylbutyrate on muscle metabolism during resistance-exercise training. *Journal of Applied Physiology, 81,* 2095-2104.

Nissen, S. L., Panton, J., Wilhelm, R., & Fuller, J. C. (1996). The effect of beta-hydroxy beta-methylbutyrate (HMB) supplementation on strength and body composition of trained and untrained males undergoing intense resistance training. *Experimental Biology,* Conference Presentation Abstract.

Ostaszewski, P., Kostiuk, S., Balasinska, B., Papet, J., Glomot, F., & Nissen, S. (1996). The effect of the leucine metabolite b-hydroxy b-methylbutyrate (HMB) on muscle protein synthesis and protein breakdown in chick and rat muscle. *Journal of Animal Science, 74,* 138.

Pritchard, N., & Kalra, P. A. (1998). Renal dysfunction accompanying oral creatine supplements. *Lancet, 351,* 1252-1253.

Rasmussen, B. B., Volpi, E., Gore, D. C., Dennis, C., & Wolfe, R. R. (2000). Androstenedione does not stimulate muscle protein anabolism in young healthy men. *Journal of Clinical Endocrinology and Metabiology, 85*(1), 55-59.

Rubinstein, M. L., & Federman, D. G. (2000). Sports supplements: Can dietary additives boost athletic performance and potential? *Postgraduate Medicine, 108*(4), 103-112.

Segura, R., & Ventura, J. L. (1988). Effect of L-tryptophan supplementation on exercise performance. *International Journal of Sports Medicine, 9*(5), 301-305.

Seltzer, S., Stoch, R., Marcus, R., & Jackson, E. (1982). Alterations of human pain thresholds by nutritional manipulation of l-tryptophan supplementation. *Pain, 13,* 385-393.

Stearns, D. M., Wise, J. P., Patierno, S. R., & Wetterhahn, K. E. (1995). Chromium picolinate produces chromosome damage in Chinese hamster ovary cells. *FASEB, 9*(15), 1643-1649.

Stensrud, T., Ingjer, F., Holm, H., & Stromme, S. B. (1992). L-tryptophan supplementation does not improve running performance. *International Journal of Sports Medicine, 13,* 481-485.

Storlie, J. (1991). Nutritional assessment of athletes: A model for integrating nutrition and physical performance indicators. *International Journal of Sport Nutrition, 1,* 192-204.

Stricker, P. R. (1998). Other ergogenic agents. *Clinics in Sports Medicine, 17*(2), 283-297.

Sturmi, J. E., & Diorio, D. J. (1998). Anabolic agents. *Clinics in Sports Medicine, 17*(2), 261-282.

Sullivan, J. A., & Anderson, S. J. (Eds.). (2000). *Care of the Young Athlete.* Rosemont, IL: American Academy of Orthopaedic Surgeons and the American Academy of Pediatrics.

Teman, A. J., & Hainline, B. (1991). Eosinophilia-myalgia syndrome. *Physician Sports Medicine, 19,* 81-86.

Terjung, R., Clarkson, P., Eichner R., Greenhaff, P. L., Hespel, P. J., Israel, R. G., et al. (2000). American College of Sports Medicine roundtable: The physiologic and health effects of oral creatine supplementation. *Medicine and Science in Sports and Exercise, 32,* 706-717.

Van Koevering, M. T., Dolezal, H. G., Gill, D. R., Owens, F. N., Strasia, C. A., Buchanan, D. S., et al. (1994). Effects of b-hydroxy b-methylbutyrate on performance and carcass quality of feedlot steers. *Journal of Animal Science, 72,* 1927-1935.

Vukovich, M. D., Costill, D. L., & Fink, W. J. (1994). Carnitine supplementation: Effect on muscle carnitine and glycogen content during exercise. *MSSE, 26,* 1122-1129.

Wallace, M. B., Lim, J., Cutler, A., & Bucci, L. (1999). Effects of DHEA vs androstenedione supplementation in men. *Medicine and Science in Sports and Exercise, 31*(12), 1788-1792.

Wyss, V., Ganzit, G. P., & Rienzi, A. (1990). Effects of l-carnitine administration on VO2 max and the aerobic-anaerobic threshold in normoxia and acute hypoxia. *European Journal of Applied Physiology, 60,* 1-6.

Bibliography

Burns, R. D., Schiller, M. R., Merrick, M. A., & Wolf, K. N. (2004). Intercollegiate student athlete use of nutritional supplements and the role of athletic trainers and dietitians in nutrition counseling. *Journal of the American Dietetic Association, 104*(2), 246-249.

Kleiner, S. M. (1999). Counseling athletes with nutritional concerns. In R. Ray & D. Bjornstal (Eds.), *Counseling in sports medicine* (pp. 227-255). Champaign, IL: Human Kinetics.

Shifflett, B., Timm, C., & Kahanov, L. (2002). Understanding of athletes' nutritional needs among athletes, coaches, and athletic trainers. *Research Quarterly for Exercise and Sport, 73*(3), 357-363.

Winterstein, A. P., & Storrs, C. M. (2001). Herbal supplements: Considerations for the athletic trainer. *Journal of Athletic Training, 36*(4), 425-432.

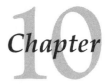
Chapter

PSYCHOSOCIAL ASPECTS OF CHILD AND ADOLESCENT SPORTS

Jason J. Stacy, MD
Joshua Scott, MD, FACSM
Jeffrey A. Guy, MD

Chapter Objectives

- ❖ Provide an overview of youth sports in the United States.
- ❖ Discuss the principles of normal growth for children.
- ❖ Discuss specific problems associated with participation in youth sports.
- ❖ Discuss appropriate intervention strategies to address special problems associated with youth sports.
- ❖ Discuss the role of the athletic trainer and other allied health professionals in supporting adolescent athletes.

NATA Educational Competencies

Psychosocial Intervention and Referral Domain

1. Explain the potential need for psychosocial intervention and referral when dealing with populations requiring special consideration (to include, but not limited to, those with exercised-induced asthma, diabetes, seizure disorders, drug allergies and interactions, unilateral organs, physical and/or mental disability).

Risk Management and Injury Prevention Domain

1. Explain the precautions and risks associated with exercise in special populations.

At no time in American history has the influence of sports been greater. Easy availability to television has made the viewing of all kinds of athletic events possible for the average family in the United States. Because of the popularity of professional and collegiate sports with the public, the retail business of marketing sports has become a multibillion dollar industry. The saturation of sports marketing, coupled with more easily available recreational athletic leagues, has significantly increased participation in organized athletics. Nowhere has this increase in sports participation been more significant than in the youth population. Children and adolescents in recreational and other organized athletics have exploded in numbers in the last few decades. With almost 7 million adolescents participating in high school sports and over 30 million children participating in an organized sport, individuals younger than age 18 make up the majority of athletes in American athletic leagues (Metzl, 2002). At increasingly younger ages, children are becoming involved in team and individual sports in their communities. Overall, this has led to many beneficial effects for children but has also introduced special problems, both physical and psychological. These problems must be identified and confronted by the athletic care provider. As one of those health care providers, athletic trainers develop a close working relationship with many of these young athletes. It is in this setting that athletic trainers must be well prepared to engage in the psychosocial aspects of child and adolescent sports.

History

The structure of physical activity and sports has changed significantly for children. It has moved from that of a spontaneous and unstructured environment with very little adult involvement to a much more organized and "grown-up" arena (American Academy of Pediatrics, 2001). There are many benefits to this organization of play, including supervision, enforcement of safety and rules, and the opportunity for all children to get equal time "in the game." However, organization has the potential to shift the goals of participation from the social interaction, neurodevelopment, and simple love of the game to that of competition, discipline, and adult demands (American Academy of Pediatrics, 2001).

With these increases in organized athletic participation in the latter part of the last century comes a surprising decline in the physical activity of both children and adolescents. More television channels, video games, and sometimes unsafe neighborhoods are just a few of the factors that have moved children inside to play. This relative inactivity has been reflected in the obesity epidemic among our nation's children. The results of the 1999 to 2002 National Health and Nutrition Examination Survey revealed that 16% of children ages 6 to 19 are overweight, indicating a 45% increase since the same study one decade before. Another 15% were at risk for becoming overweight with a BMI for age in the 85th to 95th percentiles (National Center for Health Statistics, n.d.). There is little doubt to the benefit of regular aerobic exercise in preventing obesity in both the pediatric and adult population. However, despite a growing number of children participating in sports, a large percentage of overweight children are losing this battle. Steps have been made at both the local and national levels to work toward a healthy and fit population of children and adolescents in this country. Engaging these young people in exercise while maintaining the relaxed and comfortable atmosphere of recreational sports should be the focus.

Preadolescent participation in organized sports is a relatively new phenomenon in the last few decades. These younger competitors are particularly susceptible to the demands that adults can impose, causing significant psychological stress on the athlete. The overbearing parent, coach, or even teammate is an all too familiar presence on our nation's courts, fields, and arenas. Also, events such as triathlons, weight lifting, and long distance races that used to be off limits to young athletes are now more easily accessible. These more intense competitions can require training that is beyond some children's capabilities both physically and mentally.

Normal Development

Normal growth and development of the child and adolescent can be broken down into several large categories. Motor, language, visual, auditory, emotional, and cognitive skills are some of the major functional domains of neurodevelopment. All of these skills are constantly developing in the progression of the athlete from childhood to adolescence, and a wide range exists of what is considered normal development for a child.

Gross motor skills develop rapidly in the first several years of life. Most children can walk alone by 12 months of age and can run by 18 months of age (The Harriet Lane Handbook). By 2 to 3 years of age, the child is able to run well, hop, and crudely throw and catch a ball. By the age of 5, most children are able to jump and skip. Balance improves significantly as children acquire these skills. Most children are able to throw a ball and hit a target by school age. However, children younger than 6 or 7 years are naturally farsighted and may have trouble tracking objects or judging their speed (Patel, Pratt, & Greydanus, 2002). Due to these normal developmental issues, experts recommend children do not begin organized sports until the age of 6 years.

With school-aged children, aged 6 to 10, some gender differences are noted. Girls are capable of skipping and catching a ball earlier than boys. Boys are able to kick a ball and jump with greater ability than girls (Patel et al., 2002). By age 10 to 11, most children have mastered primary motor skills and are able to perform complex movements such as hitting a ball with a bat.

In early adolescence, the disparity of gross motor development is most noticeable due to the wide range of pre- and postpubertal athletes. Gross motor skills are refined during this time period. Increases in muscle mass, strength, and agility contribute to the adolescent athlete excelling in coordination of body and mind. For most females, gross motor skills do not advance past the age of 14, whereas gross motor development in males continues through late adolescence (Patel et al., 2002).

Although the vast subject of childhood development is beyond the scope of this chapter, it is important to understand that both physical and psychological readiness have a profound impact on sports participation. Providers should be sure to educate parents and coaches about what children are capable of doing at certain ages. For example, although 6- and 7-year-old children can understand the general concept of soccer, adults should not expect the children to follow instructions to play one specific position and wait for the ball to be passed to them. Instead they all seem to "swarm" and follow the ball wherever it goes. This is a normal phase of growing and children should not be disciplined when playing in this manner.

Participation

Unfortunately, sport participation often precedes sport developmental readiness when children are thrust into organized "play" too early. The prodigal child athlete is often glorified on television, and professional sport "superstars" are getting younger as the enticement of million dollar contracts become available. Because of this exposure, some parents are starting to involve their children in competitive athletics not only for the wrong reasons but also far too early in life. These child and teenage athletes often have difficulty coping with the very adult lifestyle of competitive athletics. This can lead to simple disinterest in their sport or to more serious problems such as depression and drug addiction. Obviously, the majority of the millions of children and adolescents playing sports in this country will not go on to play professionally, and most are playing for the simple fun of the game. However, problems arise when too much emphasis is placed on winning, and the usual positive effect that the sport has on a child's self-esteem can become a negative one (Stricker, 2002).

When children become old enough to understand the rules and concepts of team sports, it is then important to group them with peers that are similar both physically and mentally. As discussed previously, all children develop at different rates and each has his or her own strengths and weaknesses. A 10-year-old prepubertal boy may play with 10- to 12-year-olds that are much more physically mature in a recreational football league age group. This not only can lead to serious injury but can also have a negative impact on self-esteem and the enjoyment of playing. Girls who are stronger or equal in strength to boys of their age may have trouble competing in physical sports with those same boys after puberty. Therefore, children may participate in co-ed sports until they reach puberty without increased risk of injury or inequities in motor or muscle development. Physical and cognitive maturity is more important that chronological age when determining peers for a child in sports (Patel et al., 2002).

Some experts even go so far as to recommend the use of height and weight as guidelines for participation in youth leagues, as opposed to age, to prevent injury. The classic example is the boy who excels in sports where size and strength development are most important due to his early maturity and significant strength advantage over the other athletes. He may be the same age as another athlete but superior in strength and ability. Not only does this situation increase the likelihood for injury to the smaller athletes, but it may cause a setting of high expectations for the developed individual due to his early success. These high expectations may lead to perceived failure once the others catch up in growth and maturity if the athlete no longer dominates play. When an athlete's self-worth is derived primarily from athletic success, the loss of that success can be debilitating to his or her psyche.

For girls, reaching puberty may actually have the opposite effect on performance. In many women's sports, girls will experience detrimental effects from the physiologic changes that occur during puberty. Women actually increase their percent body fat at the expense of lean muscle mass during puberty. This may lead to an associated decrease in sports performance. Coaches, parents, and athletes must be educated that poor performance is often related to the physiologic changes of puberty rather than a lack of motivation. It is important to discourage extreme attempts to counteract some of these normal changes. Pathologic behaviors can occur that may lead to eating disorders and problems associated with the female athletic triad when athletes restrict calories and engage in over-exercising (Harris, 2002). Further discussion of the triad is beyond the scope of this chapter.

Special Problems

OVERBEARING ADULTS

Because younger athletes are at a risk for developing anxiety or stress-related "burn out," it is important for parents and coaches to keep the organized sport focused on the children's goals to have fun and not the adults' goals to win. Although most children and adolescents will develop a competitive spirit, which is healthy, the added pressure from adults to "win at all costs" can be detrimental to the child athlete. The reaction and personal development that stem from a loss of a game can be just as important as those that come from winning (Patel, Pratt, & Greydanus, 2003). The athletic trainer must be able to recognize, approach, and deal with the overbearing coach or parent of an athlete. The athlete subsequently may become depressed, angry, or even apathetic about participation. These situations can be very difficult to deal with for a health care provider in youth athletics and, unfortunately, these problems occur too often.

As the primary health provider for the athletes, one must realize the complexity of the motivating factors positively and negatively affecting performance in young athletes. These factors also affect the provider's ability to give care. One of these factors, which can occur at both extremes, is the parental expectations for health care in athletics. In the past, injury advice tended to be "stay off it until it gets better." Currently many athletes, families, and coaches are eager to push the situation to get the athlete back on the field as soon as possible. Some push their children and feel they should play despite an injury, while others may hold their children out due to unfounded concerns of reinjury despite adequate rehab. An athletic trainer is in the position to positively affect the outcome because he or she understands the risks of returning too soon but also understands the importance of sports in the young person's life. The athletic trainer must look out for the athlete's best interest by weighing the risks of prolonged inactivity versus early return. Usually, the best position is to be an advocate for the child's safety, making sure that the sport participation remains fun. This is a central goal to children's athletics that is much too often overlooked.

Sport Specialization

Previously, it was commonplace for high school athletes to play four sports competitively in 1 year; however, many young athletes are currently engaging in year-round participation in a single sport. Although this practice may appear to develop sport specific skills at an earlier age, many overuse injuries are occurring. In addition to the physical harm this causes, these children often lose interest in a sport that they once enjoyed due to increased pressure being placed upon them at an early age (American Academy of Pediatrics, 2000). The current recommendation is to limit specialization in children younger than 12 years of age. The health care provider should be an advocate for the mental and physical health of athletes by educating parents and coaches about the adverse effects of sport specialization.

Depression

Depression in the child is particularly dangerous because many children lack the knowledge or capacity to deal with true depression. MDD will affect 2.5% of children and 8.3% of adolescents at any given time (Lagges & Dunn, 2003). These episodes can last usually 6 to 7 months and have symptoms ranging from fatigue, changes in appetite, trouble sleeping, and mood changes to somatic complaints such as headaches or stomach aches. Feelings of worthlessness or guilt may precede suicidal thoughts or attempts particularly in adolescents (Lagges & Dunn, 2003). Loss of interest in playing sports or failing grades may be present in the depressed child athlete. It is important for athletic trainers to pay particular attention to any child who they feel may be suffering from depression. Seeking professional help is extremely important for children and adolescents who have MDD, and it is any adult's responsibility involved in their care to help them do so. Immediate care must be sought for any child with either suicidal or homicidal thoughts or attempts. Psychiatric inpatient treatment is usually needed in these cases to reduce the risks of adverse outcomes. Children may be particularly poor at expressing their feelings, and approaching the depressed child can be difficult. It is imperative to make the child's parents and coach aware of the problem and to seek help from a trained counselor or physician. Most children and adolescents who suffer from MDD will have a repeat episode within 2 years after treatment (Lagges & Dunn, 2003).

Milder forms of depression that might not meet diagnostic criteria for true major depression should not be overlooked. Children and adolescents often have incredible stresses and changes occurring in their young lives. Many times, sports are a stable component in their lives, and an injury or other limitation from participation can lead to loss of this physical outlet. In the absence of the stress relief and positive self-esteem that athletics provide, an athlete may begin to experience similar depressive symptoms to those mentioned above. A provider who has close contact with the athlete may notice problems or hear about issues from teammates. As with depression, early recognition and treatment are key. Talking about the problem may be beneficial and further measures may be made with cross training or finding ways for the individual to be involved with the sport without actual participation until the injury resolves.

Substance Abuse

Substance abuse with recreational drugs, alcohol, and tobacco is a large problem in the child and adolescent population. The national survey conducted in 2005 by the Substance Abuse and Mental Health Services Administration found that 27.7% of children aged 12 to 17 were currently using or had used illicit drugs. Specifically 17.4% of these children used or had used marijuana, 10.5% inhalants, 9.9% pain relievers, 3.9% hallucinogens, 3.4% stimulants, 3.0% tranquilizers, 2.3% cocaine, and 0.2% heroin. This problem simply does not disappear when the child becomes an athlete. Although some studies have shown the protective effects that sports participation has on recreational drug use, the sheer numbers of child and adolescent athletes ensures that a statistical number will be involved in substance abuse (Arvers & Choquet, 2003). The psychological effects of substance abuse are extremely detrimental to the athlete. Mood swings and lack of interest in sports or previous activities can be a sign of substance abuse. Athletes that are involved in the abuse of drugs or alcohol must be confronted carefully but directly in order to ensure their safety. Involvement of their family, coaches, and peers is important to gain the support needed to help the athlete to a complete recovery. Even occasional drug or alcohol use can have a deleterious effect on the athlete's health and performance. Approaching the child or adolescent and telling him or her that his or her athletic performance is suffering from drug abuse may sometimes be the best way to confront him or her. Perceived loss of athletic ability may be more important to the athlete at this stage of development than any health risks in the future. However, if a concern exists and the athlete refuses to respond, referral to the proper health care professionals is indicated to ensure the health of the athlete.

ERGOGENICS IN YOUNG ATHLETES

Doping with anabolic steroids and other performance-enhancing substances has been a major issue in professional sports in recent years. However, the use of doping to improve performance with illegal and legal supplements is not limited to professional or collegiate athletes. Children as young as middle school ages have admitted to taking anabolic steroids to improve performance, look better, and appear bigger and stronger. One study showed that 2.7% of middle school students admitted to taking anabolic steroids despite half of the users knowing that these substances were bad for their health (Faigenbaum, Zaichkowsky, Gardner, et al., 1998). A study in 2001 of adolescent users of creatine found that 74% used to enhance performance while 61% used to improve appearance (Metzl et al., 2001). Adolescent users can be particularly susceptible to the perceived need to abuse steroids, especially when participating in sports that emphasize physical attributes or appearance. Use is associated with eating disorders, other substance abuse, poor self-esteem, depression, and even suicide (Irving, Wall, Neumark-Sztainer, et al., 2002).

Athletic trainers must be wary of warning signs of steroid use in children and adolescents. These can vary from very subtle changes in personality, rapid physical changes in size, acne, and hair loss to severe anger and violence that manifest on or off the field. As with any substance abuse, it is important to address these concerns with the athlete in a nonthreatening but direct manner. Athletes may also deny any abuse for fear of getting in trouble, so often teammates, parents, and coaches need to be approached if the concern is valid. It is important that the healthcare provider understand the serious effects of many of these supplements. Studies have shown the "Just Say No" model does not work with ergogenics because some agents such as anabolic steroids do work. In order to maintain an athlete's trust, one must educate the athlete about the serious side effects while acknowledging the potential for benefits. Again, it must be stressed that the athlete's health and best interest are kept in mind when confronting such problems.

OVERWEIGHT IN CHILDHOOD

The Center for Disease Control and Prevention (CDC) uses the term *overweight* rather than "obesity" to describe the condition in children and adolescents. There are two classifications: overweight (BMI greater than 95th percentile for age) or at risk for overweight (BMI from 85th to 95th percentile). Recent trends estimate the number of overweight persons age 6 to 19 have tripled since the 1960s (Fowler-Brown & Kahwati, 2004). This epidemic has serious consequences for the health of the American public because overweight children become obese adults and obesity has been linked to many serious health problems, including diabetes mellitus, hypertension, heart disease, and more. Young people also realize the risk of these diseases at an early age, plus they experience more psychosocial issues than a more normal sized individual. Lower self-esteem, depression, isolation, further inactivity, and binge eating can occur. Therapy for this problem is best when it is multifaceted. It is beneficial to encourage young people to be physically active whether in organized sports or not. Involvement of the family is also a necessary component. Providers should educate the family about diet and exercise, encourage them to make a change, and make sure they realize permanent lifestyle changes must be made to lead to slow, gradual weight loss. It may also be helpful to ask for the help of a registered dietician or even a psychologist if the psychological problems are significant. As health care providers for young athletes, athletic trainers should be proactive to encourage physical activity as a major force in the prevention of children becoming overweight.

HARASSMENT

Sexual harassment has become more of a recognized issue in the past few decades. Since Title IX of the Educational Amendment Act was introduced in 1972, the number of participating girls in organized recreational, high school, and collegiate sports has increased dramatically (Metzl, 2002). With the increasing numbers of female participants, there came more reports of sexual harassment in sports from coaches, teammates, and even officials. From problems that range from the reduction in playing time based on gender to blatant sexual advancements, the female athlete is subject to a wide variety of sexual harassment. As with many such problems, voicing a concern or reporting harassment may also be a problem as this may also put the athlete at risk for verbal or even physical abuse (Greydanus & Patel, 2002; Patel et al., 2003). An athletic trainer or responsible adult has the responsibility to the athlete to prevent such abuse or report it when it happens.

Although less common, athletic trainers must also be aware that young male athletes can be victims of sexual assault by coaches or other teammates. Hazing appears to be more common among sports teams today, although the perceived increased frequency may be due to increased reporting. These incidents can be detrimental to an individual's psychological development and should not be allowed or tolerated by coaches, athletic trainers, and athletic directors. Steps should be taken to prevent occurrence, and punishment must be significant. Policies regarding sexual abuse are established at most institutions. Once an event is suspected, athletic trainers must be sure to act quickly and discretely to alert the proper authorities.

ATHLETES WITH DISABILITIES

It is widely recognized that athletic participation is a positive experience for those individuals with disabilities. Not only are there physical benefits, there are psychosocial benefits to reap for athletes and families of athletes with disabilities. Even though contact sports are not advocated, many positive social experiences occur from participation in sports. Isolation is often a problem for families of children with disabilities that can be improved through sport participation. Athletes and families have increased opportunities to interact with others and share similar experiences, which may develop a connection to the community. Participation can enhance personal motivation, foster independence, improve coping abilities, allow athletes opportunity for social comparison, foster competitiveness and teamwork, and build self-esteem (Patel, 2002). It is important for athletic trainers to view and treat these individuals as people and athletes rather than victims of a disease. With proper help and supervision, all individuals should be able to gain the positive effects of athletic participation.

Conclusion

Organized sports participation for America's children and adolescents can have a profoundly positive impact on their physical and mental health. Teaching skills like cooperation, social interaction, and sportsmanship are just some of the added cognitive benefits of sports beyond the obvious physical benefits. In an age where video games and cable television compete with exercise and physical play for a child's attention, we must continue to impress the value of athletics. However, as with any health care provider, it is the job of the athletic trainer to become an advocate for the mental and emotional well-being of the child as he or she grows with competition. Due to the many hours spent together, athletic trainers and young athletes develop a unique relationship. Athletic trainers often get to know their athletes extremely well. This intimate relationship enables an athletic trainer to assess for both physical and psychiatric problems in athletes better than other health care providers. Athletes may view their athletic trainer as a role model, confidant, and friend. This position places significant responsibility on the athletic trainer. He or she may be the first to identify psychiatric problems, or often athletes may approach their athletic trainer to inform him or her when they have a problem. In this role, an athletic trainer does not need to know how to treat specific psychiatric disorders, but he or she must be aware of changes in athletes' personalities and signs of problems, then know when, where, and how to react and seek help.

All children are different in their growth and development, and it is important to be patient with them as they develop both mentally and physically. Child athletes should not be treated as "little adults," and care must be taken so that they understand and appreciate their sports. The push for physical fitness among our nation's children is important but must not come at the expense of mental or emotional fitness. Working in combination with coaches, parents, and other health care professionals, the athletic trainer is an integral part in achieving this goal.

Chapter Exercises

1. A 14-year-old male who is the starting running back for the high-school football team has been suspended from football practice for skipping school. When he returns to football practice, he seems disinterested in playing. His teammates comment that his grades are failing.

   - What concerns do you have for this athlete?
   - How would you approach the athlete?
   - How would you approach the coach or parents?
   - Make sure to follow up with the athlete, parents, and coach within the next 1 to 2 days.

2. A 7-year-old girl is on the recreational gymnastics team. She enjoys gymnastics, but you note that she becomes quiet and does not want to participate when her mother comes to practices. At competitions, the mother cheers loudly when the girl does well but publicly scolds her if she does not win.
   - What concerns do you have for this child?
   - What developmental milestones has the child achieved to handle this situation?
   - How would you discuss your concerns with the mother?
   - How would you discuss your concerns with the coach?

3. A 10-year-old boy, who plays on the 10- to 12-year-old little league baseball team, is slightly under-developed for age, clumsy, and mildly overweight. He does not run as fast as the other team members. The coach constantly yells at him despite the child trying to do whatever is asked of him.
   - What are the possible short-term and long-term psychosocial problems for this child?
   - How would you approach the parents?
   - How would you approach the coach?
   - What is developmentally appropriate for this child pre- and postpuberty?

4. A 17-year-old rising senior basketball player, who has aspirations of playing basketball on the collegiate and professional level, has recently asked you about dietary and hormonal supplements. He currently makes borderline passing grades in average classes and has expressed that basketball is the only way he will ever make it in life.
   - What are the risks of supplements and performance-enhancing drugs?
   - What immediate and long-term concerns do you have for this athlete?
   - What adjustment risks does this athlete have if he does have the opportunity to play at the collegiate level?

5. A 16-year-old junior on the girl's varsity tennis team at a local high school tells you that her assistant coach has been approaching her in ways that make her uncomfortable. He makes sexual jokes and has groped her on two occasions when they were alone.
   - What is the definition of sexual harassment?
   - What would you tell this athlete?
   - How would you deal with confronting the coach?

6. A close family friend asks for your advice at a social gathering. She tells you she is interested in helping her 8-year-old son with mild cerebral palsy get involved in athletics. She wishes to ask you a few questions.
   - Will her son need a preparticipation physical from his physician?
   - What sorts of advantages can she expect from exercise in her son with a disability?
   - Are there limitations as far as the sports available for her son to play?

References

American Academy of Pediatrics. (2000). Intensive training and sports specialization in young athletes. Committee on Sports Medicine and Fitness. *Pediatrics, 106*, 154-15.

American Academy of Pediatrics. (2001). Committee on sports medicine and fitness and committee on school health organized sports for children and preadolescents. *Pediatrics, 107*, 1459-1462.

Arvers, P., & Choquet, M. (2003). Sporting activities and psychoactive substance use. *Annals of Internal Medicine, 154*(Spec No 1), S25-S34.

Bravo, A. M. (2000). Developmental milestones. In G. K. Siberry & R. Iannone (eds.), *The Harriet Lane Handbook* (15th ed., p. 194). St. Louis, MO: Mosby.

Faigenbaum, A. D., Zaichkowsky, L. D., Gardner, D. E., et al. (1998). Anabolic steroid use by male and female middle school students. *Pediatrics, 101*(5), E6.

Fowler-Brown, A., & Kahwati, L. C. (2004). Prevention and treatment of overweight in children and adolescents. *American Family Physician, 69*(11), 2591-8.

Greydanus, D., & Patel, D. (2002). The female athlete: Before and beyond puberty. *Pediatric Clinics of North America, 49*, 553-580.

Harris, S. S. (2002). Developmental and maturational issues. In J. C. Puffer (Ed.), *20 common problems in sports medicine*. New York, NY: McGraw-Hill.

Irving, L. M., Wall, M., Neumark-Sztainer, D., et al. (2002). Steroid use among adolescents: Findings from project EAT. *Journal of Adolescent Health, 30*(4), 243-252.

Lagges, A., & Dunn, D. (2003). Depression in children and adolescents. *Neurologic Clinics, 21*, 953-960.

Metzl, J. (2002). Expectations of pediatric sport participation among pediatricians, patients and parents. *Pediatric Clinics of North America, 49*, 497-504.

Metzl, J. D. (2001). Creatine use among young athletes. *Pediatrics, 108*(2), 421-425.

National Center for Health Statistics. (n.d.). *Prevalence of overweight among children and adolescents: United States, 1999-2002*. Retrieved June 13, 2007, from http://www.cdc.gov/nchs/products/pubs/pubd/hestats/overwght99.htm

Patel, D. R. (2002). The pediatric athlete with disabilities. *Pediatr Clin North Am, 49*(4), 803-827.

Patel, D. R., Pratt, H. D., & Greydanus, D. E. (2002). Pediatric neurodevelopment and sports participation. *Pediatric Clinics of North America, 49*, 505-31.

Patel, D. R., Pratt, H. D., & Greydanus, D. E. (2003). Behavioral aspects of children's sports. *Pediatric Clinics of North America, 50*, 879-99.

Stricker, P. (2002). Sports training issues for the pediatric athlete. *Pediatric Clinics of North America, 49*, 793-802.

Substance Abuse and Mental Health Services Administration. (2006). *Results from the 2005 national survey on drug use and health: National findings* (Office of Applied Studies, NSDUH Series H-30, DHHS Publication No. SMA 06-4194). Rockville, MD: Author.

Psychosocial Issues and Trends for the Athletic Trainer

Daniel B. Kissinger, PhD, LPC, NCC

Chapter Objectives

- ❖ Examine psychosocial issues related to physical health.
- ❖ Examine psychosocial issues related to psychological health.
- ❖ Examine psychosocial issues related to lifestyle choices.
- ❖ Examine athletes/patients from a holistic perspective.
- ❖ Examine gender issues impacting athletes/patients.

NATA Educational Competencies

Psychosocial Intervention and Referral Domain

1. Describe the psychosocial factors that affect persistent pain perception (i.e., emotional state, locus of control, psychodynamic issues, sociocultural factors, and personal values and beliefs) and identify multidisciplinary approaches for managing patients with persistent pain.

Medical Conditions and Disabilities Domain

1. Describe and know when to refer common psychological medical disorders from drug toxicity, physical and emotional stress, and acquired disorders (e.g., substance abuse, eating disorders/disordered eating, depression, bipolar disorder, seasonal affective disorder, anxiety disorders, somatoform disorders, personality disorders, abusive disorders, and addiction).

Professional Development and Responsibility Domain

1. Describe the theories and techniques of interpersonal and cross-cultural communication among athletic trainers, patients, administrators, health care professionals, parents/guardians, and other appropriate personnel

Participation in athletics is intricately woven into the fabric of our society. Too often, however, success or failure in athletic competition centers on a win/loss record. As a result, many outside the athletic realm base an athlete's merit solely on their athletic acumen or, in many cases, on their most recent performance(s). This restricted view fails to consider that athletes do not train and perform in a vacuum absent of regular societal pressures. In reality, athletes at all competitive levels are exposed to different degrees of stressful psychosocial factors, both from within (i.e., teammates, coaches) and outside of (i.e., spectators, media) the competitive arena. Exposure to any of these psychosocial stressors can create a variety of problems for athletes, such as predisposing the athlete to injury, impeding their athletic performance, and even reducing postinjury rehabilitation success (Wiese-Bjornstal & Shaffer, 1999). Thus, it is unsurprising to see the close relationship in the sports literature between psychosocial stressors and the prevention and treatment of sport injuries.

The central aim of this chapter is to provide athletic trainers with a conceptual framework for understanding the range of psychosocial factors present within the athletic environment. The psychosocial dimensions of sport injury suggested by Wiese-Bjornstal and Shaffer (1999) will be used as a template for addressing psychosocial factors within the athletic environment. Specifically, these include the physical, psychological, environmental, and sociocultural dimensions of sport. However, more attention is given to the psychological and sociocultural dimensions. This is because sports medicine training programs tend to focus primarily on the physical and environmental dimensions of sport injury and less on the psychological and sociocultural domains (Wiese-Bjornstal & Shaffer, 1999). Discussions in each section are intended as an introduction to the multitude of potential psychosocial factors inherent within each dimension. As such, the information presented should not be construed as a review of the extant literate in each area.

Physical Dimension

In the context of the physical dimension of sport, potential psychosocial factors often center on the athlete's physical characteristics such as age, experience, physical conditioning, muscle structure, overtraining, and physical fatigue (Wiese-Bjornstal & Schaffer, 1999). Refusal to address psychosocial stressors could have significant implications for an athlete, including, but not limited to, an increased vulnerability to injury and declines in athletic performance. For instance, aside from the structural damage done to the body, physical injuries have been linked with an increased susceptibility to a litany of negative events and mental disorders (Andersen, Denson, Brewer, & Van Raalte, 1994; Begel, 1994; Calhoun, Ogilvie, Hendrickson, & Fritz, 1998; Cogan, 1998). These may include an increase in tension, confusion, hostility, loneliness, fear, or irritability (Leddy, Lambert, & Ogles, 1994; Macchi & Crossman, 1996; Udry, Gould, Bridges, & Beck, 1997). In the case of overtraining, athletic trainers need to monitor for potential burnout and overuse injuries that are often the hallmark of athletes who seek to maintain optimal athletic performance levels (Gould, Udry, Tuffey, & Loehr, 1996). Consequently, the ability to integrate appropriate physical treatment regiments with psychological strategies is crucial "if complete or holistic recovery is to occur" (Ford & Gordon, 1998, p. 80).

Another important, but less-publicized threat to an athlete's physical (and by extension, mental) health involves the dangers associated with sexually transmitted diseases (STDs). Recent estimates by the CDC (n.d.) suggest that 19 million people are infected annually with sexually transmitted diseases (STD) and infections (STI). Nearly half of those cases are youths between the ages 15 to 24 (Weinstock, Berman, & Cates, 2004), which clearly encompasses the vast majority of athletes at the high school and intercollegiate levels. Even more unsettling is the fact that acquiring any STD increases the chances of acquiring HIV (Human Immunodeficiency Virus), the precursor to Acquired Immunodeficiency Disease Syndrome (AIDS) (Clark, 1997). For continuity purposes, the psychological effects of STDs will also be addressed in this section.

As is the case with many other diseases, the psychological implications associated with STDs are significant. Notable emotional reactions of those diagnosed with STDs include disbelief, skepticism, shame, embarrassment, anxiety, a sense of being "dirty," anger, guilt, and depression (Dwyer & Niemann, 2002; Masters, Johnson, & Kolodny, 1995; Ross, 1999). Additional sources of stress related to an STD diagnosis often involve the emotional turmoil associated with having to disclose their diagnosis, modify their sexual behaviors, maintain safe sex practices, deal with fears of sexual expression, worry about hygienic issues, and deal with the thoughts of acquiring another STD (Masters et al., 1995; Ross, 1999). Still others may experience relational problems (Dwyer & Niemann, 2002; Hedge, 1996; Huber, 1996; Masters et al., 1995; Ross, 1999; Serovich, 2000, as cited in Long, Burnett, & Thomas, 2006). Physically, these issues may even manifest as premature ejaculation, low sexual desire, erectile failure, vaginismus, or orgasmic disorders (Ross, 1999).

Unfortunately, the current discourse surrounding sexual health issues is often insufficient in athletic environments, rendering athletes vulnerable to an increased risk of contracting an STD. One reason for the reluctance to discuss sexually related issues may be the stigma associated with STDs, as having an STD is often viewed as a direct result of promiscuity. Despite this avoidance, there is evidence that students have significant concerns about sexual health matters. For example, in one study of student athletes, Flint (1999) uncovered that their reluctance to engage in discussions on sexual matters often masked a deeper level of concern about sexual health issues. Thus, while sensitivity to appropriate boundaries is important (see the Environmental Dimension section on p. 280), athletic trainers should remain sensitive to the fact that, while uncomfortable at times, information on the types, symptoms, and implications of STDs should be considered relevant to the overall treatment needs of the athlete.

Psychological Dimension

Although the core role for athletic trainers remains the prevention and care of injuries and illness, they often represent the "first line of defense" when psychological conditions manifest within an athletic context (Ray, Terrell, & Hough, 1999). Thus, when coupled with their proximity to athletes, athletic trainers are often "ideally situated to assist with the psychological as well as physical sequelae of injury" (Ford & Gordon, 1998, p. 80). In order to conceptualize the full range of emotional issues facing athletes, sports medicine professionals (Ray et al., 1999) draw from the career counseling literature. Specifically, they suggest integrating the four counseling functions of providing social support, providing information, helping with goal setting, and encouraging effective decision making (Holland, Magoon, & Spokane, 1981) with "screening for more serious psychoemotional problems and referral to mental health professionals" (Ray, Terrell, & Hough, 1999, p. 7). The importance of having such a framework is clear as studies suggest that mental health issues among athletes are "at rates equal to and sometimes greater than the general population" (Brewer & Petrie, 1996, p. 269). In the context of sports medicine, three psychological factors have been shown to predispose athletes to injury. These include personality, history of stressors, and coping resources (Wiese-Bjornstal & Shaffer, 1999).

This grouping of factors evolved out of the Stress Response Model of athletic injury (Andersen & Williams, 1988; Williams & Andersen, 1998). Given the parameters of this introductory chapter, only a limited amount of empirical support is offered for each construct. It is important to remember, however, that it is the unique blend of these three constructs that should be considered when assessing the athlete's response to a distressing event such as an athletic injury.

Several personality factors have been identified that are considered influential to how one conceptualizes stressful events and, ultimately, on their vulnerability to the effects of stress. These include self-concept, introversion or extroversion (i.e., shy or outgoing), psychological hardiness, sensation seeking, competitive trait anxiety, and locus of control (Wiese-Bjornstal & Shaffer, 1999). When combined with situational factors, these personality factors are thought to often have a direct bearing on an athlete's cognitive, psychological, and behavioral reactions to an injury (Wiese-Bjornstal & Shaffer, 1999).

The second category involves the athlete's history of stressors. Williams and Roepke (1993) categorize history of stressors into life stress (i.e., major life events) and daily hassles (i.e., problems in daily living). Researchers have shown the existence of relationships between high stress levels and injury frequency and that injury risk increases in proportion to the degree of life stress the athlete is experiencing (Williams & Roepke, 1993; Williams & Andersen, 1998, as cited in Wiese-Bjornstal & Shaffer, 1999). Williams (2000), for instance, found relationships between athletic injury and both high life stress events (i.e., divorce, career change) and significant sports-related events (i.e., academic eligibility, injury status, conflict with coach/teammate). Additionally, it is important to remember that positive life stressors, such as receiving an athletic scholarship or winning an elite athletic event, could trigger a negative stress response (Williams & Roepke, 1993). In some cases, these responses could increase an athlete's vulnerability to a mental illness (American Psychological Association, 2000).

Coping resources constitute the third major category of psychological factors known to impact an athlete's stress response (Andersen & Williams, 1988). These include the athlete's personal resources and social support systems (Wiese-Bjornstal & Shaffer, 1999). In the context of athletics, several entities often lend support. For example, teammates, coaches, team physicians, athletic trainers, and personal friends often come together to support injured athletes (Ray & Wiese-Bjornstal, 1999; Robbins & Rosenfeld, 2001; Wiese, Weiss, & Yukelson, 1991). The emotional support generated through these social support networks is widely recognized as beneficial in terms of the prevention and treatment of athletic injuries (Brewer, Jeffers, Petitpas, & Van Raalte, 1994; Hardy, 1992; Larivaara, Vaisanen, & Kiuttu, 1994; Petrie, 1992; Sachs & Ellenberg, 1994, as cited in Wiese-Bjornstal & Shaffer, 1999) and postinjury rehabilitation (Robbins & Rosenfeld, 2001). One study showed that athletes even perceived athletic trainers as providing more support than either their head coach or assistant coaches, providing further evidence of the positive effect support from athletic trainers can have on postinjury rehabilitation and the athlete's overall health (Robbins & Rosenfield, 2001). These findings lend credibility to the notion of athletic trainers serving as intermediaries between the athlete and parents, physicians, or coaches when an injury prevents or limits the athlete's involvement in competition (George, 1997). On the other hand, the absence of a strong support system or personal coping strategies could exacerbate an athlete's risk for injury (Smith, Smoll, & Ptacek, 1990). In short, athletic trainers should recognize that effective social support networks and coping strategies are integral to maintaining the overall health of athletes experiencing physical and emotional distress.

In a related vein, sports medicine scholars endorse the parallels between sports teams and family systems (Zimmerman, 1993; Zimmerman & Protinsky, 1993). The usefulness of the systemic paradigm also extends to athletic trainers, especially in terms of understanding their role as an "integral member of the athletic health care team" (George, 1997, p. 361). Consider the following definition of a family system by noted counseling scholars Goldenberg and Goldenberg (2004, p. 3):

> In a family system, ...each [family] may be considered a natural social system, with properties all its own, one that has evolved a set of rules, is replete with assigned and ascribed roles for its members, has an organized power structure, has developed intricate overt and covert forms of communication, and has elaborated ways of negotiating problem solving that permit various tasks to be performed effectively.

In other words, the systemic perspective highlights that athletes do not function independently of their teammates, but in fact are part of "a set of interacting units or component parts that together make up a whole arrangement (i.e., team) or organization (college or university)" (Goldenberg & Goldenberg, 2004, p. 513). For comparison, consider the interrelationships between those of a family system and an intercollegiate athletic team:

> A student athlete is part of a social system (team) that has created a set of rules (team rules), has assigned rules (i.e., eligibility requirements, team curfews, practice schedules), roles (i.e., first team, reserve team, statistician), an established hierarchy (coach, assistant coach, team captain, team member, athletic trainers, etc.), includes specific forms of communications (hand signals, oral play calling, playbooks,) and incorporates specific problem-solving techniques (eligibility standards for student athletes, suspensions or dismissal, study halls, team dress codes, etc.) that provide discipline for the team so victory can be attained.

For another example, consider the following vignette.

In the fourth quarter of your university's first bowl game in 5 years, an unexpectedly intense rainstorm occurs. Unfortunately, the equipment manager forgot to pack the cleats that would provide better traction for poor field conditions. As a direct result of poor traction, an athlete is injured. Being the head athletic trainer, you consult with the athlete's position coach and notify him of your refusal to give medical clearance for the athlete to return to the game. The position coach relays this information to the head coach, forcing the coach to make immediate changes to the game plan. Although the team was ultimately victorious, it is learned that the athlete's injury is career threatening, drastically altering the immediate fortunes of the team and the athlete's dream of becoming a professional athlete.

Conversely, a systemic perspective may also provide insights into some of the less productive qualities of athletic teams (or even support networks). For example, family systems have an innate affection for equilibrium. In the family counseling literature, this trait is defined as homeostasis, or the tendency to maintain balance within the system. Athletic trainers should remain attuned to the fact that homeostasis may not always be beneficial to the athlete. In the context of an athletic environment, homeostasis could be loosely construed as the "damage control" seen when athletic programs are faced with misconduct on the part of an athlete (or coach). Viewed in a more positive light, homeostasis could manifest as a team rallying around the athlete and providing the emotional support the player needs to surmount a situational (or longer term) stressor. Ultimately, the systemic approach provides athletic trainers and athletes alike with a useful template for understanding the interplay between psychosocial factors and the overall well-being of the athlete within the broader athletic system they share.

PSYCHOSOCIAL FACTORS AND THE PSYCHOLOGICAL WELL-BEING OF ATHLETES

Of particular interest to sports researchers are the relationships between athletic participation and a broad range of psychological and emotional issues. Studies of intercollegiate student athletes, for example, have revealed that the challenges associated with balancing optimal physical conditioning and academic performances often leaves them vulnerable to greater levels of psychological pressure and distress than nonathletes (Bergandi & Wittig, 1984; Etzel, 1989; Etzel, Pinkney, & Hinkle, 1994). This difficult balance could in turn deplete their emotional reserves (Richards & Aries, 1999) and possibly even impede their normal cognitive, social, moral, educational, and psychosocial development (Ferrante, Etzel, & Lantz, 1996). Additionally, a number of studies show the range of issues that could befall athletes when their emotional and psychological needs are challenged.

Raglin (2001) noted that "intensive physical training routinely results in mood disturbances and decrements in performance in athletes who exhibit positive mental health profiles off-season or during periods of easy training" (p. 877). In other words, the strain of intensive practices and competition may lead to declines in mood and performance that are unlikely to occur out of season or during periods of less intense training. Research on intercollegiate student athletes has also uncovered relationships between negative emotional experiences and mental disorders (Begel, 1994; Andersen, Denson, Brewer, & Van Raalte, 1994; Cogan, 1998) such as increases in tension, confusion, hostility, loneliness, fear, or irritability (Leddy et al., 1994; Macchi & Crossman, 1996; Udry et al., 1997).

Numerous other studies on intercollegiate athletes reveal a wide range of other problematic areas for athletes. These include problems with the following:

- Substance abuse (Heyman, 1986; Parham, 1993)
- Identity (Nelson, 1983; Parham, 1993; Petitpas & Champagne, 1988)
- Self-esteem (Heyman, 1986)
- Personal competence (Parham, 1993)
- Academics (Heyman, 1986; Nelson, 1983; Parham, 1993)
- Career issues (Baillie, 1993; Chartrand & Lent, 1987; Gabbard & Halischak, 1993; Nelson, 1983)
- Interpersonal relationships (Heyman, 1986; Parham, 1993; Ryan, 1989)
- Depression and anxiety (Brewer, Petitpas, & Van Raalte, 1999).

In short, athletes are faced with multiple stressors on both the macro and micro levels, both of which have been shown to increase an athlete's vulnerability to injury (Williams & Andersen, 1998; Williams & Roepke, 1993). Unfortunately, the manifestation of these issues may be subtle, even imperceptible, to athletic trainers whose professional training focuses primarily on the prevention and treatment of physical injuries. Therefore, it is vital that the athletic trainer be vigilant in his or her awareness of an athlete's exposure to and ability to effectively process potentially damaging psychological factors. It is also important to remember that avoiding or denying the emotional or psychological needs of an athlete could have broad repercussions (Benedict & Klein, 1998; Calhoun et al., 1998; Pipe; 1993). As such, athletic trainers would be particularly well served by having a template for assessing those athletes who may be (or are presently) experiencing psychological distress.

Guidelines have been developed for recognizing the presentation styles of athletes who may be experiencing psychological or emotional distress (Silver, Wortman, & Crofton, 1990). In their view, athletes experiencing psychological distress may manifest symptoms in a number of subtle ways. These could include the following:

- Denying the potential consequences of an injury
- Highlighting the difficulties they have experienced due to the injury
- Developing a negative outlook, being noncompliant with treatment
- Providing limited information about the injury or their coping strategies to the athletic trainer

While these strategies may be ineffective in rectifying problematic situations for the athlete, they provide athletic trainers with significant information relative to the athlete's level of distress, perception of events, and their coping styles. In effect, athletes unknowingly provide vital information the athletic trainer can use to help assess for impairments and integrate these concerns into the individualized treatment plan for the athlete. However, situations are bound to arise, thus necessitating a referral to a mental health professional.

REFERRAL PROTOCOL

In the sports medicine literature, the process of referring an athlete to a mental health professional is conceptualized as a five-stage process encompassing assessment, consultation, trial intervention, referral, and follow-up (Brewer et al., 1999). However, despite the fact that a proper mental health referral is an important skill for athletic trainers (NATA Education Council, 1992), studies suggest that only a small percentage of sports medicine professionals have indeed referred an athlete to a mental health professional (Larson, Starkey, & Zaichkowsky, 1996). Thus, it comes as little surprise that many athletes are reluctant to comply with mental health referrals (Brewer et al., 1994). Some may in fact feel demeaned by such a referral, especially if one considers the strong stigma still associated with mental illness (Linder, Brewer, Van Raalte, & De Lange, 1991). In fact, a number of other barriers have been identified that reduce the chances of an athlete complying with a mental health referral.

For some athletes, the sense that they will be misunderstood by the counselor serves as a deterrent (Greenspan & Andersen, 1995). Others may perceive counseling as futile (Martin, Wrisberg, Beitel, & Lounsbury, 1997). Still others may believe they can effectively manage mental illness without professional medical intervention (Linder et al., 1991). For athletic trainers, then, sensitivity to the athlete should remain a hallmark of any referral. This is especially important given the myth of invulnerability so often perpetuated in the sports domain (Begel, 1994). In order to illustrate the difficulties in identifying and referring athletes with psychological concerns, the reader is asked to consider the following short vignette and related questions:

Over the course of the last month, you, the head athletic trainer at your university, have been treating the 19-year-old freshman star quarterback for a severely sprained knee. During this time period, and especially in the 3 weeks prior, Joe has missed several sessions of physical rehabilitation with you. When he does present for treatment, you have noticed an increase in restlessness, psychomotor retardation, and intermittent tearfulness. In addition to documenting the physical rehabilitation process, you have attributed (and documented) the following statements and behaviors to Joe:

* *"I feel physically drained" on a daily basis.*
* *"I've lost 15 lbs since my injury. I'm just not hungry."*
* *"I feel worthless not being able to help my teammates."*
* *"I feel hopeless when I think about life without football."*
* *Poor sleep, averaging 3 to 4 hours per night the last 3 weeks.*
* *Loss of interest in schoolwork and social activities.*
* *Isolated from teammates and friends, comes to treatment alone instead of with other teammates.*
* *Increasingly noncompliant with scheduled treatment.*

Discussion Questions
  1. *What pertinent issues do you feel are present in this case?*
  2. *Would you make a referral to a mental health practitioner in this case?*
       * *If so, what led you to the decision to refer to a mental health professional?*
       * *If not, what led you to the conclusion not to refer to a mental health professional?*

To nonmental health professionals, there may be a tendency to explain away this constellation of signs and symptoms. For example, it may seem logical to attribute the weight loss to muscle deterioration from missed strength training sessions or the sense of worthlessness to missing the camaraderie he experienced as a member of a team. In this case, however, the symptoms and time frame suggest this athlete is experiencing significant emotional distress. More seriously, the athlete's expression of hopelessness is a "red flag" requiring immediate further assessment for suicide risk. Overall, the combination of depressive symptoms, time frame, and statements of hopelessness suggest this athlete may be experiencing a clinically significant depressive episode and should be referred for further assessment by a mental health professional.

While there are several clinical issues present in the above vignette (i.e., diagnostic criteria, crisis intervention response), it does illustrate the need for athletic trainers without mental health training to have a framework for identifying emotionally or psychologically "at-risk" athletes. One strategy for assessing at-risk athletes is to evaluate their presentation styles. Petitpas & Danish (1995), for example, provide a set of criteria for identifying potential at-risk athletes. More specifically, they suggest that sports medicine professionals pay particular attention to athletes who do the following:

- Demonstrate an excessive preoccupation with returning to their sport after an injury
- Are in extreme denial of the negative effects of an injury
- Express guilt about their inability to contribute to the team
- Express arrogance about previous athletic success
- Isolate or withdraw from prior social support networks

Another strategy for increasing an athlete's compliance with a mental health referral was developed by Glick and Horsfall (2001). The following strategies, which were originally suggested for sports psychiatrists, are clearly amenable for use by athletic trainers:

- Appealing to the competitive nature of the athlete by reframing counseling as a "performance enhancement" strategy for the mind
- Differentiate the needs of the "person" from the "athlete"
- Appeal to the athlete's self-interest by reframing the rationale for the counseling referral as an opportunity to address skill enhancement, quality of life, or financial status from a different perspective
- Collaborate with consumer organizations such as Alcoholics Anonymous (AA) and/or Narcotics Anonymous (NA) when substance-related issues are present or suspected
- Recognize the importance of the therapeutic alliance for increasing the chances of compliance with the counseling referral and counseling professional
- Monitor "athletic envy" or hero worship by the athletic trainer, which could result in ineffective or inappropriate treatment and poor treatment outcomes
- Monitor for coercion
- Recognize the presence and importance of a multidisciplinary perspective when assessing the needs of an athlete. For example, collaborate with coaches to address the needs of the client

In summary, this section provided a solid foundation for understanding the interplay between the physical and psychological domains. Several studies illustrated reasons why athletes may be reluctant to comply with a mental health referral. Conversely, several suggestions were made that could assist athletic trainers when a mental health referral becomes necessary. Ultimately, however, it should be remembered that the provision of intense psychological interventions should always remain the domain of trained counseling and psychology professionals (Heil, 1993).

Environmental Dimension

Environmental factors are said to encompass the physical and social domains of athletic competition (Wiese-Bjornstal & Shaffer, 1999). Examples of these environmental factors range from the physical conditions of the athletic environment (i.e., playing conditions, training/rehabilitation setting) to interpersonal relationships with those closely associated with the athlete's ultimate success (i.e., coaches, officials, athletic trainers). While there are numerous important variables, interpersonal relationships will receive the most focus.

Athletes at nearly every level face challenges in balancing their athletic and personal roles and responsibilities. For those at elite levels, these challenges include balancing a range of roles and responsibilities within the larger athletic domain (Duda, 2001). Athletes may have academic study hall in the morning, afternoon practices followed by team meetings, and possibly rehabilitation for a nagging injury at night. Each of these contexts holds potential psychosocial stressors. For instance, time commitments, different roles (academic/athletic), and distinct interpersonal relationships with coaches and teammates all present different potential stressors for athletes. For the athletic trainer, such commitments could potentially limit available times for postinjury rehabilitation. When these situations occur, Fisher (1990) suggests a number of possible responses including the following:

- Setting rehabilitation schedules that coincide with the athlete's schedule
- Providing athletes with more personalized attention
- Reducing peripheral irritants, such as nonessential personnel

Inherent within each of the above suggestions is the notion of effective communication. In the context of an athletic training room or clinical setting, effective communication is a core element in providing treatment. It is important to recognize that communication patterns are heavily influenced by one's personal history and gender. Thus, consistent monitoring of one's personal barriers to effective multicultural communication can enhance the entire treatment process. One of the more challenging aspects for athletes and athletic trainers alike involves the development and maintenance of healthy relationships. Student athletes in particular often face relationship challenges that are inherently different from their nonathlete peers. For example, even after a stellar athletic performance, an intercollegiate athlete may experience antipathy on campus from those who believe the resources and privileges extended to him or her as an athlete subvert the core academic mission of a higher education institution. Student athletes may also have to balance relationships with entities such as the NCAA, their college or university policy boards, their own athletic team, or even within their own athletic department (Fletcher, Benshoff, & Richburg, 2003). Yet, while several degrees of separation may exist between athletes and administrators, an athletic trainer's proximity to athletes presents a unique opportunity to monitor their ability to negotiate these inherently complex relationships and monitor for stress.

While athletes are clearly exposed to several different types and levels of relationships, few are more important than the coach-athlete relationship. Studies suggest that the interpersonal style and behavior of a coach are among the key variables impacting an athlete's psychological, emotional, and physical response to their athletic experience (Duda, 2001; Smoll & Smith, 2002). For example, in a study of female intercollegiate basketball players, athletes who exhibited high trait anxiety perceived their relationship with their coach less positively than athletes with low trait anxiety (Kenow & Williams, 1999). Essentially, studies support the importance of coach-athlete compatibility in creating positive relational dynamics (Chelladurai & Saleh, 1980; Kenow & Williams, 1999). However, this is not meant to suggest that coaches do not have the best interests of their athletes in mind. Examples of the positive effects of strong coach-athlete relationships are evident throughout the sports literature (Wiese et al., 1991). In this case, the focus on potentially negative aspects of coach-athlete relationships is done in order to remain consistent with the theme of the chapter.

SEXUAL AGGRESSION, HARASSMENT, AND APPROPRIATE BOUNDARIES

Any discourse related to the physical safety and integrity of athletes should involve an awareness of issues surrounding sexual aggression and harassment. In the general population, for example, men who adhere to traditional sex roles have been found to engage in more "verbal sexual coercion, sexual assault, and rape" (Parrot & Cummings, 1994, p. 180). In an alarming parallel, male athletes holding similar views were more likely to misconstrue sexual assault as appropriate behavior (Berkowitz, 1992; O'Sullivan, 1991). Additionally, physical dominance, which is often promoted in the context of sport, has been recognized as a key motivator for rape.

At first glance, research would seem to validate the stereotype of the aggressive (often male) athlete. For example, male athletes competing in contact sports have been found to exhibit higher levels of aggression and greater acceptance of violence than their noncontact sport peers (Brown & Davies, 1978; Kemler, 1988). This becomes even more disconcerting when combined with anthropological research that connects higher incidences of rape with cultures that have higher tolerances for violence (Sanday, 1981). However, it should be pointed out that the actual relationship between participation in athletics and sexual aggression remains unclear (Stewart, 2003). Nevertheless, the propensity within athletics to stress aggression could have significant physical and psychological implications for athletes and should always remain a treatment consideration. Consequently, athletic trainers should not fail to consider the potential for sexual abuse to occur within the athletic (and clinical training) settings.

Victims of sexual abuse often face a litany of later psychological and interpersonal problems. These problems may include, but are not limited to, (McClintock, 1989) the following:

- Negative self-concept
- Low self-esteem
- Shame about one's body
- Distorted body image
- Anxiety and guilt about sexuality
- Interpersonal distrust
- Depression
- Substance abuse
- Mistrust of internal experiences and feelings
- A drive to perfect and/or purify one's body

As is evidenced by this partial list of symptoms, the psychological implications of sexual abuse can be extremely complex and long-term. In one study, nearly 72% of women who suffered childhood sexual abuse are predicted to be revictimized in the future (Messman & Long, 1996). Ultimately, however, responses to sexual abuse are as unique as the individual. An athletic trainer who recognizes the signs and symptoms of sexual abuse can be a key factor in limiting the possibility that an athlete will continue being revictimized later in life (Messman & Long, 1996).

Unfortunately, research suggests that sexual abuse is often perpetuated in athletic environments due to the reluctance of alleged victims, the majority of which are female, to challenge the authority of a coach's power or other authority figures (Brackenridge, 1997). Part of this reluctance could be that the same social stigma that prevents athletes from seeking counseling or psychiatric treatment (Linder et al., 1991) also reduces the likelihood that a victim of sexual harassment or assault will confront the perpetrator. However, several other factors could account for their reticence to disclose abusive behaviors, including the beliefs that sports are morally good; that children and players, rather than adults and coaches, are advised to "play fair"; the notion of voluntary sport organizations as apolitical entities; and the embarrassment and fear of confronting sexual and social taboos (Brackenridge, 1997). On the other hand, the profile of a potential perpetrator often comes as a surprise. For example, within the sports realm, perpetrators often include individuals who present as well qualified for the job, are intelligent, exhibit patience, do not appear to look or act like one who abuses others, have interpersonal skills, and appear self-assured (Brackenridge, 1997).

Another area of potential stress for athletes involves issues surrounding sexual harassment. In the context of many clinical settings, athletic trainers are urged to remember that "athletic training facilities are areas where athletes receive therapy or treatments in various stages of undress, which can create opportunities for inappropriate behavior from the athlete who is the patient or from the person providing the treatment" (Velasquez, 1998, p. 173). If and when sexual harassment issues surface, athletic trainers should take immediate action to rectify the situation, as avoidance may be construed as acceptance of the inappropriate behavior (Rubin & Borgers, 1990). Suggestions for eliminating sexual harassment in the context of athletic training settings include the following steps (Velasquez, 1998):

- Maintain awareness of steps to eliminate sexual harassment prior to its exposure in the training room or clinical setting.
- Establish an institution-wide sexual harassment policy that operationalizes sexual harassment.
- Distribute the policy and disciplinary actions if repudiated by employees or athletes.
- Immediately address inappropriate behaviors or verbal statements.
- Inform *all* members of the athletic training staff of the sexual harassment policy and steps for disciplinary action.
- Clearly communicate *all* policy and procedures for dealing with sexual harassment and place information in clearly visible areas in the training room setting.

In the case of rape prevention, professionals are urged to take a three-pronged approach to stopping rape. This includes designing rape prevention programs to address denial of rape on the part of both genders, clearly stating the components of rape (Warshaw, 1988), and educating men on suitable sexual behavior (Parrot, 1990). As in the case of each prior section, athletic trainers are strongly urged to review the sports and counseling literature on abusive behaviors (sexual, physical, emotional) and their implications so any potential harm to the athlete can be mitigated and/or addressed through the proper channels.

Sociocultural Context

Athletes are often perceived as being shielded from the transgressions encountered in general society. However, careful analysis of the psychosocial factors within the sociocultural dimension reveals a complex mixture of factors that could impact the athlete. Wiese-Bjornstal and Shaffer (1999) point to the current "sport ethic endemic" as the primary risk factor that predisposes an athlete to injury (p. 24). According to Hughes and Coakley

(1991), the sport ethic refers to "a system of principles and beliefs, held predominantly by athletes, that advocates personal sacrifice, risk taking, and playing with pain to promote conformity and adherence to sport norms."

Inherent within the sport ethic are attitudes and expectations that place athletes at increased risk for injury. Cognitive and/or behavioral manifestations of the sport ethic may include denial of pain or injury during competition or avoidance or noncompliance with proper medical attention, rather than risk being seen as weak (Wiese-Bjornstal & Shaffer, 1999). Adding to this risk is the continued focus on masculine identity in athletics. In other words, male athletes who internalize or over-emphasize their masculine identity "risk becoming disconnected from their emotions, which could lead them to the literal view of their body as a weapon" (Young, White, & McTeer, 1994, as cited in Wiese-Bjornstal & Shaffer, 1999, p. 25). Although no causal relationship is evident between sport ethic and injury, athletes may still need the myths surrounding the sport ethic dispelled in order to reduce their chances of injury. Athletic trainers clearly would be in a prime position to work with athletes in this regard. However, this would require the athletic trainer to be both cognizant of the sport ethic variables at play and the fortitude to integrate appropriate interventions (i.e., psychoeducational materials, mental health referral) to ensure the holistic needs of the athlete are being addressed.

It likely also comes as no surprise that athletics are not exempt from having, or even perpetuating, biases and/or stereotypes. Consider the comments made by John Rocker, a former pitcher for the Atlanta Braves, concerning his distaste about the possibility of playing for the New York Mets:

> *Imagine having to take the [No.] 7 train to [Shea Stadium] looking like you're in Beirut next to some kid with purple hair, next to some queer with AIDS, right next to some dude who got out of jail for the fourth time, right next to some 20-year-old mom with four kids… The biggest thing I don't like about New York are the foreigners. You can walk an entire block in Times Square and not hear anybody speaking English. Asians and Koreans and Vietnameses and Indians and Russians and Spanish people and everything up there. How the hell did they get in this country? (Sports Illustrated, YEAR).*

While such overt displays of xenophobia are soundly rejected by the vast majority of society, his comments serve to remind us of the need to be sensitive to the notion that "all interactions are multicultural" (Bernard & Goodyear, 2004, p. 134). Predictably, this self-awareness is not without challenges.

Identifying personal biases is an inherently challenging task given that our biases are often internalized and grounded in historical, familial, and social contexts. According to multicultural counseling experts Sue and Sue (2003), "none of us [counselors] is immune from inheriting the images/stereotypes of the larger society, we can assume that most therapists are prisoners of their own cultural conditioning" (p. 23). Based on this view, it seems reasonable to suggest that athletic trainers are similarly constrained. As such, self-awareness becomes indispensable in combating one's own restricted worldview that could, consciously or not, perpetuate discriminatory attitudes or behaviors. In the end, combining self-awareness with culturally appropriate treatment interventions can help reduce intolerance inside (i.e., peers, coaches, administrators, clinical settings) and outside (i.e., media, academic units, boosters, fans) the athletic realm and provide a more trusting environment for athletes who need the assistance of athletic trainers.

Because of the breadth of topics that could be covered relative to the topic of psychosocial factors in sport, it is important to address, albeit briefly, that the blending of race and sport also includes a subjective mix of historical experiences and current contextual variables. Anshel and Sailes (1990) offer some guidance when confronted by such issues, noting that "explanations for racial differences in sports performance and for patterns in athletic participation emanate largely from the sociocultural fabric of the social experiences of blacks and whites" (p. 3). However, despite the conspicuousness of race in society, it is usually not the sole breeder of discord in any environment, athletic or otherwise. In essence, athletic trainers need to have an awareness of the totality of the sociocultural variables at play. In this chapter, focus is given to one well-recognized diversity issue in sport, race, and a second and less acknowledged issue, the stressors associated with sexual identity and sexual prejudice.

In the multicultural counseling arena, racial identity models have been developed to address the interactions between Blacks and Whites. Helms' (1990, 1996) Black and White Identity models are recognized as excellent mediums for addressing cognitive, affective, and behavioral responses between Blacks and Whites. Since these models have been successfully applied across numerous professional domains, it seems reasonable to assert that athletic trainers could benefit from the knowledge inherent in each model. Racial identity, for example, involves one's conception of self as a racial being and refers to one's beliefs, attitudes, and values of self as related to other racial groups (Helms, 1994). Furthermore, racial identity development refers to a "process or series of stages through which a person passes as the person's attitudes toward his or her own racial/ethnic group and the White population develop, ultimately achieving a healthy identity" (Baruth & Manning, 2003, p. 31). Thus, athletic trainers who address their own racial heritage are essentially reflecting on how their experiences interact with those around them throughout their personal and professional lives (Ivey, Ivey, & Simek-Morgan, 1997). Yet, despite the prevalence of race in our national discourse, athletic trainers should consistently challenge their views on diversity issues outside the construct of race.

In addition to race, researchers have uncovered an array of other potential stressors within the sociocultural environment of athletes. These include the sports opportunity structure, cultural norms, and appreciably different socialization patterns (Brower, 1979; Carlston, 1983; Castine & Roberts, 1974; Donnelly, 1975; Edwards, 1972; Emmel, 1977; Greendorfer & Ewing, 1981; Hopson, 1972; Leonard, 1980; McPherson, 1981; Patricksson, 1979; Phillips, 1976; Renson, 1979; Sailes, 1984; Snyder & Spreitzer, 1978). Athletic trainers, given their close interaction with athletes and affiliated personnel, must remain conscious of the litany of psychosocial stressors inherent within each of those variables. If not, intolerance and discriminatory acts within the sports environment, regardless of the medium, could weaken the pivotal therapeutic alliance (Bordin, 1979) between the athletic trainer and the athletes under their care and reduce the potential for positive rehabilitative outcomes.

Another key element within the sociocultural domain is the notion of identity, or "the partly conscious, largely unconscious sense of whom one is, both as a person and as a contributor to society" (Baruth & Manning, 2003, p. 31). Athletic trainers and others involved with the care of the athlete can benefit by conceptualizing identity as multidimensional. For example, although athletes likely hold a central athletic identity to some degree (Brown et al., 2003), they may identify with several other diversity constructs such as race, gender, or sexual orientation (to name only a few). However, given their immersion in the sports setting (i.e., practice, travel, teammates, coaches, wins, losses), athletes often develop a central athletic identity (Brown et al., 2003) that transcends even their notion of themselves as primarily a racial entity. For example, a Black male athlete who identifies exclusively with his community based solely on race might fail to consider the notion of athletic identity and the potential for the sports environment to influence identity formation (Brown et al., 2003). However, athletic trainers should recognize that this does not dismiss the fact that race is often the lens through which many interpret the level of discrimination in sports. Support for this assertion is found in studies that indicate that

Black athletes have long been stereotyped as superior athletes (Edwards, 1973; Hoberman, 1997; Jefferson, 1998; Sailes, 1996).

On the other hand, the sports domain is clearly not the genesis of all things racist or discriminatory. In fact, researchers have found that athletic environments can actually reduce the intensity of racial biases both among (Hoberman, 1984, 1997; Jefferson, 1998) and against (Ford, 1988) athletes. Others have suggested that for some, athletics actually provides some safety from biases. Ford (1988), for example, favored the notion of a "race-less" athlete whose status as an elite athlete served as a buffer from racial tensions inside and outside the athletic realm. The weakness of this view is seen in the very small percentage of the population that achieves such status. However, even for those athletes that do attain elite levels of notoriety, the general public's perceptions of their lives are often skewed by intense media coverage and the worldview of the viewer.

In a more recent study exploring perceptions of discrimination among athletes, Brown and his colleagues (2003) reasoned that competitive sports environments (i.e., the "playing field") constitute a sort of racial bias-free zone because "the playing field is a context in which athletes are typically socialized to believe race does not matter" (p. 163). As a result, athletes whose core identity is most intimately aligned with athletics may be "...color blinded' (Brown et al., 2003, p. 163) through a socialization process that focuses on competition-related norms (Jefferson, 1998; McPherson, 1984; Stevenson, 1975) like fair play, meritocracy, teamwork, and cooperation (Coakley, 1990; 1993; Lapchick, 1996; MacClancy, 1996). In other words, the relatively benign level of racial discrimination in some competitive environments may be because the "playing field" provides an environment where competition triumphs over racial discord (Brown et al., 2003). Evidence also supports the notion that athletes identify predominantly with their team (Carron, 1982; Murrell & Gaertner, 1992; Widmeyer, Carron, & Brawley, 1993; Williams & Widmeyer, 1991) ahead of other social groups, which could further reduce negative or biased experiences in the context of athletic competition.

Building further on the notion that "all interactions are multicultural" (Bernard & Goodyear, 2004), the influx of international athletes into college and professional sports will further challenge athletic trainers to meet the needs of an increasingly diverse population of athletes. In effect, an athlete's perception of biases or discriminatory practices within an athletic environment, regardless of their accuracy, could have a negative effect on the athlete's performance or compliance with rehabilitation. As a result, athletic trainers need to recognize and monitor their own cultural biases and remain sensitive to the myriad of psychosocial factors within the athletic environment and their implications for the athlete. Consider the following case:

You, a 23-year-old White male, are finishing your first month as an athletic trainer at a small college in the South. Prior to taking this position, you lived on the East Coast and attended an "Ivy League" school, where your parents covered all your tuition, housing, and extracurricular costs. You are currently assigned to the women's field hockey team, who are the perennial powerhouse in your conference. Suddenly, a prominent member of the team, a 19-year-old Asian female, screams in pain. You rush to provide medical assistance and find her badly injured. She is crying and holding on to you tightly as you help her off the field. As you attend to her, you remain focused on the injury. Once she is stabilized, you discuss a treatment schedule for the following week. After the third rehabilitation session, you begin to become concerned. She is, in your opinion, overly emotional and "just wants to talk about her life and problems instead of just doing what she needs to do to be getting better." You are uncomfortable and withdraw from conversation, especially when she addresses her experiences subsequent to her injury. In particular, you find it hard to understand her fear of not being able to play field hockey again "because it's my life," and the fact that she will not be able to pay for school because field hockey covers the part of her tuition that her loans do not cover. After 1 week of regular treatment, you are pleased to see her back competing. On the other hand, you are relieved she is not telling you "about all her problems."

Discussion Questions

1. *What issues do you see in this study?*

2. *What cultural/ethnic variables may be at play?*

3. *How might you address each of these issues?*

4. *What areas made you uncomfortable/comfortable?*

5. *What role did your gender and/or personal experience play in how you conceptualized your reaction to the different situations/statement in this case?*

As noted earlier, another population facing a multitude of potential psychosocial stressors are sexual minorities (i.e., gay, lesbian, bi-sexual, and transgendered individuals [GLBT]). In the NATA's *Code of Ethics*, the first principle states that "members shall respect the rights, welfare, and dignity of all" (NATA, 2005). Implicit within this statement is the notion that sexual minority persons (athletes) will be accorded the same degree of respect as any other group of individuals. Unfortunately, heterosexist attitudes still remain prevalent in athletics. For example, a study exploring the attitudes of intercollegiate student athletes found that athletes indicated the presence of a clear heterosexist bias versus their attitudes toward race, socioeconomic status, and geographical location (Wolf-Wendel, Toma, Douglas, & Morphew, 2001). Predictably then, functioning within a heterosexist environment could exert a tremendous psychological and physical toll on athletes who self-identify with the sexual minority population.

Research on the experiences of sexual minorities provides a range of potential stressors faced by sexual minorities. One example is the difficulty an individual may have in gauging potential responses of others to sexual identity issues. For example, responses to gay men and lesbian women can range from subtle anxiety and uncertainty to intentional acts of violence (Gudykunst & Kim, 1997; Herek, 2000). Given this potentially dangerous spectrum of responses, it is easy to envision the reluctance of many GLBT persons (athletes) to discuss their true sexual identity. The data on the experiences of GLBT persons provide support for such reticence.

Herek (1989), a top researcher of sexual minority issues, has suggested that "over 90% of gay men have been verbally abused or threatened" (p. 283). Studies on the emotional and psychological health of sexual minorities are equally disturbing. For example, higher rates of major depression, mood and/anxiety disorders, and substance abuse are noted among bisexual men and women versus their heterosexual peers (King, 2005). Equally alarming are studies that indicate 12% of gay and bisexual men have attempted suicide and 21% have developed a suicide plan (Cochran & Mays, 2000; Paul et al., 2002). Additionally, it is also important to note that significant emotional stress is often associated with the process of "coming out," or the act of disclosing one's homosexual identity to others (King, 2005), and has been associated with feelings of isolation, poor self-esteem, depression, suicidal ideation, as well as substance use (Dempsey, 1994).

Despite progress in the battle for gender equality in sports, gender effects are still seen with respect to sexual minorities. Society continues to view male athletes as the torch bearers for masculinity, while homosexual men are still all too often equated with feminine characteristics. In essence, male athletes are assumed to be heterosexual, as the notion of a homosexual man remains inconsistent with the image of an athlete (Griffin, 1998). Women have often faced the task of surmounting the "image problem" (Knight & Giuliano, 2003). Examples of heterosexist attitudes within the media include the presentation of female athletes as attractive and feminine (i.e., heterosexual) in order to retain core audiences (Kane, 1996) and the portrayal of women chiefly in the context of heterosexual relationships (Birrell & Theberge, 1994; Duncan, 1990). As a result, female athletes have faced the unenviable task of dispelling the notion that participation in athletics will alter their sexual orientation (Griffin, 1998; Hargreaves, 1994; Kane, 1996; Theberge & Birrell, 1994). Recent data suggest that men may face similar biases if they fail to sustain society's image of the "masculine" (i.e., heterosexual) athlete (Knight & Giuliano, 2003).

Athletic trainers, for their part, need to cultivate and maintain an environment (i.e., training room) that is accepting and free of biases (i.e., derogatory language, jokes). In addition, if an athlete chooses to disclose issues related to sexual identity or struggles therein, athletic trainers should recognize their boundaries of competence and, if necessary, refer the athlete to the proper mental health profession. To that end, consider the following vignette and discussion questions:

A 21-year-old senior athlete presented for a pregame taping 15 minutes late. Upon the athlete's arrival, you notice a slight smell of stale alcohol and that the athlete appears disheveled. The athlete, whom you know well, discloses the following information to you (the athletic trainer): Upon finishing a short "media day" event the prior evening, a "close friend" appeared on the athlete's doorstep and reported being sexually assaulted by a well-known member of the athletics department at your school. The alleged victim stated there was alcohol involved, but the situation was uncomfortable and embarrassing. In addition, the "friend" stated the alleged perpetrator noted, rather subtly, that his or her position in the athletics department provides access to confidential student information.

Discussion Questions
1. *What action might you take?*
2. *How do you frame the alleged encounter between the athlete's "close friend" and the alleged perpetrator?*
3. *What gender did you assign to each member of this scenario? What influenced this decision?*
4. *How might your conceptualize change if you reversed the genders of the participants?*

GENDER ISSUES

As we know, one's attitudes and beliefs are tailored through the lens of personal experience. Among the most salient of these variables is gender. Today, many embrace the notion of gender equity with regard to sport participation. However, athletic trainers need to remain cognizant of potential gender differences within the sports domain and how these could impact their work with athletes.

Several recent studies validate the importance of considering gender effects when treating athletes. Studies involving adolescent athletes, for example, provide insight into just how entrenched gender stereotypes are in society. Holt and Morley (2004) explored gender differences among boys and girls, aged 14 years, relative to the psychosocial factors associated with athletic success during childhood. Results of the study indicated early gender disparities in the conceptualization of competitive athletic environments. In particular, athletically talented girls reported less professional and international ambitions than their male counterparts and were more motivated by participation and enjoyment of the sport. The boys in the study attributed their athletic successes more often to physical factors than their female peers. The authors suggested these findings reflect a masculine world of sport where physical strength equates to a sense of authority over a particular environment (Hasbrook & Harris, 1999). Also supported was the notion of physical strength as a shield, or defense mechanism, from appearing physically vulnerable and unworthy (Coakley & White, 1992). Furthermore, this study bolsters the notion of the sport ethic suggested earlier.

In another study, Brown and his colleagues (2003) considered both race and gender in the context of the sports environment. Their study found that among White student athletes, gender was the only statistically significant predictor of perceived racial and ethnic discrimination. These findings led them to posit that White men were more agreeable to the notion that discrimination is no longer a problem in the sports domain. However, athletic trainers need to consider racial and gender effects as broadly as possible.

Gender effects have also been identified in relation to injury appraisal, coping style, and conceptualization of competitive stress (Hammermeister & Burton, 2004). In a recent study exploring the appraisal and coping styles of male and female endurance athletes, Hammermeister and Burton (2004) found that female athletes use more emotion-focused coping strategies (EFC; positive reinterpretation, emotional social support, and dissociation), while men utilize more problem-focused coping strategies (PFC). Gender disparity is also seen in the media coverage of sport and remains an important element in how athletes are perceived inside and outside the sports domain. Huffman, Tuggle, and Rosengard's (2004) exploration of Title IX's impact on gender imbalances in sport found the gender disparity seen in the coverage of athletic events is consistent between the campus and mainstream media. That is, men remain the primary benefactors of the media coverage in athletics. In short, athletic trainers need to remain cognizant of the potential gender differences in sport and the variables impacting their experiences. Failure to consider gender differences could have significant effects on both treatment outcomes and, more importantly, the overall health of the athlete. The following short vignette further illustrates this idea.

On the first Saturday afternoon of the fall semester at the local university, a 19-year-old White, junior, female gymnast, and a 19-year-old White, all-American, male football player from the same university both experience season-ending knee injuries. The following day, the local and national news media descend on the athletic department to ascertain the health and future of the football player. ESPN even used the story as the lead-in to their primetime program by suggesting a detailed analysis of the impact of the injury to the team will be forthcoming. Conversely, no coverage is given to the female gymnast's injury until the university newspaper makes brief mention of the injury in that week's university-affiliated student paper. No other details of the injury were provided.

Discussion Questions

1. *What variables do you feel are driving the distinct differences in media coverage?*

2. *What types of responses are most appropriate when athletes disclose pressures associated with their team, coach, and the media?*

3. *Respond to the following question or statement:*

   - *Male athlete: "You saw the ESPN story, right? I need to get back on the field right away. What can you do to help me?"*

   - *Female athlete: "You saw the school newspaper blurb about my injury, right? I guess my injury isn't as severe as (the quarterback's) because the alumni don't get to tailgate at our meets."*

Conclusion

Psychosocial factors occupy a unique position in the realm of athletics, with researchers having clearly shown a link between psychosocial factors and both athletic injury and postinjury rehabilitation. In this chapter, psychosocial factors were conceptualized along four dimensions. In the physical dimension, the psychosocial factors were discussed, albeit briefly, relative to their impact on the athlete's physical health. Special consideration was given to issues of sexual health due to the burgeoning prevalence of sexual health issues within the demographics of high school and college athletes. Discussion in the psychological domain involved a review of the litany of emotional and psychological implications associated with the athletic experience and provided a short review of the process for referring athletes to a mental health professional. Also, readers were introduced to the notion of treating the athlete holistically. For the environmental dimension, information was presented on psychosocial factors inherent within the physical structure of the clinical setting and the range of hierarchal interpersonal and organizational relationships encountered by athletes. Special consideration was also given to sexual behaviors and the implications for the physical and psychological integrity of athletes. Finally, a narrow review of the psychosocial factors within the sociocultural domain was outlined, with the focus on the issues and implications on issues of race and sexual identity.

Overall, this chapter clearly illustrates the tremendous potential for psychosocial factors to impact the overall health of the athlete. As a result, athletic trainers are urged to conceptualize the needs of their athletes holistically. While the information presented in this chapter is admittedly narrow in scope, there is a wealth of research on these subjects within the sports medicine, counseling, psychology, and related mental health research databases (i.e., EBSCO, PsychInfo). Athletic trainers and allied sports medicine professionals are encouraged to read deeply in that body of knowledge.

References

American Psychiatric Association (2000). Diagnostic and statistical manual of mental disorders-revised 4th edition. American Psychiatric Association, Washington, DC.

Andersen, M., Denson, E., Brewer, B., & Van Raalte, J. L. (1994). Disorders of personality and mood in athletes: Recognition and referral. *Journal of Applied Sport Psychology, 6,* 168-184.

Andersen, M.B., & Williams, J.M. (1988). A model of stress and athletic injury: Prediction and prevention. Journal of Sport and Exercise Psychology, 10, 294-30).

Anshel, M., & Sailes, G. (1990). Discrepant attitudes of intercollegiate athletes as a function of race. *Journal of Sport Behavior,* 13(2), 87-103.

Baillie, P. H. F. (1993). Understanding retirement from sports: Therapeutic ideas for helping athletes in transition. *The Counseling Psychologist, 21,* 399-410.

Baruth, L. G., & Manning, M. L. (2003). *Multicultural counseling and psychotherapy: A lifespan perspective.* Upper Saddle River, NJ: Merrill Prentice Hall.

Begel, D. (1994). Occupational, psychopathologic, and therapeutic aspects of sport psychiatry. *Direct Psychiatry,* 14(11), 1-8.

Benedict, J., & Klein, A. (1998). Arrest and conviction rates for athletes accused of sexual assault. In R. K. Bergen (Ed.), *Issues in intimate violence* (pp. 169-175). Thousand Oaks, CA: Sage Publications.

Bergandi, T. A., & Wittig, A. F. (1984). Availability of and attitudes toward counseling services for the college athlete. Journal of College Student Personnel, 25(6), 557-558.

Berkowitz, A. (1992). College men as perpetrators of acquaintance rape and sexual assault: A review of the recent research. *Journal of American College Health,* 40(4), 175-181.

Bernard, J. M., & Goodyear, R. K. (2004). *Fundamentals of clinical supervision* (3rd ed.). Needham Heights, MA: Allyn & Bacon.

Birrel S., & Theberge N. (1994). Ideological Control of Women in Sport. In D. M. Costa & S. R.Guthrie (Eds.), Women and Sport. Interdisciplinary Perspectives (pp. 341-360). Champaign, IL: Human Kinetics.

Bordin, H. (1979). The generalizability of the psychoanalytic concept of the working alliance. *Psychotherapy: Theory, Research, and Practice, 16,* 252-260.

Brackenridge, C. (1997). "He owned me basically...": Women's experience of sexual abuse in sport. *International Review for the Sociology of Sport,* 32(2), 115-130.

Brewer, B. W., Jeffers, K. E., Petitpas, A. J., & Van Raalte, J. L. (1994). Perceptions of psychological interventions in the context of sport injury rehabilitation. *Sport Psychologist, 8,* 176-188.

Brewer, B. W., Petitpas, A. J., & Van Raalte, J. L. (1999). Referral of injured athletes for counseling and psychotherapy. In R. Ray & D. M. Wiese-Bjornstal (Eds.), Counseling in Sports Medicine (pp. 127-141). Champaign, IL: Human Kinetics.

Brewer, B. W., & Petrie, T. A. (1996). Psychopathology in sport and exercise. In J. L. Van Raalte & B. Brewer (Eds.), *Exploring sport and exercise psychopathology* (pp. 257-274). Washington, DC: American Psychological Association.

Brower, J. (1979). The professionalization of organized youth sport: Social-psychological impacts and outcomes. *Annals of the American Academy of Political and Social Science, 445,* 39-46.

Brown, J. M., & Davies, N. (1978). Attitude towards violence among college athletes. *Journal of Sport Behavior, 1,* 61-70.

Brown, T., Jackson, J., Brown, K., Sellers, R., Keiper, S., & Manual, W. (2003). "There's no race on the playing field": Perceptions of racial discrimination among White and Black athletes. *Journal of Sport and Social Issues, 27*(2), 162-183.

Calhoun, J. W., Ogilvie, B. C., Hendrickson, T. P., & Fritz, G. K. (1998). The psychiatric consultant in professional sports teams. *Child and Adolescent Psychiatry, 7*(4), 791-802.

Carlston, D. (1983). An environmental explanation for race differences in basketball performance. *Journal of Sport and Social Issues, 7,* 30-51.

Carron, A. V. (1982). Cohesiveness in sport groups: Interpretations and considerations. *Journal of Sport Psychology, 4,* 123-138.

Castine, S., & Roberts, G. (1974). Modeling in the socialization process of the Black athlete. *International Review of Sport Sociology, 9,* 59-74.

Center for Disease Control. (n.d.). Trends in reportable sexually transmitted diseases in the United States, 2003 - National data on chlamydia, gonorrhea and syphilis. Retrieved July 12, 2007, from http://www.cdc.gov/std/stats03/trends2003.htm.

Chartrand, J. M., & Lent, R. W. (1987). Sports counseling; Enhancing the development of the student athlete. *Journal of Counseling & Development, 66,* 164-167.

Chelladurai, P., & Saleh, S. D. (1980). Dimensions of leader behavior in sports: Development of a leadership scale. Journal of Sport Psychology, 2(1), 34-45.

Clark, J. R. (1997). Sexually transmitted diseases: Detection, differentiation, and treatment. *The Physician and Sportsmedicine, 25*(1), 76-85.

Coakley, J. J. (1990). *Sport in society: Issues and controversies.* St. Louis, MO: C.V. Mosby.

Coakley, J. J. (1993). Socialization and sport. In R. N. Singer, M. Murphy, & L. K. Tennant (Eds.), *Handbook of research on sport psychology* (pp. 571-586). Boston, MA: McGraw-Hill.

Coakley, J., & White, A. (1992). Making decisions: Gender and sport participation among British adolescents. *Sociology of Sport Journal, 9,* 20-35.

Cochran, S. D., & Mays, V. M. (2000). Lifetime prevalence of suicide symptoms and affective disorders among men reporting same-sex sexual partners: Results from NHANES III. *American Journal of Public Health, 90,* 573-578.

Cogan, K. (1998). Putting the "clinical" into sport psychology counseling. In K. F. Hays & E. M. Stern (Eds.), *Integrating exercise, sports, movement, and mind: Therapeutic unity* (pp. 131-143). New York, NY: Hayworth Press.

Dempsey, C. L. (1994). Health and social issues of gay, lesbian, and bi-sexual adolescents. Families in Society: *Journal of Contemporary Human Services, 75*(3), 160-167.

Donnelly, P. (1975). *Need for stimulation: Some possible antecedents of individual differences and its relationship to sport involvement.* Symposium conducted at the annual Canadian Psychomotor Learning and Sport Psychology Symposium. Quebec City, Canada.

Duda, J. L. (2001). Achievement goal research in sport: Pushing the boundaries and clarifying some misunderstandings. In G. C. Roberts (Ed.), *Advances in motivation in sport and exercise.* Champaign, IL: Human Kinetics.

Duncan, M.C., & Wilson, W. (1990). Gender stereotyping in televised sports. Los Angeles, CA: The Foundation.

Dwyer, T. F., & Niemann, S. H. (2002). Counseling and sexually transmitted diseases. In L. D. Burlew & D. Capuzzi (Eds.), *Sexuality counseling* (pp. 373-394). New York, NY: Nova Science.

Edwards, H. (1972). The myth of the racially superior athlete. *Intellectual Digest, 44,* 32-48.

Edwards, H. (1973). The black athlete: 20th century gladiators for white America. *Psychology Today, 7,* 43-52.

Emmel, L. (1977). *A review of the literature of the variables affecting the success of black athletes in professional sports.* Unpublished master's theses, Mankato State University. Mankato, MN.

Etzel, E. F. (1989). Life stress, locus of control, and sport competition anxiety patterns of College student-athletes. Unpublished Doctoral Dissertation, West Virginia University Morgantown, WV.

Etzel, E. F., Pinkney, J. W., & Hinkle, J. S. (1995). College student-athletes and needs assessment. In S. D. Stabb, S. M. Harris, & J. E. Talley (Eds.), Multicultural Needs Assessment for College and University Student Populations (pp. 155-172). Springfield, IL: Thomas.

Ferrante, A., Etzel, E. F., & Lantz, C. (1996). Counseling college student athletes: The problem, the need. In E. F., A. P. Ferrante, & J. W. Pinkney (Eds.), Counseling College Student Athletes: Issues and Interventions (2nd ed.) (pp. 1-17). Morgantown, WV: Fitness Information Technology.

Fisher, A. C. (1990). Adherence to sports injury rehabilitation programs. *Sports Medicine, 9,* 151-158.

Fletcher, T. B., Benshoff, J. M., & Richburg, M. J. (2003). A systems approach to understanding and counseling college student-athletes. *Journal of College Counseling, 6*(1), 35-45.

Flint, F. (1999). Effective group health education counseling. In R. Ray and D. M. Wiese-Bjornstal (Eds.), *Counseling in sports medicine* (pp. 93-110). Champaign, IL: Human Kinetics.

Ford, J. (1988). 'Counselling, advocacy and negotiation': Response. British Journal of Social Work, 18, 57-62.

Ford, I., & Gordon, S. (1998). Perspectives of sport trainers and athletic therapists on the psychological content of their practice and training. *Journal of Sport Rehabilitation, 7,* 79-94.

Gabbard, C., & Halischak, K. (1993). Consulting opportunities: Working with student athletes at a university. *The Counseling Psychologist, 21,* 386-398.

George, F. J. (1997). The athletic trainer's perspective. *Clinics in Sports Medicine, 16*(3), 361-374.

Glick, J., & Horsfall, J. (2001). Psychiatric conditions in sports: Diagnosis, treatment, and quality of life. *Physician and Sportsmedicine, 29*(8), 44-51.

Goldenberg, I., & Goldenberg, H. (2004). *Family therapy: An overview.* Pacific Grove, CA: Brooks/Cole.

Gould, D., Udry, E., Tuffey, S., & Loehr, J. (1996). Burnout in competitive junior tennis players: I. A Quantitative psychological assessment. *Sport Psychologist, 10,* 322-340.

Greendorfer, J. S., & Ewing, M. (1981). Race and gender difference in children's socialization into sport. *Research Quarterly for Exercise and Sport, 52,* 301-310.

Greenspan, M., & Andersen, M. B. (1995). Providing psychological services to student athletes: A developmental psychology model. In S. M. Murphy (Ed.), *Sports psychology interventions* (pp. 177-191). Champaign, IL: Human Kinetics.

Griffin, P. (1998). Strong women, deep closets: lesbians and homophobia in sport. Champaign, Il. Human Kinetics.

Gudykunst, W. B., & Kim, Y. Y. (1997). *Communicating with strangers: An approach to intercultural communication* (3rd ed.). New York, NY: McGraw-Hill.

Hammermeister, J., & Burton, D. (2004). Gender differences in coping with endurance sport stress: Are men from Mars and women from Venus? *Journal of Sport Behavior, 27*(2), 148-165.

Hardy, L. (1992). Psychological stress, performance, and injury in sport. *British Medical Bulletin, 48*(3), 615-629.

Hargreaves, J. (1994). Sporting females: critical issues in the history and sociology of women's sports. New York: Routledge.

Hasbrook, C. A., & Harris, O. (1999). Wrestling with gender: Physicality and masculinity among inner-city first and second graders. *Men and Masculinities, 1,* 302-318.

Hedge, B. (1996). Counseling people with AIDS, their partners, family and friends. In J. Green & A. McCreaner (Eds.), *Counseling in HIV infection and AIDS* (2nd ed., pp. 66-82). Cambridge, MA: Blackwell Science.

Heil, J. (1993). *Psychology of sport injury.* Champaign, IL: Human Kinetics.

Helms, J. E. (1990). *Black and White racial identity: Theory, research, and practice.* Westport, CT: Greenwood Press.

Helms, J. E. (1994). How multiculturalism obscures racial factors in the therapy process: Comment on Ridley et al. (1994), Ottavi et al. (1994), and Thompson et al. (1994). Journal of Counseling Psychology, 41(2), 162-165.

Helms, J. E. (1996). Toward a methodology for measuring and assessing racial as distinguished from ethnic identity. In G. R. Sodowsky & J. C. Impara (Eds.), Multicultural assessment in counseling and clinical psychology (pp. 143-192). Lincoln, NE: Buros Institute of Mental Measurement.

Herek, G. M. (1989). Hate crimes against lesbian and gay men: Issues for research and policy. *American Psychologist, 44*, 948-955.

Herek, G. M. (2000). The psychology of sexual prejudice. *Current Directions in Psychological Science, 9*, 19-22.

Heyman, S. R. (1986). Addressing preventive interventions in rural community psychology. Journal of Community Psychology, 14(5), 7-15.

Hoberman, J. M. (1984). *Sport and political ideology.* Austin, TX: University of Texas Press.

Hoberman, J. M. (1997). *Darwin's athletes: How sport has damaged Black America and preserved the myth of race.* Boston, MA: Mariner.

Holland, J. L., Magoon, T. M., & Spokane, A. R. (1981). Counseling psychology: Career interventions, research, and theory. *Annual Review of Psychology, 32*, 279-305.

Holt, N., & Morley, D. (2004). Gender differences in psychosocial factors associated with athletic success during childhood. *Sport Psychologist, 18*, 138-153.

Hopson, S. (1972). *The socialization process of the Black athlete.* Unpublished master's thesis, Kent State University, Kent, OH.

Huber, C. H. (1996). Facilitating disclosure of HIV-positive status to family members. *Family Journal: Counseling and Therapy for Couples and Families, 4*(1), 53-55.

Huffman, S., Tuggle, C.A., & Rosengard, D.S. (2004). How campus media covers sports: The gender-equity issue, one generation later. Mass Communication and Society, 7(4), 475-489.

Hughes, R., & Coakley, J. (1991). Positive deviance among athletes: The implications of overconformity to the sport ethic. Sociology of Sport Journal, 8(4), 307-325.

Ivey, A. E., Ivey, M. B., & Simek-Morgan, L. (1997). *Counseling and psychotherapy: A multicultural perspective.* Needham Heights, MA: Allyn & Bacon.

Jefferson, S. (1998). *Pro bound: Do you have what it takes to become a professional athlete?* Queens Village, NY: Author.

Kane, B. (1984). Trainer counseling to avoid three face-saving maneuvers. *Athletic Training, 19*, 171-174.

Kane, S. C. (1996). Precompetitive anxiety, objective performance, and subjective performance as determinants of postcompetitive anxiety. Unpublished master's thesis, Springfield College.

Kemler, D. S. (1988). *Level of athletic, instrumental and reactive aggression between contact and non-contact male and female high school athletes under pre- and post-testing conditions.* Unpublished master's thesis. Southern Connecticut State University, New Haven, CT.

Kenow, L., & Williams, J. M. (1999). Coach-athlete compatibility and athlete's perception of coaching behaviors. Journal of Sport Behavior, 22, 251-260.

King, B. M. (2005). *Human sexuality today* (5th ed.). Upper Saddle River, NJ: Pearson Prentice Hall.

Knight, J. L., & Giuliano, T. (2003). Blood, sweat, and jeers: The impact of the media's heterosexist portrayals on perceptions of male and female athletes. *Journal of Sport Behavior, 26*(3), 272-285.

Lapchick, R. E. (1996). Race and college sports: A long way to go. In R. E. Lapchick (Ed.), *Sport and society: Equal opportunity or business as usual* (pp. 5-18). Thousand Oaks, CA: Sage.

Larivaara, P., Vaisanen, E., & Kiuttu, J. (1994). Family systems medicine: A new field of medicine. *Nordic Journal of Psychiatry, 48*(5), 329-332.

Larson, G. A., Starkey, C., & Zaichkowsky, L. D. (1996). Psychological aspects of athletic injuries as perceived by athletic trainers. *Sport Psychologists, 10*, 37-47.

Leddy, M., Lambert, M., & Ogles, B. (1994). Psychological consequences of athletic injury among high-level competitors. *Research Quarterly for Exercise and Sport, 4*, 347-354.

Leonard, M. (1980). *A sociological perspective of sport.* Minneapolis: Burgess.

Linder, D. E., Brewer, B. W., Van Raalte, J. L., & De Lange, N. (1991). A negative halo for athletes who consult sport psychologists: Replication and extension. *Journal of Sport and Exercise Psychology, 13*, 133-148.

Long, L. L., Burnett, J. A., & Thomas, R. V. (2006). *Sexuality counseling: An integrative approach.* Upper Saddle River, NJ: Pearson Education.

Macchi, R., & Crossman, J. (1996). After the fall: Reflections of injured classical ballet dancers. *Journal of Sport Behavior, 19*, 221-234.

MacClancy, J. (1996). Sport, identity and ethnicity. In J. MacClancy (Ed.), *Sport, identity, and ethnicity* (pp. 1-20). Herndon, VA: Berg.

Martin, S. B., Wrisberg, C. A., Beitel, P. A., & Lounsbury, J. (1997). NCAA Division I athletes' attitudes toward seeking sport psychology consultation: The development of an objective instrument. *Sport Psychologist, 11*, 201-218.

Masters, W. H., Johnson, V. E., & Kolodny, R. C. (1995). *Human sexuality* (5th ed.). New York, NY: HarperCollins.

McClintock, J. (1989). Sexual abuse and eating disorders. *National Anorexic Aid Society, 12,* 1-2.

McPherson, B. (1981). Socialization into and through sport involvement. In G. Luschen & G. H. Sage (Eds.), *Handbook of the social science of sport* (pp. 112-132). Champaign, IL: Stipes.

McPherson, B. D. (1984). Socialization into and through sport. In G. Luschen & G. H. Sage (Eds.), *Handbook of the social science of sport* (pp. 246-273). Champaign, IL: Stipes.

Messman, T. L., & Long, P. J. (1996). Child sexual abuse and its relationship to revictimization in adult women: A review. *Child Psychological Review, 16,* 397-420.

Murrell, A. J., & Gaertner, S. L. (1992). Cohesion and sport team effectiveness: The benefit of a common group identity. Journal of Sport & Social Issues, 16, 1-14.

National Athletic Trainers' Association. (2005). *Code of ethics.* Principle one recommended by the National Athletic Trainer's Association. Retrieved October 10, 2005, from http://www.nata.org/about/codeofethics.htm

National Athletic Trainers' Association Education Council. (1992). *Competencies in athletic training.* Dallas, TX: National Athletic Trainers' Association.

Nelson, W. S. (1983). How the myth of the dumb jock becomes fact: A developmental view for counselors. *Counseling and Values, 27,* 176-185.

O'Sullivan, C. (1991). Acquaintance gang rape on campus. In A. Parrot & L. Bechhofer (Eds.), *Acquaintance rape: The hidden crime* (pp. 140-156). New York, NY: John Wiley & Sons.

Parham, W. D. (1993). The intercollegiate athlete: A 1990s profile. *The Counseling Psychologist, 21,* 411-429.

Parrot, A. (1990, November). *Do rape education and prevention programs influence patterns among New York State college students?* Presented at the 1990 annual meeting of the Society for the Scientific Study of Sex, Minneapolis, MN.

Parrot, A., & Cummings, N. (1994). A rape awareness and prevention model for male athletes. *Journal of American College Health, 42*(4), 179-185.

Patricksson, G. (1979). Socialization and involvement in sport. *Studies in Educational Sciences, 31,* 240.

Paul, J.P., Catania J., Pollack, L., Moskowitz, J., Canchola, J., Mills, T., et al. (2002). Suicide attempts among gay and bisexual men: Lifetime prevalence and antecedents. *American Journal of Public Health, 92,* 1338-1334.

Pearlman, J. (1999, December 27). At full blast. Sports Illustrated, 91(25), 60-63.

Petitpas, S., & Champagne, D. E. (1988). Developmental programming for intercollegiate athletes. *Journal of College Student Development, 29,* 454-460.

Petitpas, A., & Danish, S. J. (1995). Caring for injured athletes. In S. M. Murphy (Ed.), *Sport psychology interventions* (pp. 255-281). Champaign, IL: Human Kinetics.

Petrie, T. A. (1992). Psychological antecedents of athletic injury: The effects of life stress and social support on female collegiate gymnasts. *Behavioral Medicine, 18*(3), 127-138.

Phillips, J. (1976). Toward an explanation of racial variations in top level sports participation. *International Review of Sport Sociology, 3,* 39-53.

Pipe, A. L. (1993). Wolffe Memorial Lecture. Sport, science, and society: Ethics in sports medicine. *Medical Science and Sports Exercise, 25*(8), 888-900.

Raglin, J. S. (2001). Psychological factors in sport performance: The mental health model revisited. *Sports Medicine, 31*(12), 875-890.

Ray, D. R., & Wiese-Bjornstal, D. M. (1999). *Counseling in sports medicine.* Champaign, IL: Human Kinetics.

Ray, R., Terrell, R., & Hough, D. (1999). The role of the sports medicine professional in counseling athletes. In R. Ray & D. M. Wiese-Bjornstal (Eds.), Counseling in Sports Medicine (pp. 3-20). Champaign, IL: Human Kinetics.

Renson, R. (1979). *The dynamics of the sports socialization process.* Paper presented at the National Seminar on Sport for Young School Learners, Stockholm, Sweden.

Richards, S., & Aries, E. (1999). The division III student-athlete: Academic performance, campus involvement, and growth. Journal of College Student Development, 40(3), 211-218.

Robbins, J. E., & Rosenfeld, L. B. (2001). Athlete's perceptions of social support provided by their head coach, assistant coach, and athletic trainer, pre-injury and during rehabilitation. *Journal of Sport Behavior, 24*(3), 277-297.

Ross, M. W. (1999). Psychological perspectives on sexuality and sexually transmitted diseases. In K. K. Holmes, P. P. Sparling, P. Mardh, S. M. Lemon, W. E. Stamm, P. Piot, et al. (Eds), *Sexually transmitted diseases* (3rd ed, pp. 107-113). New York, NY: McGraw-Hill.

Rubin, L. J., & Borgers, S. B. (1990). Sexual harassment in universities during the 1980's. Sex Roles, 23, 397-411.

Ryan, F. J. (1989). Participation in intercollegiate athletics: Affective outcomes. *Journal of College Student Development, 30,* 122-128.

Sachs, P. R., & Ellenberg, D. B. (1994). The family system and adaptation to an injured worker. *American Journal of Family Therapy,* 22(3), 263-272.

Sailes, G. (1984). *Sport socialization comparisons among Black and White adult male athletes and nonathletes.* Unpublished dissertation. University of Minnesota, Minneapolis, MN.

Sailes, G. A. (1996). An investigation of campus stereotypes: The myth of the Black athletic superiority and the dumb jock stereotype. In R. E. Lapchick (Ed.), Sport and society: Equal opportunity or business as usual (pp. 193-202). Thousand Oaks, CA: Sage.

Sanday, P. R. (1981). The socio-cultural context of rape: A crosscultural study. Journal of Social Issues, 37, 5-27.

Serovich, M. (2000). Helping HIV-positive persons to negotiate the disclosure process to partners, family members, and friends. *Journal of Marital and Family Therapy, 26*(3), 365-372.

Silver, R. C., Wortman, C. B., & Crofton, C. (1990). The role of coping in support provision: The self-presentational dilemma of victims of life crises. In B. R. Sarason, I. G. Sarason, & G. R. Pierce (Eds.), *Social support: An international view* (pp. 391-426). New York, NY: Wiley.

Smith, R. E., Smoll, F. L., & Ptacek, J. T. (1990). Conjunctive moderator variables in vulnerability and resilience research: Life stress, social support and coping skills, and adolescent sport injuries. Journal of Personality and Social Psychology, 58(2), 360-370.

Smoll, F. L., & Smith, R. E. (2002). Coaching behavior research and intervention in youth sports. In F. L. Smoll & R.E. Smith (Eds.), *Children and youth in sport: A biopsychological perspective* (2nd ed., pp. 211-234). Dubuque, IA: Kendall/ Hunt Publishing.

Snyder, E., & Spreitzer, E. (1978). *Social aspects of sport.* Englewood Cliffs, NJ: Prentice Hall.

Stevenson, C. L. (1975). Socialization effects of participation in sport: A critical review of the research. *Research Quarterly, 46,* 267-273.

Stewart, I. B. (2003). Effect of long- and short-acting $\alpha 2$-agonist on exercise-induced arterial hypoxemia. Medicine & Science in Sports & Exercise, 35(4), 603-607.

Sue, D. W., & Sue, D. (2003). *Counseling the culturally diverse.* New York, NY: John Wiley & Sons.

Theberge, N. (1994). Toward a feminist alternative to sport as a male preserve. In Birrell, S., & Cole, C.L. (Eds.), Women, sport, and culture (pp. 181-192). Champaign, IL: Human Kinetics.

Udry, E., Gould, D., Bridges, D., & Beck, L. (1997). Down but not out: Athlete responses to season ending injuries. *Journal of Sport and Exercise Psychology, 19,* 229-248.

Velasquez, B. J. (1998). Sexual harassment: A concern for the athletic trainer. *Journal of Athletic Training, 33*(2), 171-176.

Warshaw, R. (1988). *I never called it rape.* New York, NY: Harper & Row.

Weinstock, H., Berman, S., & Cates, W. (2004). Sexually transmitted diseases among American youth: Incidences and prevalence estimates, 2000. Perspectives on Sexual and Reproductive Health, 36, 6-10.

Widmeyer, W. N., Carron, A. V., & Brawley, L. R. (1993). Group cohesion in sport and exercise. In R. N. Singer, M. Murphy, & L. K. Tennant (Eds.), *Handbook of research on sport psychology* (pp. 672-691). New York, NY: Macmillan.

Wiese, D. M., Weiss, M. R., & Yukelson, D. P. (1991). Sport psychology in the training room: A survey of athletic trainers. *Sport Psychologist, 5*(1), 15-24.

Wiese-Bjornstal, D. M., & Shaffer, S. M. (1999). Psychosocial dimensions of sport injury. In R. Ray & D. M. Wiese-Bjornstal (Eds.), *Counseling in sports medicine* (pp. 23-40). Champaign, IL: Human Kinetics.

Williams, J., & Widmeyer, W. N. (1991). The cohesion-performance outcome relationship in a co-acting sport. *Journal of Sport and Exercise Psychology, 13,* 364-371.

Williams, J. M. (2000). How to identify and prevent injuries resulting from psychosocial factors. *Athletic Therapy Today, 5*(6), 36-37.

Williams, J. M., & Andersen, M. B. (1998). Psychosocial antecedents of sport injury: Review and critique of the stress and injury model. Special Issue: Theoretical, Empirical, and Applied Issue in the Psychology of Sport Injury, 10, 5-25.

Williams, J. M., & Roepke, N. (1993). Psychology of injury and injury rehabilitation. In R. N. Singer, M. Murphy, & L. K. Tennant (Eds.), Handbook of Research on Sport Psychology (pp. 815-839). New York: Macmillan.

Wolf-Wendel, L.E., Toma, J.D., & Morphew, C.C. (2001). How much difference is too much difference? Perceptions of gay men and lesbians in intercollegiate athletics. Journal of College Student Development, 42(5), 465-479.

Young, K., White, P., & McTeer, W. (1994). Body talk: Male athletes reflect on sport injury. Sociology of Sport Journal, 11(2), 175-194.

Zimmerman, T. S. (1993). Systems family therapy with an athlete. *Journal of Family Psychotherapy*, 4(3), 29-37.

Zimmerman, T. S., & Protinsky, H. (1993). Uncommon sports psychology: Consultation using family therapy theory and techniques. *American Journal of Family Therapy*, 21(2), 161-174.

Bibliography

Adler, P., & Adler, P. A. (1985). From idealism to pragmatic detachment: The academic performance of college athletes. *Sociology of Education, 58*, 241-250.

Baird, J.A. (2002). Playing it straight: An analysis of current legal protections to combat homophobia and sexual orientation discrimination in intercollegiate athletics. Berkeley Women's Law Journal, 17, 31-67.

Berg, J. H., & Archer, R. L. (1983). The disclosure-liking relationship: Effects of self-perception, order of disclosure and topical similarity. *Human Communication Research, 10*, 262-282.

Blanchard, W. (1959). The group process in gang rape. *Journal of Social Psychology, 49*, 259-266.

Bohnke, D. (1971). *Attitude differentials between Negro and Caucasian intercollegiate athletes.* Unpublished doctoral dissertation. Ohio State University, Columbus, OH.

Bordin, E. S. (1983). A working alliance model in supervision. *Counseling Psychologist, 11*, 35-42.

Brandt, A. M., & Jones, D. S. (1999). Historical perspectives on sexually transmitted diseases: Challenges for prevention and control. In K. K. Holmes, P. F. Sparling, P. Mardh, S. M. Lemon, W. E. Stamm, P. Piot, et al. (Eds.), *Sexually transmitted diseases* (3rd ed., pp. 15-21). New York, NY: McGraw-Hill.

Brewer, B. W., Van Raalte, J. L., & Linder, D. E. (1993). Athletic identity: Hercules' muscles or achilles heel. *International Journal of Sport Psychology, 24*, 237-254.

Brislin, R. W. (1981). *Cross-cultural encounters: Face to face interaction.* New York, NY: Pergamon Press.

Brown, R. (1976). Educational plans of black and white athletes and nonathletes. *Sport Sociology Bulletin, 5*, 57-65.

Brown, K. T., Brown, T. N., Jackson, J. S., & Sellers, R. M. (2003). Teammates on and off the field? Contact with black teammates and the racial attitudes of white student athletes. Journal of Applied Social Psychology, 33(7), 1379-1403.

Burckes-Miller, M., & Black, D. R. (1998). Male and female college athletes: Prevalence of anorexia nervosa and bulimia nervosa. *Journal of Athletic Training, 23*, 137-140.

Byme, D. (1961). Interpersonal attraction and attitude similarity. *Journal of Abnormal and Social Psychology, 62*, 713-715.

Byme, D. (1971). *The attraction paradigm.* New York, NY: Academic Press.

Collins, N., & Miller, L. (1994). Self-disclosure and liking: A meta-analytic review. *Psychological Bulletin, 116*, 457-475.

Courtland, L. (1983). An investigation of the athletic career expectations of high school student athletes. *Personnel and Guidance Journal, 61*, 544-547.

Crooks, R., & Baur, K. (2002). *Our sexuality* (8th ed.). Pacific Grove, CA: Wadsworth.

Crosset, T. W. (1999). Male athletes' violence against women: A critical assessment of the athletic affiliation, violence against women debate. *Quest, 15*, 244-257.

Crosset, T. W., Benedict, J. R., & McDonald, M. A. (1995). Male student-athletes reported for sexual assault: A survey of campus police departments and judicial affairs offices. *Journal of Sport and Social Issues, 19*, 126-140.

Cunningham, G. B. (2003). Already aware of the glass ceiling: Race-related effects of perceived opportunity on the career choices of college athletes. *Journal of African American Studies, 7*(1), 57-71.

Cunningham, G. B., Sagas, M., & Ashley, F. B. (2001). Occupational commitment and intent to leave the coaching profession: Differences according to race. *International Review for the Sociology of Sport, 36*, 131-148.

Danish, S. J. (1986). Psychological aspects in the care and treatment of athletic injuries. In P. F. Vinger & E. F. Hoerner (Eds.), *Sport injuries: The unthwarted epidemic* (pp. 345-353). Littleton, MA: PSG Publishing Company.

Doyle, M. (2002). A new dimension for the athletic training room. *Athletic Therapy Today, 7*(1), 34-35.

Duda, J. L., Smar, A. E., & Tappe, M. K. (1998). Predictors of adherence in the rehabilitation of athletic injuries: An application of personal investment theory. *Journal of Sport and Exercise Psychology, 11*, 367-381.

Dudley, A. T. (1888). The mental qualities of an athlete. *Harvard Alumni Magazine, 6*, 43-51.

Durfur, M. J. (1999). Gender and sport. In J. Saltzman Chavez (Ed.), *Handbook of the sociology of gender* (pp. 587-588). New York, NY: Kluwer Academic/Plenum Publishers.

Earle, M. V. (Ed.). (2000). *1999-00 race demographics of NCAA member institutions' athletics personnel*. Indianapolis, IN: National Collegiate Athletic Association.

Eskenazi, G. (1990, June 3). The male athletes and sexual assault. *The New York Times*, 1, 4.

Etsel, E. F., Ferrante, A. P., & Pinkney, J. W. (Eds.). (1991). *Counseling college student athletes: Issues and interventions*. Morgantown, WV: Fitness Information Technology.

Evan, V. (1978). A study of perceptions held by high school athletes toward coaches. *International Review of Sport Sociology, 13*, 47-53.

Evan, V., & Quarterman, J. (1983). Personality characteristics of successful and unsuccessful black female basketball players. *International Journal of Sport Psychology, 14*, 105-115.

Fink, J. S., Pastore, D. L., & Reimer, H. A. (2001). Do differences make a difference? Managing diversity in Division IA intercollegiate athletics. *Journal of Sport Management, 15*, 10-50.

Fisher, A. C., Scriber, K. C., Mtheny, M. L., Alderman, M. H., & Bitting, L. A. (1993). Enhancing athletic injury rehabilitation adherence. *Journal of Athletic Training, 28*, 312-318.

Franklin, G., & Platt, J. S. (1994). How cultural assumptions may affect teaching, learning, and communication in the nation's prisons. *Journal of Correctional Education, 45*(2), 86-91.

Freischlag, J. (1976). Socio-psychological perceptions of world class sprinters: Two case studies. *FIEP Bulletin, 46*, 21-29.

Geis, G. (1971). Group sexual assaults. *Medical Aspects of Human Sexuality, 5*, 101-113.

Gelman, R., & McGinley, H. (1978). Interpersonal liking and self-disclosure. *Journal of Consulting and Clinical Psychology, 46*, 1549-1551.

Gill, D. L. (2001). Feminist sport psychology: A guide for our journey. *Sport Psychologist, 15*, 363-372.

Groth, A. N. (1979). *Men who rape: The psychology of the offender*. New York, NY: Plenum Press.

Grove, J. R., Hanrahan, S. J., & Stewart, R. M. (1990). Attributions for rapid or slow recovery from sports injuries. *Canadian Journal of Sport Sciences, 15*(2), 107-114.

Gutkind, S. (2004). Using solution-focused brief counseling to provide injury support. *Sport Psychologist, 18*, 75-88.

Hanks, M. (1979). Race, sexual status and athletics in this process of educational achievement. *Social Science Quarterly, 60*, 482-496.

Hardy, C.J., & Crace, R.K. (1993). The dimensions of social support when dealing with sport injuries. In D. Pargman (Ed.). Psychological bases of sport injuries (pp. 121-144). Morgantown, WV: Fitness Information Technology.

Heyman, S. R. (1986). Psychological problem patterns found with athletes. *The Clinical Psychologist, 27*, 68-71.

Horenstein, V. D., & Downey, J. L. (2003). A cross cultural investigation of self-disclosure. *North American Journal of Psychology, 5*(3), 373-387.

Ievieva, L., & Orlick, R. (1993). Mental paths to enhanced recovery from sports injury. In D. Pargman (Ed.), *Psychological bases of sport injury* (pp. 219-245). Morgantown, WV: Fitness Information Technology.

Jones, J., & Hochner, A. (1973). Racial differences in sports activities: A look at the self-paced versus reactive hypothesis. *Journal of Personality and Social Psychology, 27*, 86-95.

Jourard, S. M., & Lasakow, P. (1958). Some factors in self-disclosure. *Journal of Abnormal and Social Psychology, 56*, 91-98.

Kleinke, C. L., & Kahn, M. L. (1980). Perceptions of self-disclosure: Effects of sex and physical attractiveness. *Journal of Personality, 48*, 191-205.

Koss, M. P. (1993). Rape: Scope, impact, interventions, and public policy responses. *American Psychologist, 48*, 1062-1069.

Lapchick, R. (2001). *Smashing barriers: Race and sport in the new millennium.* New York, NY: Madison.

Lapchick, R. D., & Matthews, K. J. (2001). *Racial and gender report card.* Boston, MA: Center for the Study of Sport in Society.

Leaman, O., & Carrington, B. (1985). Athleticism and the reproduction of gender and ethnic marginality. *Journal of Leisure Studies, 4,* 205-217.

Martin, C., & Ridgeway, A. (1975). *The personality characteristics of black female high school athletes.* Paper presented at the AAHPERD National Convention, Atlantic City, NJ.

Matveev, A. V., & Nelson, P. E. (2004). Cross cultural communication competence and multicultural team performance: Perceptions of American and Russian managers. *International Journal of Cross Cultural Management, 4*(2), 253-268.

Meyer, B. (1990). From idealism to actualization: The academic performance of female collegiate athletes. *Sociology of Sport Journal, 7,* 44-57.

Morgan, W. P. (1978). The credulous-skeptical argument in perspective. In W. F. Straub (Ed.), *An analysis of athlete behavior* (pp. 218-227). Ithaca, NY: Movement Publications.

Morgan, W. P. (1980). The trait psychology controversy. *Research Quarterly in Exercise and Sport, 51,* 50-76.

Morgan, W. P. (1985). Selected psychological factors limiting performance: A mental health model. In D. H. Clarke & H. M. Eckert (Eds.), *Limits of human performance* (pp. 70-80). Champaign, IL: Human Kinetics.

Muehlenhard, C. L., & Falcon, P. L. (1990). Male's heterosocial skills and attitudes toward women as predictors of verbal sexual coercion and forcible rape. *Sex Roles, 23*(5/6), 241-259.

Nation, J., & Leunes, A. (1983). A personality profile of the black athlete in college football. *Psychology: A Journal of Human Behavior, 20,* 1-2.

National Athletic Trainers' Association Board of Certification. (1999). *Role Delineation Study: Athletic training profession* (4th ed., pp. 1-71). Omaha, NE: Board of Certification.

Newcomer, R. R., Roh, J. L., Perna, F. M., Stilger, V. G., & Etzel, E. F. (1998). Injury as a traumatic experience: Intrusive thoughts and avoidance behavior associated injury among college student-athletes. *Journal Sport Psychologist, 166,* 104-109.

Pedersen, P. B. (1994). *A handbook for developing multicultural awareness* (2nd ed.). Alexandria, VA: American Counseling Association.

Petrie, T. A., & Russell, R. K. (1995). Academic and psychosocial antecedents of academic performance for minority and non-minority college football players. *Journal of Counseling & Development, 73*(6), 615-621.

Picou, S. (1978). Athletic achievement and education aspiration. *Sociological Quarterly, 19,* 429-438.

Ptacek, J. T., Smith, R. E., & Zana, J. (1992). Gender, appraisal, and coping: A longitudinal analysis. *Journal of Personality, 60,* 747-770

Rapaport, K., & Burkhart, B. R. (1984). Personality and attitudinal characteristics of sexually coercive college males. *Journal of Abnormal Psychology, 93,* 216-221.

Segal, M. H., Dasen, P. R., Berry, J. W., & Poortinga, Y. H. (1990). *Human behavior global perspectives: An introduction to cross-cultural psychology.* New York, NY: Pergamon.

Slavin, R., & Madden, N. (1979). School practices that improve race relations. *American Educational Research Journal, 16,* 169-180.

Smith, D., & Stewart, S. (2003). Sexual aggression and sports participation. *Journal of Sport Behavior, 26*(4), 384-395.

Stone, A. A., & Neale, J. M. (1984). New measure of daily coping: Development and preliminary results. *Journal of Personality and Social Psychology, 46,* 892-906.

Storch, E.A., Storch, J.B., Killiany, E.M., & Roberti, J.W. (2005). Self-reported psychopathology in athletes: A comparison of intercollegiate student-athletes and nonathletes. Journal of Sport Behavior, 28(1), 86-97.

Straub, W. (1975). Personality traits of black and white high school athletes in the North and South. *Psychology of Sport and Motor Behavior, May,* 101-114.

Sue, D. W., Arrendondo, P., & McDavis, R. J. (1992). Multicultural counseling competencies and standards: A call to the profession. *Journal of Counseling and Development, 70,* 477-486.

Thirer, J., & Wiecsorek, P. (1984). On and off the field social interaction patterns of black and white high school athletes. *Journal of Sport Behavior, 7,* 105-114.

Valentine, J. J., & Taub, D. J. (1999). Responding to the developmental needs of student athletes. *Journal of College Counseling, 2*(2), 164-179.

Vanden Auweele, Y. V., Cuyper, B., Mele, V., & Rzewnicki, R. (1993). Elite performance and personality: From description and prediction to diagnosis and intervention. In R. N. Singer, M. Murphey, L. K. Tenant (Eds.), *Handbook of research in sport psychology* (pp. 257-289). New York, NY: Macmillan.

Vaughan, J., King, K., & Cottrell, R. (2004). Collegiate athletic trainers' confidence in helping female athletes with eating disorders. *Journal of Athletic Training, 39*(1), 71-76.

Velasquez, B. J. (1996). *Study of sexual harassment issues in physical education and athletics at colleges and universities.* Dissertation. Middle Tennessee State University, Murfreesboro, TN. (Abstracts International 57-9700903).

Velasquez, B. J., & MacBeth, J. L. (1997). *Sexual harassment issues in athletic training and athletic.* Presented at the 48th Annual Meeting and Clinical Symposia of the National Athletic Trainer's Association, Free Communication's Session. Salt Lake City, UT.

Wells, R., & Picou, S. (1980). Interscholastic athletes and socialization for educational achievement. *Journal of Sport Behavior, 3,* 119-128.

Whitehead, U. (1976). *An analysis of the relationship between intercollegiate football participants and the extent of the feelings of alienation.* Unpublished doctoral dissertation. University of Oregon, Eugene, OR.

Wilensky, N. (1975). *Racial attitudes of athletes and musicians of three socioeconomic groups.* Unpublished doctoral dissertation. Springfield, MA: Springfield College.

Williams, J. M., Rotella, R. J., & Heyman, S. R. (1998). Stress, injury, and the psychological rehabilitation of athletes. In J. M. Williams (Ed.), *Applied sport psychology: Personal growth to peak performance* (3rd ed., pp. 409-428). Mountain View, CA: Mayfield Publishing Company.

GLOSSARY AND INTERNET RESOURCES

Glossary

addiction: A disease that interferes with the human's ability to function normally. The disease is characterized by compulsion, obsession, and loss of control.

amenorrhea: The loss of menstrual periods for 3 or more consecutive months.

anhedonia: Is one of the so-called vegetative signs of depression, meaning loss of pleasure or joy in all things.

anorexia nervosa (AN): Is used to describe individuals who refuse to maintain a minimum healthy or "normal" weight and is characterized by an intense fear of weight gain and significant misperception of body shape, size, or image.

anxiety: Is a personal experience of cognitive worry and racing thoughts, combined with some of the following physical sensations: rapid heartbeat; shallow, fast breathing; dizziness; muscle tension; chest pain; numbness; or "butterflies" in the stomach.

at risk of overweight (in childhood): Individual with a BMI greater than 85% of individuals of the same age and sex but not yet in the category of overweight.

BAC: Blood alcohol concentration.

binge drinking: This defined for males as five or more drinks; and for females as four or more drinks in any one drinking episode.

binge-eating disorder (BED): Recurrent episodes of binge eating without compensatory behaviors.

body dysmorphic disorder (BDD): Is a pre-occupation with one's appearance that goes beyond simple vanity and causes significant distress or impairment in daily functioning.

bulimia nervosa (BN): Is characterized by binge-eating episodes typically followed by subsequent maladaptive compensatory behaviors (i.e., self-induced vomiting; misuse of laxatives, diuretics, enemas, or other medications; fasting; or excessive exercise) for a period of at least twice a week for 3 months.

chemical dependence: Ingestive addiction due to the ingesting of mood-altering chemicals, involving tolerance and withdrawal syndromes.

choice theory: A theory that underlies William Glasser's reality therapy. In choice theory, the idea is that people have mental images of their needs and behave accordingly; thus individuals are ultimately self-determining (i.e., they choose). Individuals can choose to be miserable or mentally disturbed. They may also choose to determine the course of their lives in positive ways and give up trying to control others (Gladding, 2001, p. 24).

client-centered therapy: A theory developed by Carl Rogers. It falls somewhere between the original name of *nondirective counseling* and the more modern name of *person-centered counseling*. The idea of the approach is that the client, not the counselor, should direct the counseling process in terms of focus (Gladding, 2001, p. 25).

cognitive approaches to human relations: Approaches based on the theory that how one thinks largely determines how one feels (Gladding, 2001, p. 26).

cognitive triad of depression: Three elements that, according to Aaron Beck's cognitive therapy, are present in depression: negative views about self, negative views about the world, and negative views about the future.

compliance: The overall extent to which a client takes medication as prescribed and/or attends therapy.

confidentiality: An ethical concept protecting the client from the professional's unauthorized disclosure of the client's personal information and disclosures in treatment.

consultant: A resource person with special knowledge who assists individuals and groups in resolving difficulties they have not been able to resolve on their own (Gladding, 2001 p. 30).

counseling: The application of mental health psychological or human development principles through cognitive, affective, behavioral, or systemic interventions; strategies that address wellness, personal growth, or career development; as well as pathology (Gladding, 2001).

cultural intentionality: The ability to generate alternatives from different vantage points, using a variety of skills and personal qualities within a culturally appropriate framework (Ivey & Ivey, 2003).

culture: A way of living and behaving by an identifiable group of human beings; that is, a way that is characterized by a group's habits, perceptions, customs, values, language, communication style, traditions, rituals, artistic impressions, personal preferences, social rules, and worldview.

developmental counseling and therapy (DCT): A comprehensive clinical mental health approach originated by Allen Ivey for the treatment of individuals from a non-pathological, positivistic perspective. DCT suggests that the way clients understand and operate in the world is based on two main interacting systems: their levels of cognitive development and the implications of the larger social units in which clients are involved (e.g., family, community, culture) (Gladding, 2001 p. 37).

diathesis stress: Hypothesis that both an inherited vulnerability and a specific stressor are required to produce a mental disorder.

disability: Any restriction or lack of an ability to perform an activity in the normal manner or within the range normal for a human being.

DUI: Driving under the influence; operating a vehicle illegally while under the influence of mood-altering substances. Also known in some states as driving while impaired (DWI).

duty to warn: The legal responsibility a counselor has to warn others if a client is potentially dangerous to self or others (Gladding, 2001, p. 41).

eating disorders not otherwise specified (NOS): Includes maladaptive eating behavior that does not meet the criteria for either AN or BN but is still considered pathological.

ego-dystonic features: Symptoms that are in contrast to the way a client views him- or herself. These are typically easier to treat than symptoms that the client identifies with (ego-syntonic).

empathy: The counselor's ability to see, be aware of, conceptualize, understand, and effectively communicate back to a client the client's feelings, thoughts, and frame of reference in regard to a situation or point of view. Empathy operates on at least two levels: primary empathy and advanced empathy. Empathy is one of the necessary and sufficient conditions for change, along with unconditional positive regard and congruence, according to Carl Rogers (Gladding, 2001, p. 44).

ergogenic aid: Agents used to enhance athletic performance; examples include stimulants, narcotics, diuretics, or anabolic steroids.

ethanol: Also known as ethyl alcohol, the primary mood-altering substance in beverage alcohol.

ethnicity (ethnic group): A group of human beings who share in common specific physical traits, behavioral style, religious orientation, language, cultural heritage, or a common national or regional origin.

ethyl alcohol: Also known as ethanol, the primary mood-altering substance in beverage alcohol.

euthymia: A clinical term meaning neither manic nor depressed. Derived from the Greek root meaning joyous and tranquil.

exercise dependence: Used to describe individuals who demonstrate an excessive commitment to exercise, experience withdrawal-like symptoms when away from exercise, and who choose to exercise through injury.

female athlete triad: The interrelated set of pathologies affecting active women, including disordered eating, amenorrhea, and osteoporosis.

gender: "Gender is a socially created system of values, identities, and activities that are prescribed for women and men. Unlike sex, which is biologically determined, gender is socially constructed" (Wood, 2000, p. 269).

generalized anxiety: Experience of anxiety that is nonspecific, occurring frequently, and as a result of a variety of triggers, and that influences a person's overall life perceptions.

group work: The giving of help or the accomplishment of tasks in group setting. It involves the application of group theory and process by a capable professional practitioner in order to help an interdependent collection of people reach their mutual goals; the goals may be personal, interpersonal, or task-related. According to the Association for Specialists in Group Work (ASGW), group work is a broad professional practice (Gladding, 2001 p. 56).

hazing: An initiation process involving harassment, often performed on younger or newer individuals to a group.

homophobia: Irrational fear of, aversion to, or discrimination against homosexuality or homosexuals.

HOPE: A four-stage model to assist athletic trainers in understanding issues impacting their patients.

identity foreclosure: The person is committed to a particular career or life path determined by others and without exploration of other paths.

individual counseling: One-on-one counseling between a counselor and a client (Gladding, 2001, p. 62).

informed consent: The act of the client agreeing to treatment after having been provided with information about their treatment, the procedures to be used, and the probable consequences, both positive and negative.

intentional interviewing and counseling: A counselor education approach developed by Allen and Mary Bradford Ivey in which specific counseling skills are delineated, taught, learned, and used in counseling individuals.

life stress events: An individual's psychological reactions and adaptations to the occurrence of major life events (e.g., marriage, death of a loved one, divorce of parents).

life transitions: Events that occur that may or may not prompt a person to move on to another phase of life.

major depressive disorder (MDD): A mood disorder characterized by feelings of hopelessness, worthlessness, and helplessness that is often accompanied by suicidal thoughts.

Mental Status Exam (MSE): A psychological assessment tool used to determine a person's global functioning and provide indicators of potential disorders in a broad spectrum, from disturbances of the memory to hallucinations, learning disabilities, and personality disorders.

metabolic tolerance: When the body becomes more efficient in eliminating a mood-altering substance.

muscle dysmorphia (MDM): The preoccupation with body size and muscular size, shape, or definition.

neurodevelopment: Multiple processes by which an individual grows and develops a complex nervous system during embryonic development and throughout life.

overtraining syndrome (OTS): A disorder occurring among athletes characterized by many of the same symptoms as depression but differentiated by a plateau of or even decline in athletic performance despite increased training. This leads to further increases of training with even greater declines in performance, and ultimately to total exhaustion.

overweight (in childhood): An individual with a BMI greater than 95% of other individuals of the same age and sex.

panic attack: A sudden, overwhelming experience of fear or worry for no apparent reason, accompanied by chest pain, dizziness, numbness, hyperventilation, and feelings of "going crazy" or losing control. Can be cued by a specific trigger or seemingly occur "out of the blue."

performance anxiety: An intense experience of anxiety due to an upcoming performance or competition that subsides after the event is over.

perserveration: A pattern of repeated verbalizations. For example, repeating the same sentence, word(s), or phrase(s).

pharmacodynamic tolerance: When the central nervous system is less affected by a drug.

physical dependence: A condition involving the human body experiencing difficulty or medical complications when a drug is removed and no longer available to the body; can be life-threatening with substances such as alcohol and anti-anxiety medications.

prevention: The use by counselors of educational or behavioral means (e.g., instruction or rehearsal) to help clients avoid or minimize potential problems (Gladding, 2001, p. 95).

privileged communication: A legal term based on a statute that protects the client from having his or her communications discussed in court without explicit permission.

profession: A discipline that has its own unique body of literature, prescribed course of study, membership organization, standards of conduct, and ethics (Gladding, 2001, p. 96).

proof: Used to indicate the percentage of alcohol in a particular alcoholic beverage.

psychological dependence: A pattern of use of mood-altering substances, resulting in a belief that the chemical is necessary for improved functioning.

psychopathology: Disorder or dysfunction affecting a person's mental health and well-being. Examples include learning, mood, personality, and eating disorders.

psychosocial: A term that underlies Erik Erikson's theory of human development, which deals with the resolution of social crisis and the development of social competencies. The term refers to events or behaviors related to social aspects of life.

psychotherapist: A general term used to describe a helping professional who provides mental health treatment to clients. Many professionals can be described as psychotherapists. The legal qualifications for such a title vary from state to state (Gladding, 2001, p. 99).

psychotherapy: Cognitive, affective, and behavioral means of helping troubled individuals change their thoughts, feelings, and behaviors so that they reduce their stress and achieve greater life satisfaction (Gladding, 2001 p. 99).

pyramiding: Refers to increasing a steroid dose with time to lessen potential side effects.

race: A classification of human beings based on attributes that may include hair texture and color, skin color, and other physical features; a distinct human population that is often distinguished by genetic characteristics or genotypic traits, geographic orientation or distribution, and a common history.

rational emotive behavioral therapy (REBT): The theory of counseling established by Albert Ellis in the late 1950s and originally called rational emotive therapy. The emphasis of the approach is that it is people's thoughts about events, rather than the events, that are the source of emotional and behavioral difficulties. REBT focuses on helping clients change or modify their negative thoughts to neutral, positive, or mixed thoughts, and thus think more rationally and behave more responsibly with less interpersonal and intrapersonal difficulty (Gladding, 2001, p. 101).

referral: The transfer of a client to another counselor. The referral process itself involves (at least) four steps: (1) identifying the need to refer, (2) evaluating potential referral sources, (3) preparing the client for the referral, and (4) coordinating the transfer (Gladding, 2001 p. 102).

remediation: The process by which counseling procedures are implemented with the goal of correcting a situation (Gladding, 2001 p. 104).

sexual harassment: Sexual advances (i.e., touching or grabbing) or sexual comments (either joking, flirting, or abuse) that are unwanted and inappropriate.

sexual orientation: Sexual orientation is an enduring emotional, romantic, sexual, or affectional attraction to another person. Sexual orientation is different from sexual behavior because it refers to feelings and self-concept. Persons may or may not express their sexual orientation in their behaviors (www.apa.org/pubinfo/answere.html#whatis).

somatic: Affecting or pertaining to the body, as opposed to the mind or spirit.

SPORT: A five-stage goal-setting model in which the individual specifies the goal, describes the performance, organizes for the task, reality checks, and develops a timeline for reaching a goal.

tolerance: When the body becomes more efficient in eliminating a mood-altering substance, the term metabolic tolerance is accurate; when the central nervous system is less affected by the drug, the accurate term is pharmacodynamic tolerance.

wellness: A state of being that emphasizes good health, a positive lifestyle, and prevention (Gladding, 2001 p. 127).

withdrawal: The physical changes that occur when a substance leaves the body.

worldview (also world view): One's view of the world based on his or her cultural perspective and life experiences; one's cultural viewpoint; the way a person perceives and experiences his or her relationship to the world.

xenophobia: An unrealistic fear and disdain for immigrants or internationals from countries other than one's own; a fear of strangers who are culturally different.

References

Gladding, S.T. (2001). The counseling dictionary concise definitions of frequently used terms. Columbus, OH: Merrill Prentice Hall.

Ivey, A.E. & Ivey, M.B. (2003). Intentional interviewing and counseling facilitating client development in a multicultural society (5th ed.) Pacific Grove, CA: Thompson Brooks Cole.

Wood, J.T. (2000). Communication theories in action: An introduction (2nd ed.). Belmont, CA: Wadsworth.

Internet Resources

Al-Anon and Alateen: www.al-anon.org

Al-Anon worldwide listings: www.al-anon.org/meetings/international.html

Alcoholics Anonymous World Services, Inc.: www.alcoholics-anonymous.org

Alcoholics Anonymous Resources Online, includes Alcoholics Anonymous table of contents (Alcoholics Anonymous Big Book online version): www.aa.org/bigbookonline

Alcoholics Anonymous meetings online: www.aa.org/en_find_meeting.cfm

Cocaine Anonymous World Services, Inc.: www.ca.org

Cocaine use self test: www.ca.org/literature/selftest.htm

Gamblers Anonymous: www.GamblersAnonymous.org

Illegal drug use: www.druguse.com

Information about Marijuana: www.Marijuana-Info.org

Information about Ecstasy, Methamphetamine, GHB, and others: www.ClubDrugs.org

Information on HIV/AIDS and drug use: www.HIV.drugabuse.gov

Motivational interviewing information: www.motivationalinterview.org

National Clearinghouse for Alcohol and Drug Information (NCADI): www.ncadi.samhsa.gov

National Center for Drug Free Sport, Inc.: www.drugfreesport.com

National Collegiate Athletic Association: www.ncaa.org

National Council on Gambling: www.ncpgambling.org

National Institute on Alcohol Abuse and Alcoholism (NIAAA): www.niaaa.nih.gov

National Institute on Drug Abuse (NIDA): nida.nih.gov

National Institute on Drug Abuse for Teens, The Science Behind Drug Abuse: www.teens.drugabuse.gov

Narcotics Anonymous: www.na.org or www.wsoinc.com

NA-Way magazine: www.naway/naway-toc.htm

Olympic Movement: www.olympic.org/uk/index_uk.asp

Partnership for a Drug-Free America (PDFA): www.drugfreeamerica.org

Rational Recovery Systems: www.rational.org/recovery

Secular Organization for Sobriety: www.sossobriety.org

SMART Recovery: www.smartrecovery.org

Substance Abuse and Mental Health Services Administration (SAMHSA), Department of Health and Human Services: www.samhsa.gov

Training iformation and resources: www.mid-attc.org

Twelve-step chatroom: http://stepchat.com

Twelve Steps: www.al-anon.org/steps.html

Twelve Traditions: www.al-anon.org/traditions.html

Web of Addictions: www.well.com/user/woa

INDEX

WAIT
...There's More

Special Tests for Orthopedic Examination, Third Edition
Jeff G. Konin, PhD, ATC, PT; Denise L. Wiksten, PhD, ATC; Jerome A. Isear, Jr., MS, PT, ATC-L; Holly Brader, MPH, RN, BSN, ATC
400 pp, Soft Cover, 2006, ISBN 10: 1-55642-741-7, ISBN 13: 978-1-55642-741-1, Order# 47417, **$39.95**

Special Tests for Orthopedic Examination has been used for 10 years by thousands of students, clinicians, and rehab professionals and is now available in a revised and updated third edition. Concise and pocket-sized, this handbook is an invaluable guide filled with the most current and practical clinical exam techniques used during an orthopedic examination. This Third Edition takes a user-friendly approach to visualizing and explaining more than 150 commonly used orthopedic special tests, including 11 new and modern tests.

Athletic Training Exam Review: A Student Guide to Success, Third Edition
Lynn Van Ost, MEd, RN, PT, ATC; Karen Manfre, MA, ATR; Karen Lew, MEd, ATC, LAT
272 pp, Soft Cover, 2006, ISBN 10: 1-55642-764-6, ISBN 13: 978-1-55642-764-0, Order# 47646, **$44.95**

Preparing for the BOC Certification exam is the turning point in the road to a successful career for all athletic training students. A user-friendly, organized, and well-established study guide is essential to preparing for this all-important process. Thousands of students have been successfully guided through the exam process with *Athletic Training Exam Review: A Student Guide to Success*—now available in an expanded and revised Third Edition.

Clinical Skills Documentation Guide for Athletic Training, Second Edition
Herb Amato, DA, ATC; Christy D. Hawkins, ATC; Steven L. Cole, MEd, ATC, CSCS
464 pp, Soft Cover, 2006, ISBN 10: 1-55642-758-1, ISBN 13: 978-1-55642-758-9, Order# 47581, **$36.95**

Athletic Training Student Primer: A Foundation for Success
Andrew P. Winterstein, PhD, ATC
256 pp, Soft Cover, 2003, ISBN 10: 1-55642-570-8, ISBN 13: 978-1-55642-570-7, Order# 45708, **$42.95**

Quick Reference Dictionary for Athletic Training, Second Edition
Julie N. Bernier, EdD, ATC
416 pp, Soft Cover, 2005, ISBN 10: 1-55642-666-6, ISBN 13: 978-1-55642-666-7, Order# 46666, **$31.95**

Athletic Training in Occupational Settings
Susan Finkam, MS, ATC, LAT, CEA
168 pp, Soft Cover, 2004, ISBN 10: 1-55642-632-1, ISBN 13: 978-1-55642-632-2, Order# 46321, **$44.95**

Clinical Pathology for Athletic Trainers: Recognizing Systemic Disease, Second Edition
Daniel J. O'Connor, PhD, ATC; Louise Fincher, EdD, ATC, LAT
432 pp, Hard Cover, 2008, ISBN 10: 1-55642-770-0, ISBN 13: 978-1-55642-770-1, Order# 47700, **$47.95**

Special Tests for Neurologic Examination
James R. Scifers, DScPT, PT, SCS, LAT, ATC
250 pp, Soft Cover, 2008, ISBN 10: 1-55642-797-2, ISBN 13: 978-155642-797-8, Order# 47972, **$39.95**

Psychosocial Frames of Reference: Core for Occupation-Based Practice, Third Edition
Mary Ann Giroux Bruce, PhD, OTR; Barbara Borg, MA, OTR
432 pp, Soft Cover, 2002, ISBN 10: 1-55642-494-9, ISBN 13: 978-1-55642-494-6, Order# 34949, **$53.95**

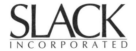